Seizures and Epilepsy in Childhood

A Johns Hopkins Press Health Book

Dr. John M. Freeman is Lederer Professor of Pediatric Epilepsy and Director of the Pediatric Epilepsy Center at the Johns Hopkins Medical Institutions. He is also an Honorary Life Director of the Epilepsy Foundation and Honorary Life Director of the Abilities Network / Epilepsy Association of the Chesapeake Region.

Dr. Eileen P. G. Vining is Associate Professor of Neurology and Pediatrics and Deputy Director of the Pediatric Epilepsy Center at the Johns Hopkins Medical Institutions. She is a former chair of the Professional Advisory Board of the Abilities Network / Epilepsy Association of the Chesapeake Region.

Ms. Diana J. Pillas is the Coordinator-Counselor of the Pediatric Epilepsy Center at the Johns Hopkins Medical Institutions and former President of the Abilities Network / Epilepsy Association of the Chesapeake Region. She is a former Vice-President of the Epilepsy Foundation.

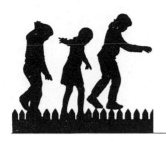

Seizures and Epilepsy in Childhood
A GUIDE

Third Edition

John M. Freeman, M.D.
Eileen P. G. Vining, M.D.
Diana J. Pillas

The Pediatric Epilepsy Center
The Johns Hopkins Medical Institutions
Baltimore, Maryland

The Johns Hopkins University Press
Baltimore and London

Illustrations in Chapters 1, 2, and 9 by Timothy H. Phelps,
    M.S., F.A.M.I.

The Johns Hopkins University Press
2715 North Charles Street
Baltimore, Maryland 21218-4363
www.press.jhu.edu

ISBN 0-8018-7050-X
ISBN 0-8018-7051-8 (pbk.)

Library of Congress Cataloging-in-Publication Data will be found at
the end of this book.

A catalog record for this book is available from the British Library.

Note to the Reader

This, the third, edition of our book continues to embody our approach to seizures and epilepsy in general. Although originally written for parents, the philosophy of this book is equally applicable to physicians, and to every person who cares for individuals with seizures and epilepsy.

The book was not written about you or about your epilepsy. It was not written about your child. It was not written about your patient. While we believe in and practice its philosophy, we adjust our approach to suit each individual's particular need and each family's situation. Obviously we would not treat a patient without first learning a great deal more about him or her, and so an individual's treatment should not be based solely on what is written here. Treatment must be based on a dialogue between you and your physician, between the physician and the patient's family. Our book is written to help you with that dialogue.

Contents

Part Two   Diagnosing Seizures and Epilepsy

Part Three   Treating Seizures and Epilepsy

Figures and Tables

Figures

Tables

Foreword to the Third Edition
by Trish Marlow, *a parent*

While sitting in our living room playing, our three-year-old daughter Alyssa had her first seizure. From there we began a sometimes frightening, confusing, and arduous journey of medical tests, an array of medications and hospitalizations. We received conflicting advice and often confusing reports from physicians. I sought more knowledge than physicians could impart to me during office visits.

After being on our journey for a few years I acquired the book *Seizures and Epilepsy in Childhood*. I quickly devoured the information it contained. The book provides many definitions and explanations of terms associated with seizures and epilepsy and is written in an easy to understand format. It offers detailed information about medical tests and treatment options. It equips parents with questions that they may wish to ask their child's physician. The book provided us with a wealth of invaluable information. We continue to use it as a guide through the complex medical options available to our Alyssa.

I highly recommend that every physician who diagnoses a child with seizures also offer this book to parents. To parents of children with seizures the book will prove to be a valuable guide through the medical process and a help through the emotional trials of having a child who has seizures.

We are grateful to Dr. Freeman, Dr. Vining, and Diana Pillas for their dedication to the research and treatment of children who have seizures.

Foreword to the Second Edition
by Jim Abrahams, *a parent*

For a parent there is no such thing as a gentle entry into the world of epilepsy. One day your child has his first seizure. From there it is terrifying, agonizing, devastating. It's not intellectual. We cope using whatever innate coping skills we have been given. Eventually we learn that information is only forthcoming on a sort of need-to-know basis. We learn to drum the word *prognosis* from our vocabulary. We make lists of questions to ask during our rushed audiences with our physicians, but we are so naïve as to the complexity of the disease that our questions often miss the mark and so frazzled by our emotions that logical processing of answers is all but impossible. So much of what we are told is too complicated. So much seems vague. The alternatives seem so limited. The ground rules seem so different.

Like everyone else, this was our experience when our son Charlie's seizures began—a dizzying procession of seizures, drugs, and references to complicated diagnostic and surgical procedures. For a while I would follow Charlie's neurologist around on his rounds, trying to figure out what was happening to our son. For a while, as a measure of my desperation, I would actually take his beginning dose of his next new drug (I weighed 170 pounds; he weighed 20 pounds), so I could try to feel what it was doing to our son.

In the midst of this uncharted sea, finding a resource like *Seizures and Epilepsy in Childhood* provided a true beacon. For months it lived as a constant companion on our nightstand. Answers are given, alternatives explained, vocabulary defined. Nothing is sugarcoated, but everything is written on a level we can understand. In an area of medicine that is more art than science, the science is spelled out. Mechanisms are defined, technology explained, hard facts are leveled—and, in our case, the ketogenic diet was found.

If you have a child with epilepsy, *Seizures and Epilepsy in Childhood* will be an invaluable ally.

Foreword to the First Edition

by Tony Coelho, *Former Congressman from California,*
Vice-President of the Epilepsy Foundation of America

Being a parent is a wonderful experience that is full of challenges. We share in our child's joy over each accomplishment and we hurt—sometimes even more than our child—over the frustrations and challenges of growing up. During emotionally challenging times, children look to their parents not only for empathy and understanding but, more importantly, for strength. The purpose of this book is to equip parents with knowledge and strength to help their children meet, tackle, and control the challenges of epilepsy.

I have a special interest in this subject, because I have epilepsy. When I first started having seizures, almost thirty years ago, my parents did not have the resources to learn the truth about this disorder. My condition went undiagnosed and untreated for several years, but, thankfully, my seizures were infrequent enough to allow me to enjoy a college career. It was only after graduation, as I prepared to enter the Catholic priesthood, that my epilepsy was diagnosed and that I first encountered the stigma of being labeled an "epileptic." As I reeled from the disappointments of being denied admission to the seminary, losing my driver's license, and not being able to find a job, my parents were sharing in my hurt. But because epilepsy was misunderstood, they could not provide me with the strength I so desperately needed during that critical time.

Happily, both the field of medicine and the public perception of epilepsy have changed dramatically since I was a child. There are now excellent resources for people with epilepsy, and Johns Hopkins has pulled together the best of the best in this comprehensive guide.

As a parent, you know that epilepsy poses a challenge for you and your child. Many boundaries, however, are due to self-imposed limits and are not caused by epilepsy. As I learned about the disorder, I realized that the list of things I *could* do was infinitely longer than the list of things I could not do. Once that fact was realized, I decided that there were very few limits brought about by my epilepsy. I went on to pursue a career, was elected to Congress, and am now tackling a new challenge in the field of investment banking.

Mine is an epilepsy success story because of many circumstances for which I am grateful. But I am not the exception, for every day parents and children work together to face the challenges of epilepsy. With resources such as this book, parents will be well prepared to face this challenge and provide their children with love, strength, and the knowledge they need to live a full life.

Preface

The Parent

"It was the most frightening experience of our lives. We heard a noise; I guess it woke us up. We rushed into Caroline's bedroom, and there she was—choking, thrashing around. We thought she was going to die. We'd never seen a seizure and didn't know what it was. By the time the ambulance arrived, the seizure was over and she was sleeping. In the hospital they did all the tests, but they couldn't find any reason for the seizure. I thought the doctor must not be any good. Of course, there was a reason! Why couldn't they find it? The doctor put her on medicine, and she became a terror. She was sleepy all the time, and her personality changed from that of a lovely, affectionate little girl to that of a whiny brat. But even that was better than when the seizures came back. Her doctor tried her on many different medicines, changing them every few weeks. We were afraid to let Caroline go outside. We watched her every moment. We were frantic. We didn't know what was happening. Our child was changing before our eyes; she just wasn't Caroline any more.

"It wasn't until we worked *with* your medical team that we began to be more comfortable with what was going on. We learned about epilepsy and what was happening to Caroline. We began to understand seizures and their treatment and to be less impatient with you doctors. We found ourselves becoming less overprotective, and the old Caroline began to come back. Gradually, the seizures came under control; she hasn't had one for almost four years now. Your group has taught us to be part of Caroline's team. You've taught us the importance of working with you to control her seizures. You've helped all of us deal with our fears. Caroline is doing well in school, and you've enabled us to resume a normal life.

"Parents can't cope with all these things by themselves; they need help. We needed to understand seizures, to understand the effects of the medications, but most of all we needed help to understand all the things that were happening to our child and to us. We needed your help so that we could allow our child to grow up to be as normal as possible and live with her epilepsy. We, as parents, couldn't do it ourselves. In your book, try to tell them what you told us."

The Teacher

"I thought I knew enough about epilepsy. We had covered it in our training, and fortunately I had never had a child with epilepsy in my class. When Nancy had a seizure I was terrified. It wasn't one of those 'daydreaming-like' spells that we had been taught to look out for. She let out a cry, fell to the floor, and turned blue. I thought she had stopped breathing. The room was in chaos. The children were frightened. I didn't know what to tell them. The ambulance came and took her to the hospital.

"Nancy was back in school two days later, no different than before; but I, and the class, thought we had been changed forever. I was planning to move her desk to the front where I could quickly get to her; Barbara, her friend, was going to escort her to the bathroom; Enid volunteered to carry her books and accompany her through the halls and on the stairs. Everyone agreed to watch her on the playground. We had planned to have the nurse help me explain what had happened. Fortunately we didn't need to do any of these things. Nancy's mother told us that she had read this book and that Nancy had only a small chance of having another seizure. She wasn't to be treated any differently than before. The local epilepsy affiliate came and gave a 'Kids on the Block' presentation about seizures and epilepsy, and we realized that it didn't have to be a big thing."

The Physician and the Nurse

"I saw Nancy in the emergency room. It was a busy day. We obtained the CT scan, got the blood work, and admitted her to the hospital. The MRI was done the next day. The parents had myriad questions, but there just was not enough time to answer them. Our floor nurse suggested that they read this book."

. . .

We've heard these stories often. Parents frequently come to us for a second opinion, and we see children who have had seizures and have been started on treatment by other physicians. What we find is that the diagnosis and medication are generally correct but that the parents, and even older children, still are seeking to understand. Seizures have not been fully explained. Fears and myths have not been dispelled. The future looks bleak to them. Sometimes parents lack understanding because those in the emergency room are too busy for a detailed discussion. Sometimes the discussion takes place at a time when everyone is too frightened to hear and understand the explanations. The most important thing we offer is perspective. While we help the family to understand the science and psychosocial aspects of seizures, we also help them focus on the whole child, not just on the child's seizures. We want everyone to realize how their reactions to the seizures may be distorting the family relationships. We want to help the child and the family to *live with epilepsy.*

Living with epilepsy means learning to live with uncertainty. It means learning to assess the risks and the benefits of many different aspects of the child's life. "Can he swim?" "Does she need medication?" "Can we stop treatment?" Living with epilepsy also means keeping the seizures in perspective. It means realizing that seizures are usually only a small fraction of the life of a person with epilepsy. Living with epilepsy means avoiding handicapping your child. It means maximizing your child's assets and adjusting to the limitations, if any. Living with epilepsy may involve a struggle to find the best medication to control your child's seizures, to find optimal medical care. It may mean battling the school system or other bureaucracies to get the help your child needs. It means rediscovering the joy of having a child who is learning, playing, and developing.

Over many years, we have worked as a team to develop a positive approach that incorporates both the medical science and the social science of seizures. This positive approach, which emphasizes what a child or adolescent *can* do rather than what he or she can't do, allows families to understand the many ramifications of epilepsy and to accept and cope with their children's seizures. This book was written to make this approach available to all families who have a child with seizures or epilepsy. Living with epilepsy will not always be easy. It will vary with the child and the child's problems. But using an optimistic approach and keeping epilepsy in perspective will make living with epilepsy better.

Since we wrote the first edition of this book, many people who have had their questions answered by it have called us just to say thank you. We have learned that many of the families we follow find that having the chance to read the book, seek answers to their questions, and digest the answers at leisure provides a more complete approach to resolving their natural anxiety. This book is not meant to replace a discussion with your physicians, but rather to supplement that important discussion. Indeed, many physicians have told us that they give the book to parents, or tell them how to get a copy. Parents have given the book to teachers, caregivers, and even their physicians. It is used as such a supplement in our own clinical practice. It is meant to help you understand epilepsy and its treatment and to help you formulate questions for your physician so that you can be a more informed participant in your child's care.

Acknowledgments

This book is the product of a team that has worked together for more than twenty-five years. We have learned from each other. The words and ideas no longer belong to any one individual. We have also learned from the many parents and children who have been part of our clinic as both patients and friends.

In some ways this book is part of a long tradition of comprehensive care for children with epilepsy and their families begun at Hopkins in the 1930s under Dr. Samuel Livingston. This book's message echoes the title of one of his first books, *Living with Epilepsy*. However, our comprehensive, caring approach to epilepsy is partially due to the parents of our patients, who have helped to form our attitudes, and to their children, who have taught us what it is like to live with seizures.

It is a better book because of the many friends who have read, edited, and commented upon it. We give our deep gratitude to all of them for their generous contributions.

We were particularly grateful to Jeannette Hopkins, who set the original manuscript free. We are also deeply grateful to Jackie Wehmueller and Anne M. Whitmore, editors at the Hopkins Press, who further improved the subsequent editions.

The enthusiastic reception of the earlier editions has confirmed the need for a book like this and has encouraged us to publish this updated and expanded third edition. To all the parents who have called us to express appreciation and with suggestions for improvements, our grateful thanks.

**Seizures and Epilepsy
in Childhood**

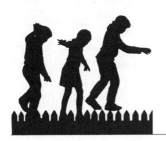

Introduction

We see many families whose children have had a single seizure and many others whose children have epilepsy who come to us for a second opinion. There are common themes among all of these families. One theme is that the family and child are focused on the seizure or seizures; they are unable to look at the whole child and the bigger picture. Their life and their child's life have become centered primarily on the seizures. A second theme is that the families and children are overwhelmed by the mythology of epilepsy, by the fear of future handicap or retardation. Few families understand what seizures are and what they are not. They come seeking to understand what has happened and what is likely to happen.

Many physicians, even those very knowledgeable about seizures, epilepsy, and their treatment, focus on these medical aspects and do not put epilepsy in the proper perspective of the whole child and family.

We believe that no child's life should be defined by seizures. No one is "an epileptic." The seizures and epilepsy are usually only a small portion of the child's life. We believe that to put them in perspective you must understand the brain, seizures, and how to cope with epilepsy. You must understand the mythology and how different it is from reality. Only with this understanding can you avoid handicapping your child, prevent his being handicapped by others, and allow him to reach his full potential. That is why we have written this book. While primarily for parents, it is also a book for everyone with seizures and for all who are touched by seizures—families, teachers, and health professionals.

1

We hope this book will reassure you that 70 to 80 percent of children who do have epilepsy can have their seizures completely controlled with medication and can function as normally as everyone else. Many of these children will, after a time, stop taking medicine and will have outgrown their epilepsy. For the smaller percentage of parents whose children's epilepsy has not been completely controlled or whose children have other disabling conditions, we hope our book will help you and them to function as normally as possible and to maximize their assets and minimize their disabilities.

Parents come to us with many fears: "Will my child be all right?" "Will he swallow his tongue?" "Will she die?" "Does she have a brain tumor?" "Will he be retarded?" "Can he ever lead a normal life?" "Can seizures ever be controlled?" "Can I ever leave her alone?" "Will medication make him an addict?" All of these thoughts—and more—run through the mind of a parent whose child has had a seizure. The children themselves have similar fears: "My God! Is this going to happen again?" "What will my friends think?" "Will I ever be able to ride my bike again?" "Can I go to college?" "Can I ever drive?" "Will I be able to get married?" "What about children?"

Before we can help you to deal with these fears and put epilepsy in perspective, we must debunk the mythology. Both terms, *epilepsy* and *seizures,* carry the myths and misconceptions of centuries past, when people who experienced them were thought to be possessed by witches and were confined in special colonies or shunned. They saw a child suddenly "seized," losing control, falling to the floor, his body jerking. A few minutes later this child was back to normal. What could have caused this to happen? It must have been some outside force! The devil? Not so long ago people believed this. We now know that seizures come from electrical disruptions in the brain.

Also part of the mythology, many people still believe that epilepsy and seizures are always devastating, that they will continue to recur, that they will get worse, that the brain will be damaged, and that their child might become handicapped, retarded, or even die. Now we know that only a small percentage of children who have a single seizure have a second seizure. We also now know that most children who have had several seizures, who by definition have epilepsy, will still have their seizures controlled with medication, that most children outgrow their seizures and can be taken off medication. Only a minority of children with epilepsy will have difficult-to-control seizures. Most children with seizures are absolutely normal all or virtually all of the time, except during the seizure.

The myths persist because epilepsy remains a hidden condition. People see only the small percentage of children who are severely handicapped and who have seizures. The vast majority, whose seizures are well controlled and who function normally, do not advertise that they have epilepsy. If your neighbor's child has seizures and is doing well, you may never even know that he has epilepsy. Only if that child has a seizure when his friends are around do they become aware of his epilepsy. His friends' parents may say, "I never knew he had epilepsy. He looks so normal!" "I thought that all children with epilepsy were retarded." "The only child I knew with seizures was in a wheelchair and never went to school." If we want to combat these old myths and prejudices, children with epilepsy and their families have to be far more comfortable and open about the disorder. Only then will the public understand that most people with epilepsy are just like themselves. Seeing only children who are disabled, you get the wrong impression. You may have no idea that most children who have epilepsy encounter no problem as a result of their seizures.

You can handicap your child if you continue to believe the myths. Most individuals with epilepsy *can* function normally, becoming exuberant children, vigorous adolescents, and productive adults who are free of seizures altogether. Yet we still see children who are handicapped by parental overprotection. You will have to learn what protections are reasonable and realistic, and which restrictions will simply handicap your child. Avoiding overprotection will require that you understand not only seizures but also your reaction to them, your child's reaction, and the reactions of others. You need to work actively to prevent seizures from becoming a handicap. In most cases, you can succeed.

Society's misperceptions and prejudices can handicap your child. The Epilepsy Foundation, the national voluntary organization for people with epilepsy, has done a wonderful job over the past decades of informing the public of the truth about epilepsy and about people with epilepsy. EF has attempted to dispel the prejudice embodied in the term *epileptic*. But prejudice can't be wholly eliminated with words and information alone. Prejudice must be fought by example as well. To overcome your prejudice truly, you have to play with a child who has epilepsy, you have to go to school with him, live with him, and come to realize that he is a child, just like any other, with his own strengths,

Who's got epilepsy?

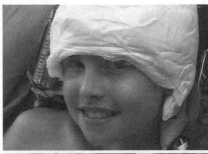

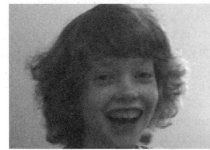

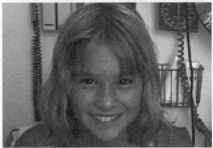

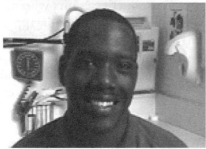

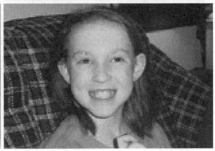

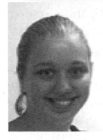

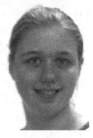

All these bright young people!

weaknesses, peculiarities, and personality. He just happens to have seizures.

Not every child or adult with epilepsy will avoid handicaps. Some are handicapped by brain damage from head trauma, infection, or the other multiple causes of epilepsy. Others are handicapped by mental or motor impairment. Some are handicapped by their difficult-to-control seizures, despite many new medications. For all persons with epilepsy, better understanding and services continue to be needed and will improve their lives. In many areas local Epilepsy Foundation affiliates can provide information, resources, and programs. They can be an important source of support for families of children with epilepsy.

If your child believes in the mythology, she can handicap herself. If she allows herself to be overprotected, if she believes she can't do things because of her seizures, then she will be unable to reach her full potential. Just as you must allow her to take risks, so she must be willing to try new things. It requires self-esteem, courage, and determination for her to venture into the unknown, to stay at another child's house when it's possible she could have another seizure, to go to the school dance when she might be embarrassed, to apply for a job when a seizure could occur and someone might find out that she has epilepsy. Once handicapped by fear of seizures or by overprotection, it becomes difficult to break free and lead a normal life. It is far easier to prevent a handicap than to overcome it.

Helping your child to be normal will require a partnership between you and your physician. This book will help you create that. For example: your physician will do tests and may propose medication, but do not allow your physician to make all the decisions. Your doctor should be familiar with epilepsy, with the choice of medications for controlling seizures, and with their side effects. He should be willing to discuss with you the risks and benefits of each medication and of each test, but it is your job, as the parent, to be a partner in the management—to be an informed consumer. You should ask: "Why is this test being done?" "What are its risks?" "What are the risks and benefits of treatment?" As a parent, you will be your child's best advocate if you are informed and understand seizures and their treatment. You must understand what epilepsy is and what it is not. You must understand what is myth and what is fact.

We have written this book to help you understand seizures, your reaction to them, and the reaction of others. Through the stories of many of our patients we illustrate how accurate diagnosis, comprehensive treatment or management, and sensitivity to the impact of seizures can help a child and his or her family live better with epilepsy. With medical information, you will understand the many different kinds of seizures, how the brain is organized, and how it works. With knowledge of medications, you will understand your child's treatment. Only with this more complete understanding can you become a strong advocate on the team that is helping your child.

Part One

Why Do Seizures and Epilepsy Occur?

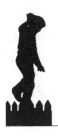

1. How the Brain Works:
Understanding Seizures and Why There Are So Many Types

A seizure *is a sudden electrical discharge in the brain which results in an alteration in sensation, behavior, or consciousness.*

Epilepsy *means recurrent seizures.*

Seizures and epilepsy are not of themselves a disease. They are the response of the central nervous system to a variety of disturbances to its inherent stability. The response of the brain to these disturbances and the type of seizures that may result depend on the type and location of the disturbance and on the many intrinsic mechanisms that serve to maintain the brain's inherent stability. The mechanisms that govern the brain's ability to respond or not to respond to the disturbances also control the nature of the response. The mechanisms controlling stability of brain activity have been likened to driving with one foot on the brake and the other on the accelerator. The vehicle's speed will depend on the multiple factors pressing on or releasing the accelerator, as well as those factors increasing or decreasing the pressure on the brakes.

For most people, the brain is like a black box, and seizures are frightening events that come from this black box like static from a radio. Thinking of seizures in this fashion reveals a lack of understanding of what is happening during a seizure. Without more knowledge, you will be relegated to accepting whatever medication your physician prescribes and hoping that he or she is correct and that the medication will stop the static.

We believe that parents and children should be participants in their own care. To be an effective participant, you must be knowledgeable about how the brain works and about how and why these temporary disturbances of the brain's function called seizures occur. Perhaps the easiest way to understand how the brain functions, and why it dysfunctions, is to look at an analogy. Society is a complex system of individual interactions, yet it is familiar to all of us and offers an understandable explanation of how the brain may work and how it may have a seizure.

Society: A Model for Disruptions and Seizures

The brain is a society of cells called neurons; it works through the interactions of individual neurons, one with another. Brief disruptions in the brain, that is, seizures, are caused by alterations in the interactions of these cells. To understand normal brain function and the disturbances of function called seizures, it may be helpful to consider another complex but more familiar structure—society, with its multiple interactions and disruptions.

We all live in "society," and that society is made up of many smaller communities: a family, a neighborhood, a church, a workplace, a town, a country. We are each members of these multiple communities. Each of us is different: male or female, black or white, young or old. Our interactions create the social environment. So, too, is the brain a society, one composed of millions of individual cells (neurons), each with its own characteristics, each with its own interactions, each influencing and being influenced by its neighbors and by its local community. The brain has many different regions or communities, and within these regions cells relate to each other in different ways. The regions also influence one another.

Throughout most brains, as within most societies, these interactions occur in a chaotic but balanced, orderly fashion, with few disruptions. But, occasionally, in a society, there are disruptions of varying magnitudes—like a holiday, a parade, an accident, a fire, a strike. Interruptions occur more often in some communities than in others; unpleasant disruptions, for example, occur more frequently in big cities with a greater diversity of people and more multiple interactions than in rural environments. After these "blips" in the normal pattern of life, the communities usually resume their previous tempos and quickly return to normal activities.

But occasionally such disruptions are more intense. Perhaps lives are lost in a fire. The community is disrupted, its ordinary functions come to a halt, it grieves, it holds memorial services. Interactions among citizens are changed, not forever probably, but for a longer period of time than if a parade had passed by. The response of the community will depend on multiple factors—its ethnic heritage, its size, its age, and the interrelationships within the community. Some disruptions spread more widely and involve larger segments of the community, the region, the country, or the entire society. A strike of bus drivers or rail workers may affect a whole region. A march for a popular cause may mobilize a community or a nation.

Similarly, within the brain, communities of cells and areas of the brain interact at their own pace—different paces for different regions of the brain. These interactions in the brain can be assessed by the EEG (electroencephalogram), a record of the minute amounts of electrical activity that brain cells give off as they relate to each other. The normal EEG appears as a series of wiggly lines, with rhythms seeming to move almost at random across the paper. The electrical activity measured varies from one area of the brain to another. But on rare occasions a "blip" appears among these wiggly lines, a small jolt of electricity, a "spike" or sharp wave (see Chapter 7). This spike is like the minor community episode, such as an automobile accident, that disrupts normal activity briefly. The brain quickly resumes its activity. Such spikes on the EEG are of little consequence. Only when these spikes recur frequently in one area of the brain is it evident that that particular community of cells is prone to disruption.

Recurrent spikes are evidence of the neurons' tendency to misfire. When enough neurons misfire at the same time, a spike can be seen on the EEG. If a sufficient number of cells misfire together, then they may make a muscle move or jerk, or they may cause a sensation. This change in behavior or movement is a seizure, a *simple partial seizure* (see page 40). Depending on where in the brain the disturbance occurs and how widespread the disruption, there may be a twitch of a muscle or a finger, a brief twinge of sensation, a jerk of the facial muscles. Each of these may be a single seizure. Sufficiently brief or infrequent, they are of no consequence. Single seizures are not epilepsy. Epilepsy is two or more seizures.

A Seizure Focus

Within society there are soapbox orators or fiery speakers who stand on street corners, trying to cause disturbances, urging people to "take action." Most people walk by. Occasionally, some people stop, listen, and then walk on. Some of the audience may get excited, but action virtually never ensues; they don't change their behavior and a demonstration does not begin. But on rare occasions, this fiery speaker arouses the surrounding crowd and a march or a demonstration occurs. It will not happen solely because he is an inspired speaker but because of the interaction between the speaker and the audience. The interaction must be sufficient to rouse the crowd to action.

Within the brain there may be tiny scars or small abnormalities which are irritating to the surrounding cortex. They may be the source of the spikes discussed above. This "focus" may act like the fiery speaker, inciting the surrounding neurons to "fire." Usually nothing happens, and the focus does not get the neurons excited; the crowd pays no attention and goes its own way ignoring the minor disruption. A seizure requires that a sufficient number of cells pay attention to the focus. Enough neurons must be recruited to fire simultaneously to alter the function in that region of the brain. A seizure thus requires the interaction of the abnormal area *and* the surrounding community of cells.

The susceptibility of surrounding neurons to interaction is termed "threshold." To understand a spike or a seizure, we must understand the level of arousal or "threshold" of the surrounding cells. If the brain's threshold is lowered it is more susceptible to the effects of the "fiery speaker," the scar, and a seizure is more likely to occur in that community of the brain. If the electrical activity from a scar interacts with mildly aroused surrounding cells, a local disturbance may appear as recurrent spikes on the EEG, but this is not a seizure. A seizure is a paroxysmal electrical discharge of neurons in the brain *resulting in alteration of function or behavior.* A spike results when a small number of neurons react simultaneously. Only if sufficient numbers of neurons are recruited does the electrical activity, seen as a spike, cause the behavioral changes that we refer to as a seizure.

The type of alteration of function or behavior that occurs in a seizure will depend on the magnitude and type of the disruption or disorganization and on the "community" of the brain in which it occurs. Local disruptions of brain function are called "partial" seizures because only part of the brain is involved. Since each area of the brain has a different function, the manifestations of an electrical disruption or seizure will differ, depending on which area of the brain is involved. When a partial seizure affects one area of the brain, the manifestations may be twitching of the thumb, hand, or face. If it affects other areas, there may be a tingling sensation, a peculiar smell, an unusual taste. In still other areas, the seizure may lead to changes in behavior—staring or alterations of awareness. All such seizures are caused by the local (contained) disruption of electrical activity.

But, as in a societal disruption, a seizure or demonstration may not remain confined to a local region. Depending on its intensity and depending on the threshold of the brain, the disturbance or seizure may become sufficiently severe to involve one side of the brain, a "unilateral" seizure, or, indeed, the whole brain and become a generalized seizure.

Just as we do not understand exactly why demonstrations begin, spread, and end in a society, we also do not yet completely understand the factors that maintain the seizure focus in the brain or the interactions with the "crowd" of surrounding neurons. How does excitement, lack of sleep, or a fever alter the threshold of the surrounding cells? What genetic and environmental factors influence the threshold? If we understood the multiple factors and interactions that cause disruptions in the brain, and the factors that cause these disruptions to stop, we could probably prevent seizures from occurring altogether. But we do not.

Why Do Seizures Occur?

Only by understanding something about the physiology of the brain—how it works—and its anatomy can we understand the many different types of seizures that can occur and consider why they happen.

The brain works on electricity, with neurons (nerve cells) communicating and interacting by discharging or "firing" tiny electrical impulses along interconnecting "wires" called axons. The electrical impulse results in the release of a chemical called a neurotransmitter from the axon's ending or terminal (Figure 1.1). The neurotransmitter then interacts with the next cell. These neurotransmitters can be excitatory, that is make the next cell more likely to fire, or inhibitory, that is cause the next cell to be less likely to fire (Figure 1.2). Each cell has many thousands of endings; some of them (excitatory) are telling the cell to say "yes" and increasing the chance of that cell's firing (like pressing on the accelerator). There are some endings on the cell that say "no" (in-

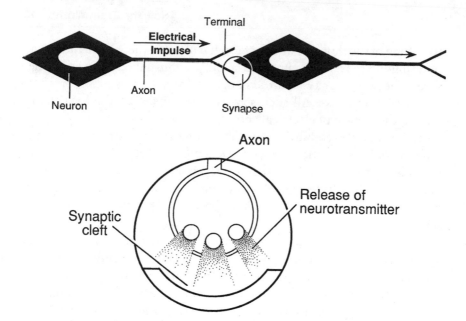

Figure 1.1 Communication between nerve cells. Neurons or nerve cells communicate by discharging electrical impulses along interconnecting axons, resulting in the release of a neurotransmitter, which floats across the space between cells (the synaptic cleft) and activates the next cell.

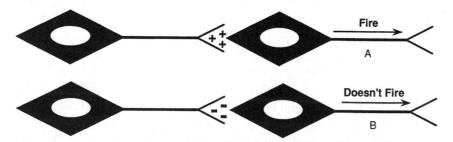

Figure 1.2 Excitation and inhibition of neuron. Some neurotransmitters, released by electrical impulse of neurons, may excite the next cell and cause it to fire (A); others inhibit the next cell and make it less likely to fire (B). The total of the excitatory ($+$) and inhibitory ($-$) impulses that influence each cell determines whether the cell will be stimulated to fire (its threshold). When the excitatory ($+$) impulses outnumber the inhibitory ($-$) impulses, the cell will fire.

hibitory), decreasing the chance of that cell's firing (like the brake). The balance of these excitatory and inhibitory impulses influences its threshold, or how readily that cell can be stimulated to fire (Figure 1.3). The increase or loss of influences saying "no" can also decrease or increase that cell's likelihood of firing.

One cell firing alone does not cause a seizure or even a movement. For a muscle movement, such as a twitch of a finger, to occur, many hundreds of cells must fire together. The process involves "recruitment" of a sufficient number of neighboring cells to fire simultaneously. If not enough cells are recruited, then not enough muscle fibers contract (shorten) to move the muscle. When you purposely move your finger, some muscle fibers on one side of the finger joint slowly contract (pull) in a coordinated fashion. The movement is controlled by the relaxation of muscle fibers on the other side of the joint (fired by different brain cells). This coordination and interaction of the different groups of brain cells that control the muscle fibers on each side of the finger joint allow you to manipulate finger movement. If, however, one group of cells in the brain fires without the controlling influence of other cells, your finger jerks or twitches. This is what happens in some types of seizures (Figure 1.4).

The brain functions normally when there is a balanced interaction

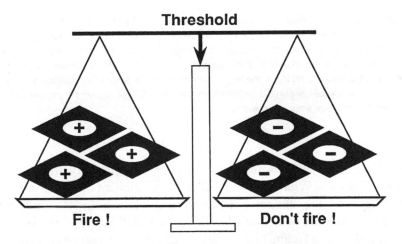

Figure 1.3 Threshold, the balance between excitatory (+) and inhibitory (−) influences. A loss of inhibitory influences or increase in excitatory influences may cause a cell to fire. Similarly, a loss of excitation or an increase in inhibition may cause a cell not to fire.

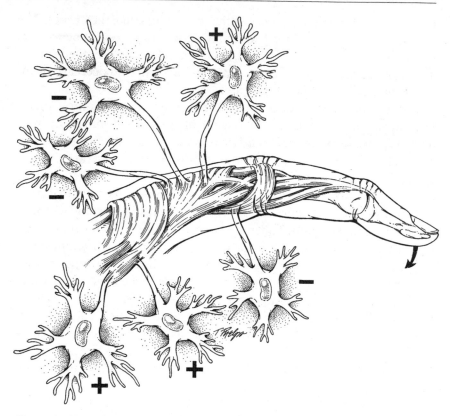

Figure 1.4 Muscle twitches and movements. Movement of a finger requires coordination of cells in the brain to achieve smooth coordination of muscles on both sides of a joint. The drawing shows a smooth downward movement of the finger, in which the contraction of the muscles on the underside, stimulated by nerve cells firing (+), is accompanied by relaxation of muscles on top of the finger, caused by nerve cells being inhibited from firing (−). In a seizure, all cells on the underside might fire suddenly, causing the finger to jerk rather than to move smoothly downward.

of many cells. When a sufficient number of cells work together, an "event" occurs. What the event will be is determined by which cells are firing. If the firing cells are in the motor area of the brain, the event may be the movement of a finger, hand, or foot; if they are in the sensory area, it may be a feeling like a tingle or a burning. In other areas it may be a taste, or a smell, or a memory. These normal human experiences occur when specialized parts of the brain are sufficiently excited.

A seizure occurs when the balance between excitation and inhibition is lost. A motor seizure, for example, happens when a sufficient number of cells spontaneously fire together and produce a sudden movement, a jerk. Not all sudden movements are seizures. A seizure is usually the result of repetitive firing of these same cells; when in the motor area, repetitive firing leads to the rhythmic, repetitive jerking of a group of muscles. Other types of seizures occur when cells from other areas of the brain fire simultaneously. The type of seizure depends on how many cells fire and which area of the brain is affected.

The truth is that we don't really know *why* a seizure occurs. We understand much about how the brain works and what a seizure is, how it happens, but not always why. We can explain how single cells fire, how they communicate with other cells, and a lot about the chemical and electrical makeup of neurons. We know that a cell's function is affected by its chemical environment. We know, for example, that oxygen and glucose (sugar) are required to keep neurons healthy and working; lacking sufficient oxygen or glucose, cells may fire abnormally and cause a seizure. Lack of blood supply to a part of the brain, such as after a stroke, can cause seizures by reducing the oxygen and chemicals necessary to keep these nerve cells functioning normally. Significant changes in important chemicals, such as calcium and magnesium, can cause seizures; so can a lack of certain vitamins. These chemical changes may provoke a disturbance in the brain, or a single seizure, by influencing the thresholds for firing, but they rarely cause epilepsy.

A high fever, a blow to the head, or an infection of the brain, such as meningitis or encephalitis, can provoke an isolated seizure by causing sufficient disruption of surrounding cells. But most seizures are the result of the *interaction* between the fiery speaker and the crowd, between the provocation to the brain and the surrounding neurons.

The Importance of Threshold

The threshold is the level of excitement at which a neuron will fire. As we have indicated, a cell's threshold is determined by the excitatory and inhibitory influences upon it. The seizure threshold is the level at which the brain will have a seizure, at which multiple cells will fire simultaneously (Figure 1.5).

Chemical factors like insufficient oxygen or low calcium can lower the threshold, as can fever, excitement, lack of sleep. In general, the

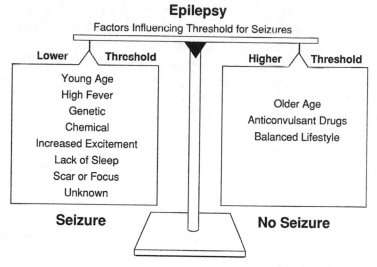

Figure 1.5 Factors influencing threshold for seizures. While genetic factors may be most important, factors such as young age and fever may lower the threshold, making a child more likely to have a seizure. Factors such as older age and anticonvulsants may decrease the chances of a seizure.

brain has a large margin of safety to protect it from misfiring. The size of this margin of safety is determined genetically. As a consequence, some people are closer to the threshold than others. In individuals with a previously low genetic threshold, fever may cause an event known as a febrile, or fever-induced, seizure. Seizures can be produced in anyone if the temperature becomes sufficiently high (107° to 108°F) and if the brain becomes sufficiently excited. In those with a lower genetic resistance or threshold, a febrile seizure may occur at a temperature of 103° or 104°. If the threshold of an individual is quite low, a seizure may occur with only slightly increased temperature, at 101° or 102°. Similarly, mild head trauma may cause a seizure in a child with a low genetic threshold, whereas it would take far more severe head trauma to cause a seizure in a child with a higher threshold.

❑ **Mrs. Circiello was driving the children to school when a truck hit the car broadside. Both children in the back seat hit their heads against the side of the** car. Tommy's friend Michael had a tonic-clonic seizure. Tommy was fine except for the bump on his head.

Why did one child have a seizure and the other not? One possibility is that Michael hit his head harder and this caused a greater disturbance in the brain. A second possibility is that, since Michael's father has seizures, Michael has inherited a lower threshold. Therefore, although his injury was the same as Tommy's, it was sufficient to trigger a seizure.

The threshold for a seizure is dependent also on age. Young children have lower seizure thresholds than adults. That is why young children are more likely to have a seizure when they get a fever and why most epilepsy begins in childhood. The increase in threshold with age may be the reason why most epilepsy that has begun in childhood is outgrown.

Emotional factors and other physical factors also influence a child's margin of safety. Excitement in response to a birthday party or a trip, or agitation caused by an argument or punishment, or anxiety during an exam may lower the individual's margin of safety and cause a seizure. So may lack of sleep in an individual whose threshold is already low. Such interactions of genetic threshold and environmental influences may explain many single, presumably "spontaneous," seizures.

Chemical changes in the blood, such as low blood sugar or low calcium levels, make neurons more susceptible to firing but are usually insufficient of themselves to produce seizures except in a "low-threshold, seizure-prone" child.

Although the margin of safety is largely determined by a child's genetic makeup, it varies from time to time and day to day depending on factors like the above. Whatever the margin of safety is at a given point in time, the threshold may be exceeded and a seizure result if there is an additional inciting influence, such as head trauma. Thus, a greater injury, a lower margin of safety, or a combination of the two may result in a seizure at a specific time. *Anyone can have a seizure if the trauma or disturbance is sufficiently great to exceed his threshold.*

On the other side of the scale (see Figure 1.5), anticonvulsant drugs, for example, increase the margin of safety and decrease the chance of a seizure's occurring. If medication is accidentally forgotten, then the margin of safety decreases, the child is closer to his threshold, and a seizure becomes more likely.

Thus, multiple interacting factors influence the susceptibility to seizures in any individual child, and their interactions may play a role in determining why seizures occur and recur at a specific time. As we learn more about the brain and its mechanisms of control we will understand more about threshold and about an individual's margin of safety. If we could increase that margin of safety, or increase the threshold, then we could better prevent seizures.

These are many of the aspects of *why* a seizure, a disruption in the brain, occurs, but where in the brain it occurs and how it spreads are equally important, because they determine the type of seizure.

Explaining to Your Child How the Brain Works

Virtually all children watch television. All have had the experience of disruption of the screen. A storm causes the picture to flicker or to briefly go off. A problem at the TV station interrupts the show. All of these are "seizures" in your TV set. This analogy is easy for most young children to understand, and it is indeed what happens during a brain seizure. We tell children that their brain is like the TV set. It works on electricity and usually plays well. If, or when, there is a brief electrical storm, the picture may become fuzzy; some people having a seizure may stop what they are doing and just seem to dream. A bigger electrical disturbance in the brain may cause a child to fall down, and people around him may be scared. But when the storm is over, the person will be fine, just like your TV set. The disruption lasts only a little while.

In explaining seizures to older children you may want to go into more detail about how the brain works and about how the spread of electricity causes different types of seizures. But, as with younger children, the important message is that these disruptions are *temporary*. Most of the time their brain works just fine. It was briefly interrupted and it will be normal. Most people are worried about the future, and in most cases, seizures that start in older, normal children will be brought under control; most will be outgrown, and usually, when your seizures are controlled you will be able to drive a car.

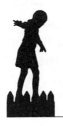

2. The Kinds of Seizure and Where They Arise in the Brain

Episodic electrical events can occur in different areas of the brain, and the type of seizure they produce will differ depending on what area is affected.

The Many Types of Seizure

❑ You heard a loud noise and ran to Johnny's room. Your son was stiff, his back was arched, he didn't seem to be breathing, and he was turning blue. Then he started shaking violently and was foaming at the mouth. Your first thought was that he was about to die!

❑ Mary was sitting with you at the dinner table when suddenly she stopped eating and stared into space. You called her, but she didn't respond. You had to call her several times. "Why does she daydream so often?" you wondered.

❑ William comes running to you with a frightened look on his face. He is pale and then has a glassy look in his eyes. You call him, but he doesn't respond. You notice that he is smacking his lips and fumbling with his clothes. Then as you hold him, he stiffens and begins to shake violently.

❑ Trina began to have jerking at the corner of her mouth. "It's just a habit," your doctor had said, but it's gotten worse. Now the jerking is there all the time and sometimes it spreads to involve the whole side of her face.

All of the events described above are seizures, and yet each differs from the others. Each may require a different evaluation by your physician. Each may require different medication. Each may have a different outcome. The type of seizure depends largely on where in the brain it starts and on the direction and speed of the spread of the electrical activity.

Seizures are divided into two major groups, "partial seizures" and "generalized seizures." "Partial seizures" (simple or complex) are also called "focal" or "local" seizures, because they begin focally—that is, in one place. It is important to identify partial seizures, because, since they begin focally, there may well indicate a problem in that specific area of the brain, one that may need special attention. The physician looks for a scar, a tangle of blood vessels, or a tumor as the cause of such seizures. If focal seizures cannot be controlled with medication, then surgery can be considered. "Generalized seizures," on the other hand, seem to start all over the brain at once. We are unable to detect either by clinical signs or symptoms, and sometimes not even from the EEG, where this widespread electrical activity begins.

Partial seizures have different implications from generalized seizures. Since they start in one particular area of the brain, they may require special evaluation; they may also require the use of particular medications or other therapy. Since the diagnosis of a seizure is based on the history of the event—the history you give—your description is critical to your physician's assessment. At the time the seizure is happening, you may be panicked and may not be a careful, dispassionate observer. If the episode doesn't recur, it was not important. If it *is* recurring, then careful observation, or better yet a home video of the event, may be invaluable. A picture is worth a thousand words to the physician who is trying to understand what has happened.

When seizures start focally, in a particular area of the brain, and when they spread slowly enough, in seconds or minutes, their onset can be experienced and witnessed or remembered, as in William's case. The onset is called the "aura" or warning, the warning that bigger things are coming.

How do focal seizures spread to become generalized? Why don't all focal seizures spread? What contains a focal seizure? If we knew the answers to these questions, we would understand far more about epilepsy than we do and be better able to prevent or limit seizures than we are. But we have few answers at the present time. Generalized seizures that appear to start in all parts of the brain simultaneously have no identifiable focal onset. We do not understand their anatomy. It does not make sense for the whole brain spontaneously and suddenly to experience a disruption. Nevertheless, in generalized seizures this is what appears to occur, causing disruptions like staring, stiffening, or shaking.

Terms Describing the Phases of a Seizure

Physicians commonly use certain special terms to describe parts of a seizure: *aura, ictus,* and *postictal.*

Aura. An aura is simply the start of a partial seizure. The frightened feeling that William experienced is called an aura if it precedes a bigger seizure. If the feeling is all that William experiences, he is said to have had an aura—a *simple partial seizure.* This may be the warning of a more widespread seizure to come. If the seizure spreads within the temporal lobe and affects consciousness, then it becomes a *complex partial seizure.* If it spreads throughout the brain, resulting in stiffening and generalized shaking, it becomes a *generalized seizure.* But with each seizure, the onset, which may be an abnormal smell, taste, abdominal sensation, or emotion (its focal beginning), is still called the aura.

Ictus. Ictus is the Latin word for "stroke" or "attack." Physicians sometimes use the word to mean a seizure. Thus, a simple partial seizure involving the hand, or a complex partial seizure, even a generalized seizure with loss of consciousness and jerking, could each be termed an ictus.

Postictal. Postictal means "after the attack" or seizure. After a person has had a seizure involving motor activity of her arm, the arm may be weak or even paralyzed for minutes or hours. This is termed a postictal paralysis, also called Todd's paralysis, after the physician who identified it. After a generalized tonic-clonic seizure, the person may go to sleep for a period. This is called the postictal state. After a partial complex seizure, the person may have postictal confusion. Each of these conditions occurs *after* the seizure is over.

Just as overexcitement and rapid synchronous firing of the neurons characterize the active phase of the seizure, so in the postictal phase the predominant activity of the brain is inhibitory. Neurons are less likely to fire. This effect helps to quiet the excitability of the cortex and stop the seizure. However, because inhibition also prevents the cells from resuming their normal activity, the person is sleepy or confused or may experience a temporary paralysis.

When observers say, "This person's seizures lasted an hour," what they really mean is that the individual had a generalized tonic-clonic seizure, which may have lasted only five minutes, but that the person then slept (was in a postictal state) for an hour. The difference between the two is important, because there is *no* danger from the postictal state. That quiescent state is simply the time necessary for the brain to recover and return to its normal functioning. If the seizure (jerking) had lasted for the entire hour, that would have been considered a medical emergency.

How Are Seizures Classified?

The Old System: "Grand Mal" and "Petit Mal" Seizures

At one time, seizures were classified into two types: big and small—in French, *grand* and *petit*. Since seizures were thought of as bad—*mal* in French—they were classified as "grand mal" and "petit mal," terms still, unfortunately, used by many patients and many physicians. It is unfortunate because they are imprecise. Many types of seizures are "big and bad," causing a patient to fall to the ground and shake. Johnny's seizure and William's seizure caused each child respectively to fall down and shake, so in the old days, both would have been called grand mal seizures. But the two seizures were different; William's seizure had a partial, or focal, beginning.

The term *grand mal* (big and bad) means different things to different people. Some people consider big a seizure that another, with worse seizures, might consider small. If one person has a spell in which he just stops and stares, as Mary did, while another, like William, has a spell in which he stares, smacks his lips, and is confused, and a third, such as Trina, has jerking of the face—are these little spells all "petit mal"? They are different types of seizures, coming from different parts of the brain, with different implications of causation, requiring different evaluation, requiring different medications, and probably having differing outcomes. Thus, the terms *grand mal* and *petit mal* are now seldom used in classifying seizures.

The New System: "Generalized" and "Partial" Seizures

An internationally accepted system of classification of seizures was adopted in 1981 (Table 2.1). This new classification separates seizures into "generalized" and "partial" (also called "focal").

Table 2.1   Seizure Classification

International classification	Old term
Partial seizures	Focal or local seizures
Simple partial (consciousness not impaired)	
• With motor symptoms	Focal motor
	Jacksonian seizures
• With somatosensory symptoms	Focal sensory
• With autonomic symptoms	
• With psychic symptoms	
Complex partial (consciousness impaired)	Psychomotor seizures
• Simple partial onset	Temporal lobe seizures
• With impairment of consciousness at onset	
Partial that secondarily generalize	
Generalized seizures	
(Convulsive or nonconvulsive)	
Absence	Petit mal
• Simple	
• Atypical	
Myoclonic	Minor motor
Clonic	Grand mal
Tonic	Grand mal
Tonic-clonic	Grand mal
Atonic	Akinetic, drop attacks
	Minor motor

Note: Adapted from *Epilepsia* 22:493–95, 1981.

Partial seizures may or may not alter consciousness or awareness, depending on where they start and which structures of the brain they involve. Partial seizures that do *not* alter consciousness are called "simple partial seizures," in the past called "focal motor" or "focal sensory" seizures. Partial seizures in which consciousness is altered or lost are called "complex partial seizures."

Generalized seizures affect the whole brain, not just one part, and they alter consciousness. In a generalized seizure, there is no obvious partial or focal onset or aura. When there is a focal onset, and the seizure progresses to involve the whole brain, it is termed a "partial seizure with secondary generalization."

Generalized seizures come in two sizes: large and small—convulsive and nonconvulsive. *Nonconvulsive* refers to alterations of consciousness but without jerking movements. *Convulsive* here means that there are muscle movements like jerking or stiffening.

Generalized Seizures

It seems intuitively obvious that the brain is unlikely to "seize" all over at one time. A seizure must start somewhere, but in most generalized seizures we cannot find a source. As technology improves, we are finding that some generalized seizures start in an area of abnormal cortex and spread so rapidly that without special techniques we cannot find the origin. Knowing that a generalized seizure starts in one place and rapidly spreads is important, however, because a source may be identifiable and the seizures may prove surgically treatable. Without an identified source, surgery is not an option.

Absence Seizures

An absence seizure, formerly called petit mal, is a very special and uncommon type of seizure. It starts suddenly and without warning. The child displays a glazed look and stares. She doesn't know what is happening and usually cannot later recall things that occurred during the seizure. Occasionally, there is a little eye-blinking or head-bobbing. The episode usually lasts just seconds, occasionally as long as fifteen seconds, and ends just as abruptly as it started. When the seizure ends, the child is immediately alert. There is *no* confusion afterward. These seizures may occur *many* times a day and are often mistaken for daydreaming.

It is usually easy for the physician to produce an absence seizure in his office by making such a child take deep breaths. Usually fifteen to thirty deep breaths (hyperventilation) will produce a typical spell. (Don't worry, exercise, such as running, swimming, or bike riding, which may make someone "out of breath," does *not* produce one of these spells. These seizures are actually more common when the child is bored or tired.)

A parent may see only a few seizures, because the brain's activity must be interrupted for more than one second before a spell is apparent. Thus, very brief electrical events (less than one second in duration) are observable only on the EEG. But, in a sense, the child's awareness may be being interrupted frequently, and the child may miss some of what is going on around him.

Occasionally a person who has these spells describes life as being "like a movie from which brief segments have been cut out." Teachers describe the child as daydreaming. Friends may call the child "spacey."

Atypical absence seizures are similar to absence seizures but may have more pronounced motor symptoms, such as tonic or clonic spells, or may have automatisms (involuntary behaviors) as seen in complex partial seizures. The EEG does not have the classic three-per-second spike and wave pattern seen in simple absence seizures. Atypical absence seizures are more commonly seen in children with a damaged nervous system and are often associated with other types of seizures.

Absence seizures may superficially be mistaken for complex partial seizures, because both involve staring. Since they may require different treatments and have different outcomes, differentiating between them may be important (see complex partial seizures, below).

Myoclonic Seizures

Myoclonic seizures (*myo* meaning muscle, *clonic* meaning jerk) are abrupt jerks of muscle groups. A hand may suddenly fling out, a shoulder may shrug, a foot may kick. Occasionally, an entire body may jerk, as in a startle response. *All myoclonic jerks are not seizures.* Myoclonic jerks can come from the spinal cord, not just from the brain. They need not be abnormal. Normal individuals who are falling asleep may suddenly experience a jerk of the body and startle awake. This is a normal phenomenon called *sleep myoclonus* and is *not* a seizure.

Myoclonic seizures (formerly called minor motor seizures) may take many different forms. They probably arise, or at least the jerk arises, from deep structures in the brain stem that control posture and tone in the body.

An abrupt increase in tone in a muscle group will cause a sudden movement of that part of the body. An abrupt increase in tone in the flexor muscles will cause the body to bend forward at the waist, the head to drop down on the chest, the arms to bend at the elbow, or the knees to come up to the chest. Any or all of these movements may occur during a myoclonic jerk or during myoclonic seizures. If they occur when a child is standing, he may suddenly be thrown to the ground, perhaps hitting his face, breaking a tooth, or cutting his forehead. If the tone is suddenly increased in the extensor muscles, the head may be thrown back, the back may arch, the legs extend, and the arms stiffen. A child who is standing may be thrown backward to the ground.

Myoclonic seizures can be serious, because they may be difficult to control and because they are often only one manifestation of a mixed seizure disorder.

Some varieties of jerks or myoclonic seizures are termed *benign myoclonus of infancy* (or childhood). They are benign because they are outgrown. The term *benign* is often easily applied in retrospect.

Myoclonic seizures are like being jolted by an electric shock. They are single jolts. On rare occasions, infants and young children may experience a *series* of these jolts, sometimes even many series per day. Such a series of myoclonic jerks constitutes a special, serious form of epilepsy called "infantile spasms" (see page 119).

Atonic Seizures

Atonic seizures, like myoclonic seizures, are sudden, single events. However, rather than a sudden increase in tone causing a movement of a joint or flexion or extension of the whole body, atonic seizures are a sudden *loss* of tone or posture. Arms, legs, or torso muscles, instead of supporting the body by their tone, suddenly go limp. The body slumps or gives way. The arms may suddenly fall, the legs give way, or the body crumple to the ground.

Atonic seizures, like myoclonic seizures, probably originate in areas deep in the brain stem that control muscle tone. Since the areas that increase tone are close to those that decrease tone, children with seizures involving sudden changes in tone may have either myoclonic or atonic seizures and often both.

Tonic-Clonic Seizures

Tonic-clonic seizures, formerly called grand mal seizures, are the sort most people think of when seizures are mentioned. The most memorable and frightening type of seizure to the observer, they are the most common seizure type in children, although not in adults, and despite common misconceptions are unlikely to result in brain damage or in death.

In a tonic-clonic seizure, the person initially stiffens and simultaneously loses consciousness (and thus is unaware of events). The stiffening is called the tonic phase and causes the individual to fall to the ground. The eyes "roll back in the head," the head goes back, the back arches, and the arms stiffen, as do the legs. This is similar to what happens during a myoclonic, extensor seizure, but this tonic phase of a tonic-clonic seizure happens more slowly. The extension is continued for what seems like an eternity but rarely lasts more than thirty seconds.

Since during this tonic (stiff) phase all the muscles are contracted, the chest muscles contract as well, and it is difficult for the person to breathe. He often turns somewhat blue about the lips and face (due as much to the face being flushed with the bluish blood of the veins as to the lack of oxygen). Saliva may cause a gurgling sound in the mouth or throat.

It is the blueness and gurgling sound that may cause observers to exclaim, "He's swallowed his tongue!" This is a common misconception. A person can't swallow his tongue, since it is attached to the back of the throat. "Quick, stick something in his mouth to keep him from biting his tongue!" someone else may advise, but this is bad advice. At the onset of the tonic phase of a seizure, the jaw becomes tightly clenched, and attempts to pry it open and put something in are likely to result in broken teeth.

After the tonic phase of a tonic-clonic seizure, rhythmic jerking begins. This is the clonic phase. The fists are tightly clenched, the arms repeatedly flex at the elbows and then briefly relax. The legs flex at the hip and knee joint in a similar fashion; the head may flex and then fall backwards. These movements are rhythmic and rapid, initially several per second, but then slowing. They are not the flailing movements or trembling often seen in imitation (pseudo) seizures. This rhythmic jerking seems to last forever, although only occasionally does it last more than a few minutes. Then the jerking becomes less severe and occurs at a slower rate, finally ceasing. The end of the jerking is usually accompanied by a deep sigh, after which normal breathing resumes.

The seizure is now over, but the child is not awake and will not yet respond. This postseizure period is the postictal state when the brain can be thought of as "exhausted" from all its activity. In reality, the brain is quite active, but its major activity is to inhibit (stop) the cells from firing. This inhibition has brought the seizures under control.

The postictal period often lasts a few minutes, longer if the tonic-clonic period has been long. If left alone, the person may sleep, but he can be aroused and may feel tired and confused. Muscles may be sore, and the tongue may have been bitten. The best course of action for an observer at this time is to be supportive and reassuring. Allow the person to rest until he is alert and able to go his own way.

A seizure occasionally may be limited to the tonic (stiffening) phase.

The tonic phase lasts for only a short while, usually less than a minute, and may be followed by a postictal sleep. A patient may on rare occasions experience a clonic seizure with the rhythmic movements previously described but without the preceding tonic phase. Management during and after the clonic seizure is identical to that after a tonic-clonic seizure.

There is no important distinction among these last three types of seizures—tonic, clonic, and tonic-clonic—formerly called grand mal seizures. Their causes are variable, their outlooks are the same, and their management with medication is identical.

Partial (Focal) Seizures and the Anatomy of the Brain

In order to understand partial or focal seizures and their many manifestations, it is necessary to understand something about the anatomy of the brain. Indeed, it was from a careful study of the events that occurred during partial or focal seizures that Dr. Hughlings Jackson, considered the father of modern understanding of epilepsy, first deduced the organization of the brain. He watched the slow spread of focal seizures (subsequently called Jacksonian seizures) from the finger to the hand to the arm and then to the face, and reasoned that these areas must be next to one another in the brain. The result was the identification of the anatomy of the motor strip (Figure 2.1).

These deductions subsequently have been confirmed by Dr. Wilder Penfield and Dr. Herbert Jasper, who, during operations to remove tissue responsible for focal epilepsy, stimulated areas of the brain with small amounts of electricity. Depending on which area was stimulated, a finger would move, a foot would jerk, the face and tongue would twitch, or a finger or lip would tingle. Even certain memories or images would be recalled. Minute electrical stimulation is used even today to "map the brain" before a surgeon removes electrically abnormal brain tissue, so that tissue important to normal function can be identified and avoided during the surgery (see Chapter 14).

As the human brain has evolved, its "thinking and processing" parts have become greatly enlarged. This "thinking" part of the brain is the cortex. The cortex has four major sections, called lobes, responsible for separate functions (Figure 2.2A). The frontal lobes are responsible for personality and memory. The temporal lobes on the left side control speech (in most people) and those on the right control subtle higher

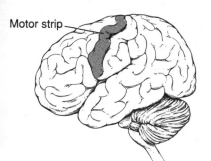

Motor strip

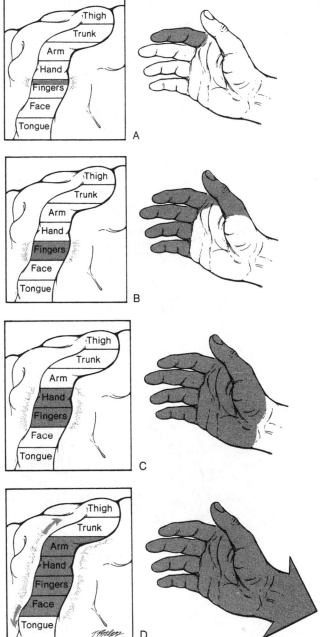

Figure 2.1 Brain, showing motor strip and progression of motor symptoms of a partial seizure. Hughlings Jackson observed the slow spread of seizures from jerking of a finger (A), to jerking of all fingers (B), to involvement of hand and wrist (C), then arm and face (D). From this spread he deduced the anatomy of the motor strip of the brain. Hence, seizures of this sort have been called Jacksonian seizures.

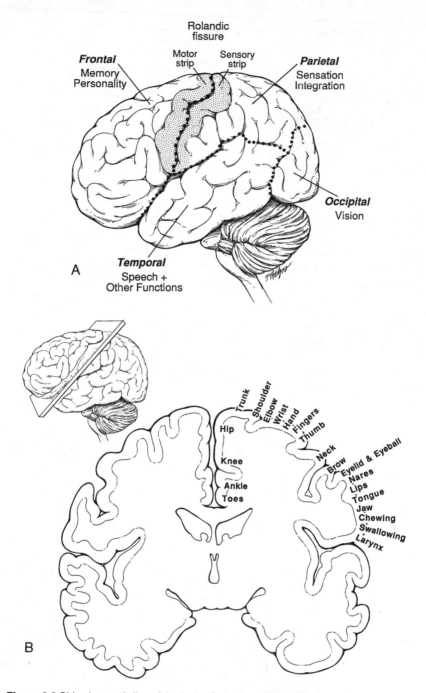

Figure 2.2 Side view and slice of the brain. Side view of brain (A) shows the major lobes and their functions and the motor and sensory strips; a slice of the brain (B) shows location of motor and sensory functions.

functions such as spatial and musical recognition. The parietal lobes contain areas for making associations and interpreting sensations, such as the ability to recognize objects placed in the hand. The occipital lobes are the site of processing visual information.

The *left* side of the brain controls movements of the *right* side of the body and receives sensation from the *right* side of the body. Thus, the left occipital lobe processes vision of things in your right field of vision, and the *right* side of the brain processes similar functions for the left side of the body (Table 2.2).

Motor and Sensory Areas

Perhaps the easiest areas of the brain to understand and explain are the motor strip and sensory strip (Figure 2.3). If a surgeon were to take

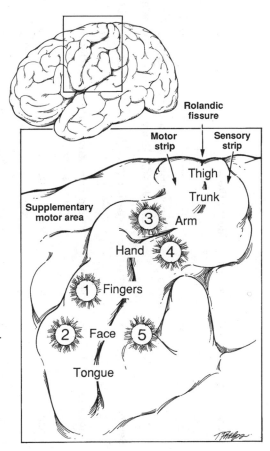

Figure 2.3 Motor and sensory areas of the brain. Electrical stimulation at area 1 causes twitching of a finger; at 2, facial movements; at 3, jerking of the arm; at 4 in the sensory strip, tingling in the hand; at 5, tingling of face or lips.

Table 2.2 Localization of Function within the Brain

Function	Area	Left side	Right side	Deficit if removed
Motor	Motor strip	Control of face, arm, and leg on right side of body	Control of face, arm, and leg on left side of body	Weakness (hemiparesis) of the opposite side
Sensory	Sensory strip	Sensation from right side of body	Sensation from left side of body	Inability to identify what is in hand, where hand is in space, whom hand belongs to, and so on
Cortical sensation	Parietal lobe	Integration of sensation from right side of body	Integration of sensation from left side of body	
Vision	Occipital lobe	Vision to the right side of the body	Vision to the left side of the body	Lack of vision of things to one side or the other
Speech	Temporal lobe	Speech (on left side in 95% of right-handed people, on left side in 70% of left-handed people)		
Intelligence, personality, sense of humor	Not lateralized or localized			

off a person's skull and the coverings of the brain to expose the motor strip of the frontal lobe and introduce a small amount of electrical current (stimulus) on the brain-surface in the finger area (area 1), the awake patient might see some twitching of the index finger of one hand. If this were done to the left side of the brain, the right index finger might twitch. Were the surgeon to move the current slightly up or down the strip, it might cause another finger to move. Moving the current to the face area (2) would cause facial movements; in area 3, the arm on the right side of the body might jerk. These movements are, in a sense, little seizures, a slight seizure induced by the surgeon's electrical stimulus.

If the electrical stimulus comes from within the brain cells themselves (rather than from a surgeon's electrical stimulus), caused for example by a scar, a stroke, or a tumor, the resulting movement would be called a seizure. If the seizure stays local (focal), it may consist of just the repeated twitch of a finger, a hand, or the face. If the seizure focus is in the sensory strip and occurs in area 4, then the patient may experience a tingling or funny feeling in the hand (on the opposite side of the body); if the seizure began at area 5, then the feeling might be in the face or lip.

Focal motor or focal sensory seizures such as these do occur. Trina's seizures (see page 21) are focal motor seizures involving the lip and face, occasionally spreading locally to involve one side of her face. Seizures may start locally, then spread slowly or rapidly to include other areas of the brain. When a focal seizure spreads to other parts of the brain, the initial movement or sensation is the aura, or warning, of bigger things to come.

The Temporal Lobes: Lateral (Outer)

The outside of the left temporal lobe is involved in aspects of speech. Someone with a problem in one of these areas may have difficulties in finding the correct word to use; the person may know the correct word and yet be unable to say it, or may be able to say words (or repeat words) but not be able to say them clearly, or may be able to talk clearly and fluently but not make sense. These are all called "expressive" problems, problems in expressing thoughts. The type of expressive problem depends on exactly which part of the speech area is involved (Figure 2.4). Abnormalities in other, slightly different areas of the temporal lobe may cause "receptive" problems, an inability to understand words or phrases, difficulties in comprehension.

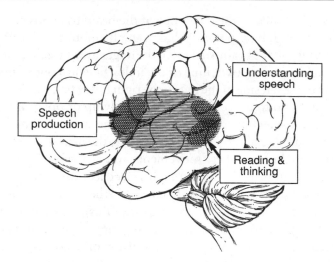

Figure 2.4 Speech and language areas of the brain. Areas in the temporal (and frontal) lobe, usually on the left side, are responsible for speech and language. Specific functions appear to lie in relatively discrete areas on the outside of the brain.

Stimulation of the left temporal cortex with small amounts of electricity can locate precisely which part of the brain is involved in each function and can simulate these difficulties. Problems in finding or saying words also occur during or following focal seizures and thus can often aid the physician in identifying where the seizure began (or remains). There is no comparable localization on the outside of the right temporal lobe except in *some* left-handed individuals.

The Temporal Lobes: Mesial (Inner)

The mesial, or middle, inner aspect of both temporal lobes is of great importance in epilepsy, since they are quite prone to damage and are frequently the source of seizures. (This area of the brain and some of its features are shown in Figure 2.5.)

Stimulation of the front of the mesial temporal lobe, or seizures originating from that part, may produce a smell, usually an unpleasant, acrid smell, often described as the smell of burning rubber. Stimulation farther back in the mesial temporal lobe may produce abnormalities of taste (bitter, metallic) or sensation in the abdomen (cramps, discomfort) or a rising sensation from the abdomen to the throat (as if nauseated).

Also in the mesial part of the temporal lobe are structures called the amygdala and hippocampus, important structures connected to areas of the brain involved with emotions, such as fear, and controlling func-

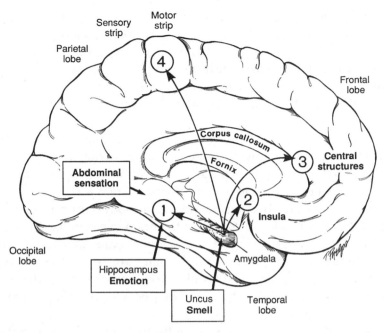

Figure 2.5 Temporal lobe, inner side, and spread of seizures. The inner side of the lobe is often involved in seizures. Change in functions during a seizure can indicate the location of the electrical discharge. The amygdala, hippocampus, and uncus are among the most important of these areas. With their many interconnections to the frontal lobe, they influence emotions, consciousness, and autonomic function. If a seizure starts in the uncus, the aura may be an unpleasant smell. It may then spread to the hippocampus (1), followed by a sensation of fear, or to the insula (2), causing abdominal sensation, then spread to other central structures (3), causing loss of awareness and a complex partial seizure, or to the motor area (4), causing a tonic-clonic seizure.

tions such as blood pressure, heart rate, and paleness or facial flushing (autonomic functions). William's seizure began with the sensation of fear, probably originating in this part of his brain and spreading to involve autonomic functions (the paleness he displayed) before becoming generalized and spreading throughout the brain. This part of the brain is also involved in storing memories. Thus, stimulation (or seizures) may produce flashbacks or memories or feelings, as if something had been seen or experienced previously (déjà vu). Electrical stimulation of these areas, or spontaneous electrical activity such as seizures, may create or recreate one, all, or any combination of these feelings and experiences.

Seizures that begin in the temporal lobes may remain focal or may spread slowly or rapidly. For example, seizures starting in the uncus (see Figure 2.5) may initially consist of just a peculiar smell (such as burning rubber). This may be the only thing that happens during a seizure, or the seizure may spread to the hippocampus (1) and be followed by a sensation of fear. The spread may be to the insula (2) and cause a rising sensation in the abdomen and chest or abdominal discomfort. Further spread to area 3 may lead to loss of awareness, with staring, often accompanied by automatic, unconsciously repeated movements, such as lip smacking, picking at one's clothes, and wandering around aimless and confused. These movements are called automatisms. Spread of the seizure from the uncus (1) to the motor strip (4) may lead to a focal motor seizure, a seizure affecting one side of the body (unilateral seizure), or to a seizure spreading throughout the brain (a generalized seizure).

Because there are so many diverse functions either in or closely connected to the temporal lobe, seizures coming from this area can have a variety of manifestations and may alter consciousness. Since they start from one area, they are "partial," but they become complex and so are termed "partial complex" seizures.

Consciousness, or awareness, is not located in any single area of the brain. A surgeon can remove half of the brain (either half) and consciousness remains intact. Loss of consciousness is experienced when either both sides of the cortex dysfunction simultaneously or when there is an interruption of the communication between the cortex and the more centrally located parts of the brain. Alterations in consciousness can be seen naturally during sleep, when the electrical activity of the cortex changes. During seizures that involve alterations in consciousness, the electrical activity of the cortex as a whole is always altered.

The Frontal Lobes

Areas of the frontal lobes other than the motor strip are less well defined; they have to do with personality, memory, anxiety, alertness, and awareness. Because there are so many connections between the frontal and temporal lobes (see Figure 2.5), it is often difficult to determine from the way a seizure looks whether the function being disrupted is in the frontal or the temporal lobe. Some areas in the supplementary motor area, near the motor strip (see Figure 2.3), seem to control the coordination of movements of groups of muscles. Electrical stimulation of, or seizures in, the supplementary motor area thus may cause the eyes, head, and body to turn away from that side and may appear to cause a brief staring and loss of awareness before some of the stereotypical seizures called complex partial seizures appear.

Other Areas of the Brain: The Occipital Lobes and Parietal Lobes

The temporal lobes and the frontal lobes are the most important in a discussion of epilepsy because they are the most "epileptogenic." We don't know why, but they seem to have a lower threshold for seizures.

Scars, tumors, and other damage in the temporal and frontal lobes of the brain are much more likely to be accompanied by seizures than damage to the occipital lobes or parietal lobes. However, just for completeness, we will briefly discuss these areas as well.

The primary function of the occipital lobe, located in the back of the brain (Figure 2.6), is vision. Messages from the retina (the back of the eyeball) are transmitted by way of the optic (eye) nerves and by a pathway (the optic radiation) to the occipital lobe, where vision is registered by the brain. Objects off to your left side (when you look straight ahead) register on the right side of your retina (see Figure 2.6), and the mes-

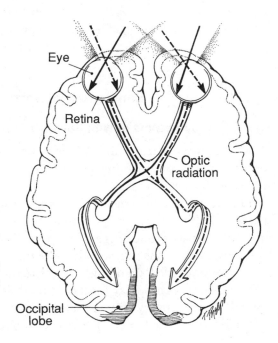

Figure 2.6 Occipital lobe, visual pathways. Vision is located in this lobe. An image on a person's right side is seen by the left portion of the retina; electrical impulses from the left side of the retina travel through the visual pathways to the occipital lobe of the cortex on the left side.

sage proceeds along the path to the right side of your brain. Images of objects on your right (when you look straight ahead) go to the left side of your brain. Vision is complex, and when one stimulates the occipital cortex electrically, the patient sees only bright lights in a random pattern. When a seizure begins in the occipital lobe—which is not common—flashing bright lights may be experienced off to the left side, if it occurs in the right cortex, or to the right side if the left cortex is involved.

The parietal lobe is where perception comes together, where much of what we sense by vision or touch achieves meaning. Here, those flashing lights become patterns constituting a formed visual image; through interconnections with the frontal lobe (where memories are stored), we are able to store the images as memories or to recall formed images as recognized faces or scenes. The posterior temporal-parietal lobe is the site where sounds heard become the pattern of words, which are recognized and remembered or given meaning by association with prior experiences stored in the frontal lobes. It is where speech that is heard becomes speech that is understood and where the sense of touch and feel of a particular object is identified as a key, a ball, or a block. Thus, the parietal lobe is called "the association cortex." It is rarely the source of seizures and seems to play little role in our understanding of the types of epilepsy. It is not, in other words, very "epileptogenic."

This basic and simplified lesson in brain anatomy should provide a better understanding of the many variations of partial seizures discussed below.

Simple Partial Seizures

With Motor Symptoms or with Sensory Symptoms

Simple partial seizures may involve movement, with jerking of the foot, face, arm, or any other part of the body. They may involve the senses, with a peculiar tingling, burning, or abnormal sensation in any part of the body. Where the jerking or sensation occurs will depend on where in the brain the electrical activity begins and how it spreads. Since motor and sensory functions are lateralized—one side of the brain controlling the other side of the body—the motor jerking or sensory feeling will be one-sided, on the side opposite the brain's activity.

Partial seizures may stay local or spread slowly up or down the motor strip or the sensory strip (see Figures 2.1 and 2.2) in a slow spread or "march" that used to be called a Jacksonian seizure.

With Autonomic Symptoms

Since a seizure may begin in areas of the brain that control involuntary functions (see Figure 2.5), it may start with the face becoming pale or flushed. The heart may begin to beat rapidly; there may be abdominal cramps and discomfort or a fullness in the chest or throat. Physicians call these "autonomic" symptoms because it is the autonomic part of the nervous system that regulates involuntary body functions like heart rate, blood pressure, and bowel function.

Since the autonomic system has to control both sides of the body simultaneously, not a single half at a time, the physician often cannot identify the side of the origin of the seizure by these manifestations alone.

With Psychic Symptoms

Seizures coming from certain parts of the brain can either trigger or stimulate emotions or stimulate the recall of prior experiences. Fear is one emotion frequently experienced alone or as the aura of a seizure, as in William's case. The emotion is often described in vague language: "I just felt scared." "I can't describe it—it's a weird feeling." "I know something's going to happen, I know it's coming." A child may not be able to describe the feeling at all, but his face may have a frightened look and he may come running to his parent and hold on tightly. But, occasionally, feelings expressed are more specific. A scene experienced in the past will be reexperienced spontaneously; voices will be heard, though often they cannot be understood. (These feelings must be carefully differentiated from the hallucination of drugs or psychiatric illness.) Occasionally a person will have the sensation of déjà vu, that he has experienced something before (even if it has not previously occurred) or that he has seen someone before; or there may be an experience of jamais vu (never seen), in which something or someone very familiar seems to be unknown.

Similar experiences may have occurred to each of us on occasion. But when they recur, when they are frequent, or when they are associated with other episodic changes in function or behavior, they may be simple partial seizures.

❑ **Olga comes running to her mother. "I've got that feeling in my hand again. I think I'm going to have another seizure." In a few moments she develops jerk-**

ing of the arm and then of the whole side of her body. What kind of a seizure is this? Where did it start in the brain? Would it have been a different kind of seizure if it had begun with jerking in the hand or foot or with autonomic or psychic symptoms?

All such events are simple partial seizures starting in one of several areas of the brain. They may or may not spread to involve other brain areas.

Complex Partial Seizures

Because the functions located in the temporal lobe and in the frontal lobe are complex, seizures beginning there can be very complex. There are, in addition, many interconnections of both frontal and temporal lobes to other areas of the brain—centrally located—that control alertness and awareness. Thus, seizures beginning in the temporal or frontal lobe may alter consciousness. If they do, they are termed "complex partial seizures."

With Simple Partial Onset

A simple partial seizure may spread quickly to the areas that affect consciousness and may result in staring, confusion, loss of alertness, or aimless movements. These are called complex partial seizures "with simple partial onset." They are simple partial seizures with a secondary spread sufficiently slow that we can recognize where they started. These seizures are most likely to begin in the temporal lobe (Figure 2.7).

With Loss of Consciousness at Onset

Complex partial seizures may not produce changes in behavior or function before alterations in consciousness occur. The child may start with a blank stare without any warning or aura, then wander around the room, pick at his clothes, do repetitive movements, and so on. Such seizures, with sudden impairment of consciousness, are likely to originate in the frontal lobe.

Distinguishing between complex partial seizures with simple partial onset and complex partial seizures with loss of consciousness at onset may be difficult or impossible. It may require careful analysis of a video-EEG, on which the instantaneous correlation of changes in the EEG and changes in behavior recorded by the video can be seen. The correct dif-

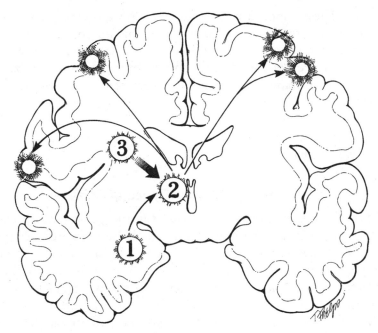

Figure 2.7 Examples of spread of partial seizures, simple and complex. If electrical activity remains confined to area 1, there is a simple partial seizure, manifested possibly by sensory, autonomic, or psychic symptoms, all functions located in the temporal lobe. If activity spreads to 2, an area that controls consciousness, alertness, and awareness, cortical function is altered and the patient stares, is confused, or wanders aimlessly—in a complex partial seizure with a simple partial onset. If the spread from 1 to 2 is so rapid that symptoms of the seizure in area 1 are not detected *or* if the seizure begins at 3 (in the frontal lobe) and spreads to 2, it will produce the same alterations in consciousness. This is also a complex partial seizure.

ferentiation between these two subtypes is not important unless surgery is being considered.

Gelastic Seizures

Gelastic or laughing seizures are a rare type of seizure which usually begins with a laugh or a giggle. The seizure may progress to other focal motor manifestations, or the child may become confused. Gelastic seizures rarely become generalized seizures. They are most commonly caused by a benign congenital tumor called a *hypothalamic hamartoma,* which is located deep in the middle of the brain (near area 2 in Figure 2.7). The gelastic seizures themselves seem to arise from within the tumor. These tumors are generally very slow growing and very difficult to remove totally without causing destruction to vital areas. Often the best course seems to be to live with the laughing seizures, use medication to prevent them from becoming more generalized seizures, and get several opinions at epilepsy centers before proceeding with surgery on the hamartoma.

Again, before a physician can classify a seizure, she must be sure that a child is actually having seizures. Therefore, diagnosis and classification go hand in hand.

Differentiating between Types of Seizure

One of the most confusing areas of classification both for physicians and for parents is differentiation between absence seizures (see page 26) and complex partial seizures (page 42). This differentiation may be important, since it may determine which medications should be used to treat your child. Further confusion comes when you try to differentiate either of these staring spells from normal daydreaming. Let us give you an example of how we try to differentiate daydreaming from seizures.

❑ **The teacher has called to say that Lisa is daydreaming in school. You have noticed some episodes of "daydreaming" at the dinner table. Does she have absence seizures? Does she have atypical absence seizures? Does she have complex partial seizures, or is she daydreaming?**

The questions your physician will want to ask you about Lisa are:

• "How frequently is she having these episodes?" Daydreaming would occur infrequently and be situational. Absence seizures may occur many times a day. Complex partial seizures rarely occur more than several times a day or a week.
• "How do these episodes begin?" While most seizures have an abrupt onset, occasionally complex partial seizures begin slowly and a warning precedes them. Daydreaming usually does not start abruptly.
• "Can you interrupt these episodes?" Daydreaming can easily be interrupted by calling the child's name or by physically touching her. Seizures, on the other hand, cannot be interrupted.

• "How long does the episode last?" Daydreaming can go on until something else catches a child's attention. Absence seizures rarely last more than fifteen seconds. Complex partial seizures may last up to several minutes.

• "What does the child do during the episode?" While daydreaming or during absence seizures, the child is likely to stare into space. During complex partial seizures, the child is likely to smack her lips, pick at her clothes, or display other automatisms.

• "What is the child like when she 'comes back?'" The child who is daydreaming or having an absence seizure will be immediately alert. The child with a complex partial seizure will usually be confused for seconds or minutes.

• "Does the child remember what was said during the episode?" While daydreaming, the child may be aware of what is happening but not pay attention. During a seizure, the child is not fully aware of what is happening around her.

• "Do the spells occur only at special times?" If they happen only, say, in math or geography class, the child is likely to be daydreaming. If they occur at random times or whenever the child is tired, they are more likely to be seizures.

With these careful observations, you and your physician can usually differentiate the type of episode.

Locating the Site of Onset

All partial seizures may at times spread to affect the whole brain. This spreading usually results in a tonic-clonic seizure. Depending on the direction of the electrical spread, however, it may result in an atonic seizure, in which a child suddenly collapses to the floor or is thrown down, or a tonic seizure, in which the child suddenly stiffens and arches his back.

The parent should carefully observe the onset of a seizure and its progression so that the physician can have an accurate history, in order to determine if there was focal onset, aura, or warning. As with focal or partial seizures, a focal onset of a generalized seizure implies a focal problem or disturbance. Generalized seizures with focal onset require an especially careful medical evaluation, because *if* these seizures cannot be controlled with medication, *and* if the focus can be identified, there may be a possibility of a "cure" of the seizures by surgical removal of the area where the seizure begins.

Now, with some understanding of the brain's anatomy, organization, and how it works, you should be better able to understand the many kinds of seizures and the different names physicians use when they describe your child's seizure or seizures. This naming is important because it will help determine the treatment for your child.

Part Two

Diagnosing Seizures and Epilepsy

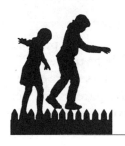

3. How We Diagnose a Seizure and Decide What It Will Mean for Your Child

Was It a Seizure?

A seizure, as we have seen (Chapter 1), is a sudden alteration in behavior or in motor function caused by an electrical discharge in the brain. It should be very easy to diagnose a seizure, since it is simply a sudden change in behavior or motor function. But sometimes it's not that simple; people have sudden changes in behavior all the time. Sometimes children faint, daydream, or fall down. How do you tell if those events are seizures?

The only way to diagnose a seizure is to take a very careful history of the event that has occurred. That's why doctors ask all those questions: What was the child doing when it happened? What was the first thing that was noticed? What happened next? What was the child doing during the episode? The doctor may ask you to demonstrate what you saw (if you saw it). Was the child trembling, making rapid movements of the arms or legs, or were the child's arms or legs jerking rhythmically? What was the child like afterward? Was she tired? Did he have a headache? Did the child wet herself during the spell? While none of these findings is specific for a seizure, the pattern may make the physician more or less suspicious that the episode was a seizure.

There is no diagnostic test for a seizure or for epilepsy. The diagnosis rests solely on the physician's interpretation of the history of the episode which occurred. Although many persons with seizures and epilepsy do have abnormal EEGs, many do not. EEGs don't tell the whole story. Many people have the frequent electrical discharges seen on the EEG. Changes in an EEG in the absence of change in a person's function are not seizures or epilepsy and should rarely be treated.

Since physicians rarely have the opportunity to see the seizure events for themselves, they must depend on the observation of parents or other witnesses to the episode. Most of these observers have never seen a true seizure and are upset and panicked by what they have seen. When they relay the information through third parties, the story can grow more lurid or lose important details. Frequently, events occur at school or when the child is with friends. The person who actually saw the event will give more useful responses if he or she is calmly questioned about exactly what happened. This is one of the reasons why the parent is such an important member of the team. The physician can't make a diagnosis without good information. Parents may need to talk to teachers, friends, or even other children who saw what happened.

Let us give you an example of how difficult it may be to determine whether a particular episode was a seizure and how we think about the episode's importance for the child's future.

❑ **Jane is thirteen years old. A nurse is cleaning her arm with alcohol in preparation for taking blood tests ordered by her physician. The nurse takes out the syringe and needle and Jane says, "Wait a minute, I don't feel well." She looks pale and sweaty, then collapses in the chair. She stiffens and has jerking of her arms and legs that lasts perhaps a minute. Was that a seizure? "Yes," the physician says, "but it was a seizure due to fainting. That is what is called 'convulsive syncope.' Jane fainted, just as many people faint when blood is taken. In some people, fainting is enough to trigger a brief seizure. It's nothing to worry about. That is not epilepsy. She'll be fine."**

That diagnosis was easy. Jane's seizure occurred because of fainting. The episode was witnessed from the start by people trained to observe carefully. They heard Jane say she didn't feel well. They saw her become pale and sweaty *before* losing consciousness. It was clear to them that Jane fainted and then had a seizure. The episode occurred in a situation in which fainting is not uncommon. But suppose Jane had been sitting in the hot sun with her friends at a baseball game when the episode occurred? Could she have been drinking beer or taking drugs? Would her friends have noted the paleness and sweating before she fainted, became stiff, and had the brief jerking movements? If they hadn't noticed the fainting and had only seen the jerking, your doctor might not have known why the seizure occurred and would have been concerned that it might recur. He could not have been as confident in saying that it was convulsive syncope.

After taking a careful, detailed history,
the physician should be able to say one of three things:

1. "That episode was clearly a seizure."

or

2. "That was clearly not a seizure. It sounds to me like a fainting spell (breathholding spell, etc.)."

or

3. "I'm not sure what that episode was. I don't think it was a seizure, but let's wait and see if it recurs. If it does recur, I want you to observe the child carefully and look for . . ."

Even if a single episode was a seizure, it may not be important to your child's future, since most single seizures do not recur or require treatment. If episodes are recurring, it should not take long for careful observation to determine their true nature. If infrequent and not interfering with the child's life, they are less important. Rare episodes will either disappear as mysteriously as they appeared, or they will become sufficiently obvious and frequent to allow proper diagnosis.

Many people have been told that their child has had a seizure and the child was subsequently treated with medication, all because of incorrect interpretation of a single event, such as fainting. When in doubt about an event or about the circumstances of it, it is usually better to wait and see if a similar event occurs. It is better to live with uncertainty than to allow yourself or your physician to be too eager to label the event and begin treatment.

If there is doubt about the nature of the event or events, whether or not your child is on medication, you should explore this further with your doctor. Even when your child clearly has had a seizure, different seizures will have different meanings for the child's future. The meaning may well depend on the context in which the seizure occurred. He may not need extensive evaluation and medication. Decisions about evaluation and treatment may depend on the circumstances in which the seizure or seizures occurred.

Provoked and Unprovoked Seizures

❑ Your child is playing outside when his friend comes banging at the door. "Come quick!" the friend shouts. "Something's happened to Bobby!" You run and find Bobby on the edge of the playground making gurgling sounds and with his arms and legs jerking. "Was that a seizure?" you ask your physician later. "It certainly sounds like one," she replies. "We have to be concerned that Bobby might have another one. If he does, then he has epilepsy—by definition." If by talking to Bobby's friend his mother learns that Bobby was climbing a tree, fell, and hit his head, the doctor might answer differently: "I think Bobby had a slight concussion and a brief seizure, what we call a 'posttraumatic seizure.' These brief seizures after a child hits his head are not uncommon and rarely recur. I think that this is what we call a provoked seizure. I don't believe he has epilepsy or will have epilepsy."

It is not the mere occurrence of a seizure but also the *circumstances* under which the seizure occurs that determine if a child is likely to have more seizures. Furthermore, the child must have two or more seizures or he does not have epilepsy.

If a child has several seizures during an episode of meningitis, or after a head injury, or with diarrhea and dehydration, or with other acute conditions, these seizures are termed "provoked" seizures or "symptomatic" seizures, ones that have a defined cause. Just as Jane's seizure after fainting was a provoked seizure, so was Bobby's after hitting his head. The acute brain disturbance that caused them will disappear or be cured and the seizure should not recur.

Although acute conditions such as a head injury or meningitis *can* cause permanent damage to the brain, and that damage *can* later lead to "unprovoked" recurrent seizures—epilepsy—permanent damage followed later by epilepsy is not a consequence of acute symptomatic seizures in children.

Episodes Often Mistaken for Seizures

Many changes in motor function or behavior are commonly mistaken for seizures. These include fainting, tics, and other sudden jerking movements, breathholding spells, migraine headaches, and episodic changes in behavior. Doctors who are aware of these types of behaviors can take a careful history and usually separate them from seizures.

Is It Fainting or a Seizure?

❏ It had been a long church service and, as usual, Rebecca had almost been late. Her alarm had not gone off, and when her mother had called her there had barely been time to get dressed. No time for breakfast. Her mother told the doctor, "The sermon was long and dull, and Rebecca remembers standing for the hymns and feeling dizzy. The next thing she remembers is waking up outside the church. She doesn't remember passing out. The paramedic who happened to be there asked me if Rebecca had epilepsy. Does she? You'll tell me the truth, Doctor, won't you?"

Fainting spells are commonly misdiagnosed as seizures. Indeed, some people have been treated for "epilepsy" for years when they had simply fainted. Fainting is caused by insufficient blood going to the brain. Since one of the brain's important activities is to maintain consciousness and posture, when the brain does not get enough blood, the person may become dizzy and slump to the floor. This decrease of bloodflow to the brain may be due to slowing of, or even brief pauses in, the heart beat. Or it may result from prolonged standing, the blood becoming pooled in the legs or in the abdomen with not enough blood available to pump to the brain. Or it could result from anemia, insufficient red blood cells to carry oxygen to the brain.

In each case, the lack of blood initially causes a paleness, followed by sweating. The person feels "lightheaded," or dizzy. The room seems to spin, and he or she slumps (not crashes) to the ground. As soon as the person is lying down, the heart does not have to pump blood up to the head, the blood supply to the brain is immediately increased, and within seconds he regains consciousness. He will usually still be pale and sweaty, may briefly be confused, and may still feel weak. Even though he has had a change in motor function and consciousness, he has not had a seizure, since that change was not caused by abnormal electrical activity in the brain.

Fainting can precede and cause a seizure, as in Jane's case, or occur without a seizure, as we have seen in Rebecca's story. Fainting spells may occur when someone has gone too long without eating, when someone gives blood, or occasionally because of insufficient sleep or extreme tension or anxiety or overventilation due to anxiety. In individuals who have low blood pressure, fainting can be brought on by standing up too fast.

One often unrecognized cause of fainting is lack of salt.

❏ Elsie was a long-distance runner. At fifteen she led the cross-country track team's championship team. She was running at least five miles a day until the day she passed out in the shower. Because Elsie's sister had epilepsy, her mother was sure that Elsie had had a seizure. When seen by her physician Elsie was rail thin. Her exam was normal except for her pulse, which was a runner's 55 beats per minute, and her blood pressure, which was quite low at 90 over 65. Instead of ordering an MRI and an EEG, her physician asked about her eating habits. Because of her father's high blood pressure, the family added no salt to their cooking and Elsie avoided salt. Else was salt depleted, and the hot shower had caused her blood pressure to drop further. After adding salt to her diet. Elsie felt better, her blood pressure registered 110 over 80 at her follow-up examination, and she had no more episodes of fainting.

When we understand the circumstances and the sequence of events, we should be able to distinguish easily between convulsive syncope (seizures with fainting) and other seizures. The preceding paleness and sweatiness described are typical of fainting but not of seizures. Wetting oneself is more common during seizures than after fainting but can occur in both situations. On the other hand, any person who bites his tongue may be having a seizure, but someone who faints does not bite his tongue.

When the sequence of events is unclear, the physician will probably want to wait before making a diagnosis, since it is better to be uncertain than to label the event a seizure. If the child continues to have these episodes, either the nature of the spells will become clear or further tests will be indicated to determine the appropriate diagnosis and treatment. An EEG *does not* differentiate between fainting and seizures unless an episode occurs when the EEG is running.

Fainting spells are not considered seizures unless they are accompanied by stiffening or jerking. If they are accompanied by stiffening or jerking, they are considered provoked seizures but are not considered serious, since they are unlikely to recur except in similar circumstances. They are not considered epilepsy and do not respond to medications used to treat epilepsy. This convulsive syncope or convulsive fainting has no more meaning than the fainting episode itself.

Is It Daydreaming or a Seizure?

❑ "Phillip has become forgetful," you tell your doctor. "The other day we were cleaning up the yard, and I asked him to pick up a pile of leaves. He just went on raking up the leaves. I shouted at him a second time, but he ignored me. I got mad, but when I went over to him he claimed he hadn't even heard me. He seems to be doing that a lot lately."

"It could be a lot of things," your physician replies. "As you know, adolescents often have selective hearing. It could be that he was listening to his Walkman, or daydreaming, or just tired of being nagged. Could he be taking drugs? Since you say that he has been having a lot of these things, I suppose that they could be seizures, the kind we call absence or petit mal. Let me get him to overbreathe (hyperventilate) a little bit and see if we can produce a spell."

A teacher may describe a child as "daydreaming a lot" or as "not paying attention." Or, on occasion, a child herself may report that she is missing short segments of her lessons or brief parts of a TV program or video game. Without seeing a staring spell, it will be difficult to interpret such brief events. Such spells can often be precipitated by hyperventilation in the physician's office; if an episode can be made to occur, the physician can see the spell and interpret for herself.

Daydreaming can be very difficult to differentiate from the brief lapses in attention caused by absence seizures. (We discuss this in Chapter 2.) However, daydreaming is common in situations which are boring or when a child is tired, whereas absence seizures can occur at any time. Absence seizures may be seen at mealtimes and interrupt a conversation or eating, situations in which a child is unlikely to daydream. Daydreaming can usually be interrupted by calling the child's name or touching the child. Absence seizures cannot be interrupted.

Tics

❑ "Joshua started these funny movements a couple of weeks ago, Doctor. It's just in his face. He sort of makes these funny faces, not all the time, but they're getting more frequent. I've yelled at him to stop. They drive me crazy. He'll stop for a little while and then do it again. Now he's started jerking his shoulder and grunting. Do you think he's getting epilepsy?"

Tics, like seizures, are sudden, paroxysmal movements. They are usually quicker movements than seizures themselves. While they most commonly affect the head and face, they may affect other parts of the body as well. Unlike seizures, they can be voluntarily controlled for periods of time. A tic may be simple, so that the movement looks like a twitch of a muscle or group of muscles, or it may be a complex pattern of movements. Unlike seizures, the recurrent movements are stereotyped. Seizures rarely look exactly the same from episode to episode because of the variations in spread of the electrical activity in the brain. But most tics are reproduced exactly and should, therefore, be easy to identify. Medications can be used to treat severe tics, but they are different from those used to treat seizures.

Myoclonic Jerks

❑ **"We were lying down together on the couch, watching TV, and Carl was just dozing off, when suddenly he had this big jerk, like a seizure. His arms and legs went out like he was struck by a jolt of electricity. Then he was awake, and just like nothing had happened. This is the third one of these I've seen in the past few months. This isn't epilepsy, is it? I'm worried because Carl's uncle has epilepsy."**

Myoclonic jerks are sudden movements, usually of an arm, leg, or both arms or legs, often occurring just as an individual is falling asleep. These are called "sleep myoclonus," and they are common and normal. Myoclonic jerks during waking hours are less common, but unless frequent they should be of little concern. Frequent myoclonic jerks can be a form of epilepsy (see Chapter 2).

Breathholding Spells

❑ **"Susie used to be such a good baby, but now she's got 'the terrible two's.' First, she started with temper tantrums, crying when she didn't get her way. Then she began to hold her breath and turn bluish, and I'd just pick her up and she would settle down. But now something different is happening, and I'm scared. Yesterday she was running and tripped and bumped her head. She started to cry, then she just held her breath and couldn't breathe. She turned blue, then she became stiff and arched her back and started to jerk all over. I'm sure she had a seizure."**

Have you ever noticed that when your child cries hard she will often exhale and seem to hold her breath for a long time before taking another breath? This is normal, even when the delay before the next breath seems interminable. For reasons that are unclear, some children hold their breath longer than others and turn blue or stiffen their bodies and arch their backs or even lose consciousness. This is a "breathholding spell." In a few children, at the end of the breathholding, a seizure may occur with stiffening and occasional jerking.

The blood has lost some of its oxygen while the child is holding her breath, and that is why she turns blue. With insufficient oxygen, the child loses consciousness. If the lack of oxygen is severe or if the child's seizure threshold is low, a seizure may be provoked.

A breathholding spell is virtually always caused by minor trauma, like a fall or bump, or by frustration when, for example, a toy is taken away or the child is punished. In such cases, stiffening and jerking are always preceded by crying and breathholding. Seizures of epilepsy, on the other hand, are virtually *never* brought on by such trauma or frustration and are *never* preceded by similar crying. Breathholding episodes, even when accompanied by seizures, do not need to be treated with anticonvulsant medicine, and they do not respond to such medication.

Typical breathholding spells do not require any laboratory examination. Treatment of breathholding spells consists of carefully explaining their benign nature to the parents and reassuring them that the child will not die, does not need resuscitation, and will outgrow the spells. When the oxygen level drops, the child will automatically start breathing again on her own and the brain will be protected. While very frightening to the parent, breathholding episodes will *not* result in brain damage.

Sometimes these breathholding spells can be aborted or prevented by diverting the child's attention. Also, since the crying and frustration that cause these spells are reinforced by parental overprotection in fear that a spell will reoccur, behavioral modification should be taught to the family by the physician or by a behavioral psychologist. Parents should learn to ignore the crying, reward the child's good behavior, and not reward the tantrum and breathholding with attention and concern. The spells will probably then decrease in frequency and the child will outgrow them without long-term consequences as the central nervous system matures.

There is a second form of these spells that is misnamed "pallid breathholding spells," usually occurring after trauma such as a bump on the head. The child suddenly stops what he has been doing, turns pale, and may fall down. Occasionally the child will then arch his back and, rarely, experience jerking movements. Such spells are not preceded by crying, breathholding, or turning blue. They are caused by "vaso-vagal syncope," the medical term for fainting. It occurs because of over-activity of the normal reflex that slows the heart rate. If the heart beat slows sufficiently, not enough blood is pumped to the brain and the child loses consciousness and stiffens. These "pallid breathholding spells" are the infancy and childhood counterpart of fainting when blood is drawn. The slowing of the heart rate can often be reproduced in the physician's office by pressing on the child's closed eye. If a child has an overactive vagal nerve reflex, the physician will hear a dramatic slowing of the heart rate, at times even a brief pause between heart beats. If an EKG (electrocardiogram) is running at the time, the in-creasingly longer interval between heart beats can be documented.

Although they are frightening, pallid spells are usually benign and will be outgrown. Only rarely, when the spells are quite frequent, is it necessary to consider treatment. But treatment should not be with an-ticonvulsants, because these spells are not seizures. The appropriate medications are those that block the action of the vagus nerve and pre-vent the slowing of the heart.

Migraine Headaches

❏ **"Lisa has been having headaches for a year or more, Doctor, but these past few months they've become more frequent. Now she has one several times a week, and she is missing a lot of school. She says that they are all over her head but mainly start behind her eyes. She has to come home from school and feels sick to her stomach. She usually goes to bed and wants the lights off be-cause they bother her eyes. Sometimes she will throw up, and then she feels better. She sleeps for a few hours and then is fine. She hasn't had any seizures for almost two years now, but the headache is like the ones she sometimes had after her big seizures. Do you think she could have migraine? I used to have mi-graine attacks when I was young."**

Migraine headaches are not uncommon in children, but they often do not resemble adult migraine. They rarely are unilateral or associated with warnings (auras) such as flashing lights or unilateral sensory symp-toms. Migraine headaches in children may build up as pounding headaches, with nausea, and sometimes with vomiting. The child usu-ally tries to avoid light, goes to his room, lies down, and goes to sleep. Such headaches typically last for hours. In children these headaches are usually bilateral. This kind of an attack is not like a seizure, but the episode is sometimes confused with a seizure when the headache component is less severe or when nausea and vomiting are less prominent.

Migraine commonly occurs in families, hence there appears to be a genetic predisposition. Longer duration of the episode and nausea suggest migraine. The presence of other seizures may indicate, however, that the headaches are related to a seizure (epileptic cephalgia). The headache of the migraine attack and the headache after a seizure can be similar, since both are caused by dilation of blood vessels in the brain.

The EEG may be abnormal both in persons with migraine and in those with seizures; therefore, the EEG is an unreliable procedure for deciding which kind of episode has occurred. In some instances, it may not be possible at all to differentiate between migraine headaches and headaches related to seizures. Indeed, as noted, migraine and seizures may coexist. Migraine is more common in those individuals and families with a history of seizures, and seizures are more common in those with a history of migraine. If the doctor thinks these events are more likely to be seizures, he may suggest a trial of anticonvulsant medication; a good response to these drugs suggests that the events were, indeed, seizures. If the doctor thinks these are more likely migraine attacks, he will prescribe antimigraine drugs. Again, a good response to this medication will suggest that he was right. Migraine has been known to respond to some anticonvulsants, but it is doubtful that seizures will respond to medications now used to treat migraine.

Paroxysmal Behavioral Disturbances

❑ "Peter has been a terror for years now. We've had him to several psychologists, and we're on our third psychiatrist. Now he's in a residential school for further evaluation. Something has to be done to control these outbursts before he kills someone. They did an EEG, and now they say that this is epilepsy because the EEG is abnormal. I've read about epilepsy, and Peter has never had a seizure. It's just that when someone frustrates him, or does something he doesn't like, he erupts like a volcano. There's no controlling him. He hits and bites and punches. I'm afraid he'll hurt somebody. Gradually he'll calm down and act as if he's sorry. Could this be epilepsy? I almost hope so, since then we'll have medicine to treat him."

Sudden outbursts of bizarre, often violent behavior are not uncommon among emotionally disturbed children and also among those who are mildly or moderately retarded. Psychiatrists often ask their neurological colleagues if such episodes can be seizures. *The answer is virtu-ally always no!* Studies have shown that violence that appears to be in-tentional almost never occurs during a seizure. If a child is restrained or threatened during the confusion that commonly occurs after the seizure, he may react in a combative but random fashion. In this post-ictal, that is, postseizure, confused state, the child does not mean to fight back or even understand what he is doing.

Episodic behavioral outbursts are almost always precipitated by an event or by frustration. Seizures never are. Seizures usually have a post-ictal state in which the child is tired or confused. Behavioral outbursts often do not. However, the EEG is virtually never helpful. An EEG ob-tained between seizures or behavioral episodes may be either normal or abnormal and, therefore, does not differentiate seizures from behavioral outbursts. Spikes on an EEG (see Chapter 7) can be observed in children who never have seizures.

Repeated episodic behavioral changes, in the absence of obvious seizures, are virtually never seizures and, therefore, do not respond to anticonvulsants.

Rare patients have confused even the best neurologists. In these cases, trying to capture the episode on video-EEG monitoring (see Chapter 7) may be the only method of ascertaining what is a seizure and what is not. It is worth noting that the same individual may experience behavioral problems and seizures also.

Nonepileptic Seizures (Psychological Seizures, Pseudoseizures)

Psychological symptoms may cause intentional or subconscious episodic alterations in function or in consciousness that are mistaken for seizures but are *not,* in fact, of electrical origin and hence are not seizures. Although they may closely imitate seizures, such nonelectrical episodes are "pseudoseizures" or "psychological seizures." Pseudo-seizures are not any less important than real seizures; they are just dif-ferent. They are *not* imitation seizures to be dismissed. They are not in the child's imagination. They are not to be punished or rewarded. They are that child's unspoken cry for help and should be considered impor-tant and addressed by a psychiatrist or a psychologist.

❏ **"I'm glad we finally got an appointment with you. Leslie's schoolwork is deteriorating, and the medications do not seem to be helping her seizures. Ever**

since our divorce she has had seizures, and her doctors have tried every combination of medication. Nothing has helped. Every time she spends a weekend
at her father's house she has a seizure. She falls to the ground, flails her legs
and arms, and doesn't respond when we shout at her. I know that her EEG is abnormal. Isn't there something you can do to help? Is she a candidate for
surgery?"

Does Leslie really have seizures? It's hard to be sure. Her doctor
might ask for a more precise description of the "flailing." He would
want to check to see what abnormalities, if any, appear on the EEG. He
would be suspicious that the episodes occurred only at her father's
house and began after the divorce.

As with seizures, pseudoseizures require therapy, but therapy that is
quite different from that used for "true" electrical seizures. Our first approach would be to take a much more careful history of the events that
occurred and the circumstances under which they occurred. We would
also take a separate history from Leslie. "Were you taking your medicine at your father's house? Do special things cause these episodes, for
example an argument or a fight? Depending on our sense of this story,
we would try to decide whether these were real seizures or pseudoseizures.

Since Leslie is having problems in school, and since the medications
for presumed seizures have been ineffective, we would probably decrease her medication slowly. We would also inquire about symptoms
of depression that might be affecting her schoolwork and causing pseudoseizures. If the episodes continue despite counseling, we would need
to observe an episode and the simultaneous electroencephalogram to
see if the episode in question is accompanied by electrical discharge
from the brain. Video-EEG monitoring can, at times, be crucial in separating true electrical seizures from nonelectrical pseudoseizures. An
EEG taken during a seizure will virtually always reveal an abnormality. EEG abnormalities found between episodes do not mean that the
episodes in question are seizures.

It is important to remember that a child may have true seizures *and*
pseudoseizures. It is vital to know *which is which* so that medication
can be adjusted to control any true seizures and psychological counseling initiated to eliminate the pseudoseizures.

The Physician's Evaluation

A careful, detailed history should enable the physician to say that an event was *not* a seizure or *was* a seizure. If neither conclusion is clearly demonstrated, the physician should confess, "I'm not sure what that episode was" but be reassuring.

1. *If the episode was not a seizure,* it will not require a CT scan or an MRI. It will not require an EEG. Depending on the nature of the episode, it may not require any further evaluation. It should be treated with reassurance and the physician's assessment of what the incident was: fainting, sleep myoclonus, daydreaming.

2. *If the episode clearly was a seizure,* the physician should be reassuring and point out:

- The seizure may not be important to the child's future and may not need further testing or treatment.
- Most single seizures in children do not recur.
- After a single seizure most children do not require a CT scan or an MRI.
- After a single seizure most children do not require medication.

3. *If the physician is not sure what the episode was,* then either:

- It will recur, in which case careful observation should help the physician establish the nature of the episodes.
- It will not recur, in which case it was not important.

Thus, after a single episode the diagnosis is rarely important, since regardless of the nature of the episode, the management is the same—reassurance of child and family and observation of the child. If the episodes recur often, it should not take long to establish their true nature. If they are infrequent and are not interfering with the child's life, they are less important. Rare episodes will either disappear as mysteriously as they appeared, or they will become sufficiently obvious and frequent to allow proper diagnosis.

If first episode clearly was a seizure, physician should:

Ask about circumstances, including

- acute illness
- remoteness
- duration of episode

Consider possible causes, including

- fever
- metabolic factors
- stroke
- infection
- tumor

Reassure the family that in 70 percent of cases,
seizures do not recur.

If seizure recurs, physician should:

Get a good history.

Tell the family what to watch for.

The child who has clearly had a single seizure needs appropriate test-ing to determine the cause if:

- the child is, or has been, sick; or
- the child has a progressive neurologic problem; or
- the child has remaining neurologic deficit.

When the child has a seizure out of the blue, without any of the above conditions, then:

- The child does *not* need a CT or MRI.
- The child does *not* need blood work.
- Some physicians believe that the child does *not* need an EEG.

The child who has not had a seizure, or whose episode was unclear, does *not* need testing, for there is no test that will tell you if the event was a seizure or not. Careful observation, watching and waiting—Tinc-ture of Time—is often the best approach.

The EEG does not diagnose or rule out seizures.

Remember:

• Almost 10 percent of all individuals will have a single seizure at some time during their lives, most often in childhood.
• Of those who have a single seizure, 50 to 75 percent will never have another.

For such reasons, it is not necessary for you or your physician to be overly concerned about the future just because your child has had one episode, even if that episode was a seizure.

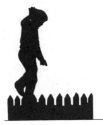

4. How We Evaluate and Think about a First Seizure

Since a seizure may be the sign of an acute disturbance of the nervous system, every child with a first seizure or suspected seizure should be seen immediately by a physician, who will search for a cause that may require urgent treatment.

The first thing your physician will want to know is if your child has a fever. The causes of a seizure in a child who has a fever may be quite different from the causes in a child who has none (Table 4.1).

Febrile Seizures

❑ **The car screeches to a stop at the emergency room entrance. The mother rushes in with a small infant in her arms. "I thought my baby was dying," she sobs. "I was holding him and giving him his bottle, and all of a sudden he felt very warm to me, like he had a fever. Then his eyes rolled back in his head, he got stiff and started to jerk all over. I gave him mouth-to-mouth resuscitation, and then the jerking stopped. We just got in the car and rushed over. He's sleeping now. Is he going to be all right?"**

Most first seizures in a child less than five years of age will be what are called "febrile seizures," seizures brought on by fever. These are the most common seizures of childhood and occur in 3 to 4 percent of children. Uncommon during a child's early months, they reach their peak at about eighteen months and are, in general, outgrown by the time a child is five years old. When a young child has a seizure *and* a fever, it

Table 4.1   Potential Causes of a First Seizure

With fever
   Febrile seizure
   Meningitis (viral, bacterial)
   Encephalitis (viral)
   Unknown (idiopathic)
Without fever
   Unknown (idiopathic)
   Chemical imbalance (dehydration, excess fluids, calcium, magnesium)
   Trauma
   Tumor
   Vascular malformation, stroke

Note: Seventy percent of first seizures in children are of unknown cause. Also, causes vary with the child's age.

is urgent that he be seen by his physician to be certain that this seizure is not due to *meningitis,* an infection in or around the brain caused by bacteria or by viruses, or encephalitis, an inflammation within the brain itself that is usually the consequence of a virus. In the past, bacterial meningitis was a killer of young children, but now, with modern antibiotics *and* with early diagnosis, most children with meningitis can recover without disability. Most viral infections of the brain are mild and do not need to be treated; for the few severe viral encephalitic infections, treatments are being developed.

When your child is seen by your physician, the doctor will, of course, want to take a careful history and perform a careful physical and neurologic examination. The physician will look for the cause of the fever in the ears, throat, perhaps the urine, and he may want to check the blood count. He will consider meningitis and, depending on the child's age and how sick he looks, may consider a lumbar puncture (spinal tap) to check for infection in the fluid around the brain and spinal cord. A spinal tap sounds frightening, but it is an easy and virtually risk-free procedure in children.

The child who has a first seizure with a fever does not necessarily need special x-rays or brain scans.

Fever lowers the brain's threshold for seizures and thus may provoke them. Indeed, as noted earlier, a seizure can be induced in anyone if the person's temperature is sufficiently high. Young children have a lower seizure threshold anyway, and thus are more susceptible to a seizure when a rapidly rising fever further lowers this already low threshold. This is the reason why such seizures tend to occur in young children. The threshold gradually increases over the first years of life as the brain becomes more mature, which is why these infants and young children outgrow the tendency to febrile seizures as they grow older. Febrile seizures are very uncommon after age five or six.

Susceptibility to febrile seizures appears to have a genetic base. Certain families tend to be prone to such seizures.

These three factors—the lower threshold of the infant (ages three months to two or three years), the height and rapidity of rise of the fever, and the genetic threshold—all three in combination may lower the seizure threshold sufficiently to cause a seizure: A higher fever or more rapid rise in fever may be required to induce a seizure in an infant without a family history of seizures; a lower fever in an infant with such a family history may be enough. In an older child, whose threshold is higher, a high fever may be sufficient with a family history of seizures (febrile or afebrile) but insufficient without a family history of seizures.

The first seizure with fever can be terrifying to a parent. Occasionally the seizure may be mild and brief (no more than slight slumping and loss of consciousness, or a rolling of the eyes back in the head), but often there is stiffening, a jerking, and loss of consciousness. Nine out of ten febrile seizures last only a few minutes, usually fewer than fifteen, but even brief seizures seem to last a lifetime to parents who have never seen a seizure before and who believe that their child is choking, or swallowing his tongue, or even dying.

What Should You Do during a Seizure?

A child who is having a seizure should be placed on her side and protected from sharp objects. Tight clothing should be loosened.

• Do not try to put anything in your child's mouth—she will not swallow her tongue.
• Do not restrain your child's movements.

Most of these seizures will stop on their own in a few minutes. If one seizure lasts more than ten to fifteen minutes, or if the seizure is repeated two or more times, call an ambulance or take your child to the emergency room yourself or to your doctor's office. If the child is still having a seizure, the physician will want to give medication to be sure that the seizure stops promptly.

The child does not *necessarily* have to stay in a hospital just because she has a fever and has had a seizure. The decision about hospitalization is a judgment to be left to you and your physician.

Most children with febrile seizures will recover from the seizure very quickly (within an hour) and can usually return home. Children with meningitis or encephalitis may have a varying course—from a mild illness to one that is severe or even fatal—and probably will need to stay in the hospital for a period of time.

After the Seizure Is Over

If the seizure has stopped, the physician will want to find the cause of the fever and hence of the seizure. Because it is the physician's first responsibility to assure that the fever and seizure are not caused by meningitis, he will examine the child. If the child is more than two to three years of age, clinical examination can determine this. If the child is under one year of age or if there is any question about meningitis, a spinal tap should be performed to rule out the presence of this infection.

Your doctor will probably recommend other tests to search for the source of the fever that triggered the seizure. In the young child with a first seizure with a fever, tests for other causes of the seizure are rarely helpful, however. If the child has recovered from the seizure and is running around the doctor's office, as is true after most febrile seizures, further testing with scans and EEGs is rarely helpful. The physician can best try to calm your own fears by giving you information about seizures of this kind.

Questions You Will Ask

You will have many questions about febrile seizures, among them these:

"Will he have more seizures?"

Only 25 to 30 percent of children who have had one febrile seizure will ever have another. If the first febrile seizure occurs in the first eighteen months of life, occurs in the first hour of an illness with only moderate fever, and if there is a family history of febrile seizure, then that child may have a high chance (greater than 80%) of having another febrile seizure. If the child has none of these risk factors, the chances of recurrence may be as low as 10 percent.

Chance of Recurrence after One Febrile Seizure

Overall, chance of recurrence is 25–30%.

If first seizure occurs

> before 18 months of age,
> in the first hour of an illness,
> without high fever, *and*
> in family with history of febrile seizures,

chance of recurrence may be as high as 80%.

However, a child who has a second seizure has about a 40 percent chance of having a third, and after a third, also a 40 percent chance of having a fourth. But only 9 percent of children with febrile seizures do have three or more.

"The doctor says that since the fever came after the seizure, it wasn't a febrile seizure."

Fever (or illness) can trigger a seizure in someone who has a low threshold. When a child has a first seizure, it may not be possible to tell whether it was a febrile seizure or a first nonfebrile seizure merely triggered by the fever. Since neither will be treated—because it was a first seizure—it makes little difference. The chance of another one remains about 25 percent.

"What will happen if he does have another?"

Nothing is likely to happen to your child as a result of febrile seizures.

- There is *no* evidence that recurrent febrile seizures damage the brain.
- Children who have febrile seizures *do not* develop mental retardation as a consequence of the seizures.
- These children do *not* develop cerebral palsy as a result of these seizures.
- There is *no* evidence that these children have an increased chance of having learning disabilities.

Children who have one, two, or even three or more febrile seizures grow up just like children who have never had such seizures. Virtually the *only* consequence of a febrile seizure is an increased chance of having another febrile seizure.

"With the first seizure I called 911 and they took John to the emergency room. I was there most of the day while they did the tests. Do I have to call 911 with every seizure?"

No. Calling 911 with the first seizure was the natural thing to do. You didn't know what was happening to your child. Now that you have read this book, you know that most seizures will end on their own. Your child will be fine in a short time. You only have to call for help *if* the seizure lasts longer than five to ten minutes. Long seizures may require medication to stop the seizure, and that medication should be given in the emergency room.

"What about a seizure that lasts more than thirty minutes? Will it recur?"

Only one in ten febrile seizures lasts more than thirty minutes, and most of those prolonged seizures are the initial seizure only. A child who has had a prolonged first febrile seizure is no more likely to have a second seizure than if the first seizure was short. But if the first seizure was long and the child does have a second seizure, then the second seizure may also be prolonged.

"Can't these seizures be prevented?"

Yes, certain medications can markedly decrease the chance of another febrile seizure, but there are risks as well as benefits. You will have to weigh the risks of the medicine and the benefits of avoiding another febrile seizure against the risks of having another seizure.

Phenobarbital is the most effective medication for preventing recurrence of febrile seizures, although it is ineffective when the child already has the fever. If it is given on a daily basis in sufficient quantities, there will be a marked decrease in the chance of another seizure. The amount of phenobarbital in the blood should be checked periodically to be sure that there is enough. But beware of its side effects.

"Should medication be given to prevent another seizure?"

Unfortunately, there is no current treatment without risks of side effects. Medications such as phenytoin (Dilantin) and carbamazepine (Tegretol) do not prevent febrile seizures. Sodium valproate (Depakene), when taken daily, is as effective as phenobarbital in preventing recurrences, but in this very young age group there is also a high risk (as high as one in 800) that sodium valproate may cause severe, even fatal, liver disease. As a consequence, we rarely recommend sodium valproate for the prevention of febrile seizures.

Phenobarbital produces side effects, especially in infants and young children. Many children (20–40%) who take phenobarbital will become hyperactive or will develop behavior problems or disturbances of sleep. For more than half, the side effects are sufficiently severe that the phenobarbital has to be discontinued. Even more important, there is also evidence that phenobarbital may decrease intelligence and negatively affect learning.

There is evidence that diazepam (Valium), given by mouth or rectally when the child has a fever, decreases the chances of another febrile seizure. This may be useful if a child lives at a great distance from medical care or if there is concern about a prolonged febrile seizure. However, given intermittently like this, diazepam causes sleepiness and irritability, and one study showed that parents often did not give the medicine in time to prevent another seizure. Either they did not recognize that the child was sick before the seizure occurred, or they did not detect the fever, or the child was at the day care center and the medicine was at home. In short, while Valium, if given at the onset of illness, *can* prevent febrile seizures, it seems to cause more burden on the parents than it relieves. (However, if a child's first seizure lasted more than 10 to 15 minutes, it may be useful to have Valium or Diastat* on hand to use if the child has a second seizure *and* that seizure lasts more than 10 to 15 minutes.)

Since there is increasing information that the chance of recurrence of seizures is low and the consequences of recurrence few, there is increasing consensus among physicians to avoid recommending any continuous medication. We only consider continuous medication in the very rare instance of a child who has many seizures with fever, and rarely use intermittent Valium for prevention of recurrences.

"What is the chance of my child's developing epilepsy?"

Epilepsy is defined as two or more recurrent seizures that are not provoked by fever. Febrile seizures do not cause epilepsy. The chance that

*Diastat, an expensive form of rectal Valium, is convenient and stable even when not refrigerated. For occasional use it may be preferable.

epilepsy will develop is slightly higher in a child who has had a febrile seizure than in one who has not, but not much greater (see Table 4.2).

Of children who have had a febrile seizure, more than 98 out of 100 will never have epilepsy.

The risk factors for epilepsy's developing in a child who has had a single febrile seizure are:

- if the first febrile seizure was prolonged (more than 15 minutes);
- if the seizure was one-sided or focal;
- if there were two or more seizures during that initial episode;
- if there is a family history of epilepsy;
- if the child has a neurologic disorder, such as cerebral palsy, or if his development had been delayed before the seizure.

A child who has a febrile seizure but none of these risk factors has approximately one chance in 100 of later developing epilepsy. A child

Table 4.2   Risks Associated with Febrile Seizures

Type of risk	Percentage of risk
Risk of	
Mental retardation	No greater than
Cerebral palsy	in children without
Learning problems	febrile seizures
Death	
Risk of epilepsy	
If there were no febrile seizures	0.5
If there was 1 febrile seizure	2.0
Risk of epilepsy after one febrile seizure with risk factors*	
0 risk factors	1.0%
1 risk factor	2.5%
2 or more risk factors	5–10%

*Risk factors:
  Seizures longer than 15 minutes
  Two or more on same day
  Family member with epilepsy
  One-sided seizure

with one factor has a 2.5 percent chance, and a child with two or more risk factors has a 5 to 10 percent chance of epilepsy. Thus, in the worst situation, a child who has all three risk factors would have only one chance in ten of experiencing multiple nonfebrile seizures.

"Isn't there anything that can be done to reduce even these small risks?"

There is no evidence that the risks of developing epilepsy increase, even if your child has more febrile seizures. There is also no evidence that placing your child on medication after a febrile seizure will reduce the risks of later epilepsy.

Think positively! Your child has a 70 percent chance of *not* even having a second febrile seizure. His chances of not developing epilepsy are greater than 90 percent.

Evaluation of the Child with a First Seizure without Fever

Now let's talk about the evaluation of a child who has had a first seizure *without fever.*

If your child clearly has had a seizure, your first question, and indeed that of your physician, should be "Why? What caused it?" Since a seizure is the result of a disturbance of normal brain function and since there can be many different types of disturbances, there are many different causes of seizures.

One type of disturbance is acute, usually only temporary, and while capable of causing a single seizure (a single provoked seizure), rarely causes recurrent seizures. Since some of these causes—such as infection or trauma—could require urgent treatment, your physician will concentrate on them at the time of your child's first seizure.

Most first seizures without fever are of unknown cause.

While not knowing a cause for the seizure is frustrating, the diagnosis of an *idiopathic* seizure (a seizure of unknown cause) is the best possible diagnosis for your child. A diagnosis of idiopathic seizure is an occasion for considerable optimism. It means that your doctor hasn't found a serious cause. More than half of first seizures are idiopathic. Idiopathic seizures are likely to be completely controlled with medication and are likely to be outgrown. If there is a single such seizure, your child does not have epilepsy.

Causes of Nonfebrile Seizures

• Trauma
    Birth trauma
    Head trauma
• Tumor
• Structural problems
• Vascular problems
    Stroke
    Abnormal blood vessels

• Metabolic conditions
    Low blood sugar
    Low calcium
• Infection
    Meningitis
    Encephalitis
• Idiopathic (of unknown cause)

Seventy percent of nonfebrile seizures are idiopathic, meaning we don't know the cause. Of all the causes of seizures, these are the most likely type in an otherwise normal child. Idiopathic seizures are also the kind of seizures most likely to respond to medication and to be outgrown.

Evaluation of a child who has had a seizure but no fever depends on many factors: the age of the child, the type of seizure, how soon after the seizure the child is seen, and whether the child has returned to normal. The frequency of various causes of seizures changes with the age of the patient (see Figure 4.1). After taking a careful history, the physician will look for general physical abnormalities. Abnormalities of the heart's rhythm or rate may lead to a lack of oxygen to the brain; other heart disease may lead to strokes or seizures. Lung problems can cause brain infection. High blood pressure can cause seizures, as can acute or chronic kidney disease. Some birthmarks provide evidence of problems in the brain that may cause seizures, so your physician will look carefully at your child's skin. Brain tumors and cancer are rare causes of seizures in children.

Your doctor will also want to concentrate on the child's neurologic function and on your child's development, to detect any *new* neurologic abnormality that might suggest a stroke, infection, or tumor requiring treatment, to verify that there is *no* abnormality, or to document old neurologic abnormalities for comparison with future examinations.

A careful neurologic exam does not necessarily require a neurologist. If your physician is concerned about some of the findings or discovers suspicious abnormalities, he may want to refer you to a specialist, a child neurologist. Decisions about testing and treatment similarly

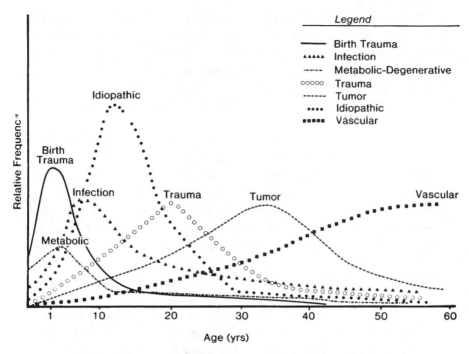

Figure 4.1 Relative frequency of causes of new onset seizures from birth to sixty years.

do *not* require the opinion of a child neurologist. Your pediatrician or family physician *and* this book should help you with your anxiety.

"You mean that's all there is? You tell us our son has had a seizure and you're only going to talk to us and examine Peter. Aren't you going to do any tests?"

The physician's appropriate response to that question is, "There is no laboratory test for a seizure. The diagnosis of a seizure depends on your description of what happened." Some tests can be of help in looking for a cause of the seizure. Certain tests help the physician rule out other peculiar episodes that simulate seizures. He may want to do an electrocardiogram if he is concerned about abnormalities of heart rate or rhythm. He may order blood tests if he suspects anemia, diabetes, or other chemical problems. But the diagnosis of a seizure itself can only be made by direct observation of the spell by a physician or by his careful interpretation of the observations of others.

Remember, as we discussed in Chapter 3, at the end of this detailed history, the physician can say, "That was a seizure" or "That was not a seizure. It was . . . ," or often she will say, "I'm not sure what that was." If the doctor (and you) are certain that it was not a seizure, then usually no further evaluation is necessary. If you and she are not certain, then no work-up need be done, either. Wait to see if it happens again. If you and your doctor think the event was a seizure, even then no further evaluation may be needed. Seventy percent of first seizures never recur. Tests such as EEGs or brain scans do not tell you if it was a seizure.

The most common tests performed when a child has had a seizure are an EEG and a CT (computerized tomography) or MRI (magnetic resonance imaging) scan. Some people think that a brain wave test, an electroencephalogram (EEG), will diagnose epilepsy, but *an EEG does not diagnose a seizure unless a seizure occurs* during *the EEG.* The EEG may, however, be very helpful in suggesting the appropriate treatment of children with seizures. A CT or MRI scan may, in the proper circumstances, be useful in searching for the cause of the seizure, but a brain scan does not itself diagnose epilepsy. Nor does it rule it out. Although these tests may be useful in determining the cause of a seizure, both EEGs and scans can be normal in the child who has had a seizure and either or both may be abnormal in a child who has not had and never will have a seizure. A detailed discussion of these tests is in Chapter 7.

Just as after a first febrile seizure, after a first afebrile seizure you will have many questions: "Will it recur?" "Can it be prevented?" "What are the risks of prevention?" The remainder of the book will address these questions for you.

Yes, there is some risk of another seizure's occurring. There are medications that may prevent further seizures, but they entail risks. Therefore, let's begin by discussing risks and benefits.

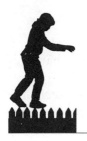

5. Decision Making: Assessing Risks and Benefits after a Nonfebrile Seizure

"When are you going to start Frank on medication? What are its side effects?"

"Now that Joyce has had a seizure, how long before I can allow her to ride her bike again?"

"Billy was going to go on a trip out west this summer. Should I put down the deposit? Will he be able to go?"

Life is full of risks and benefits. We take risks for ourselves and for our children every day. Although no one would ever do it, the safest place to raise a child is in a padded cell. In that cell the child could not be injured when he fell down, tumbled from a tree, or crossed in front of a car. Your child would be safe! But you would be sorry. Clearly, a child raised without risk would be a very abnormal child. Living, therefore, is best seen as a series of assessments of the relative importance of risks and benefits. Making decisions about which risks (costs) to take for which benefits is what we all do subconsciously all the time.

Risk-benefit analysis involves weighing the good against the bad. On the good side of the scale, we calculate the chance of a benefit and the worth of the benefit. A small chance of winning a large amount of money in the lottery may be "worth it" and outweigh the risk involved in losing a small amount of money. Worth has different meanings in different situations and to different people. Achieving "worth" or "winning" always involves some risks and consequences that must be weighed against the potential benefits.

Medicine is a series of risk-benefit analyses. In the past, physicians tended to do all of the analysis for you and recommended what you should do—whether your child should take medication and what medications he should take. This approach is much easier for the parent, and perhaps for the doctor as well, since it doesn't involve as much time and discussion. With the advent of a more medically sophisticated public, however, the patient and the family are, and should be, more closely involved in the decision-making process. The physician will still weigh the risks and the benefits and make recommendations on the basis of his assessment, but you as parent should weigh them as well. The risks of what he recommends are *your* risks (or your child's), not his, and the benefits that accrue, accrue to *you or your child*. Your evaluation of the worth of the benefits or the consequences of the risks may differ from your physician's.

Some decisions in medicine are clear and easy, others are more difficult. If your physician thinks your child has appendicitis, not operating could lead to a ruptured appendix and infection resulting in, at least, a severe illness and, at worst, death. The risks of operating are small with modern anesthesia, but there is a small risk of death and of infection with any operation. Comparing the risks of surgery with those of not operating, virtually anyone would recommend surgery. But suppose the signs of appendicitis are not clear and there is only some tenderness in the child's abdomen. Your doctor might postpone surgery because the risks of an operation might be greater than the risks of waiting. As the child is observed, the time may come when the risks of waiting would outweigh the risks and consequences of surgery.

As we talk about the risks and benefits of the decisions you will now have to make about your child and her seizure management, keep in mind that

• there will be risks and benefits to each decision you make *or don't make;*
• these risks and benefits will vary greatly in their consequences and in the magnitude of the consequence, both good and bad;
• the risks and benefits are *yours and your child's,* not your physician's; and
• frequently there are no "correct" or "incorrect" decisions. In many situations, different people will come to different decisions. Whatever decision is made or not made, there are always consequences, and they must be assessed in advance as far as is possible.

Decision Making

Goal: The outcome which the patient
or family finds most desirable

Step 1: The chance of each outcome is
estimated by the physician.
Step 2: The desirability of each outcome is
valued by the parent or patient.

| Likelihood of outcome | × | Desirability of outcome | = | Value |

No one can accurately predict the future. Consequences are not always foreseeable. Therefore, you and your physician must always make the best decision possible without feeling guilty if things don't work out the way you planned.

Whether or Not to Use Medicine

The first decision you face may be whether to treat your child after a first nonfebrile seizure.

At one time, physicians believed that a single seizure was the first sign of epilepsy and that a person who had one seizure would inevitably have more. Therefore, after the first seizure they prescribed medication to prevent the recurrence that was "bound" to occur. Today, we, like many other physicians, do not believe this.

We have learned that after a single "big" generalized tonic-clonic seizure of unknown cause the chance of recurrence may range from 10 to 50 percent, depending on a number of factors. Children with a first big seizure and a normal EEG appear to have a low risk of recurrence. Children with an abnormal EEG may have a much higher risk of recurrence. Children with staring spells—absence or partial complex seizures—are likely to have, or to have had, recurrent seizures. The first seizure of this type rarely comes to the attention of the parent or the physician. The same is also true for myoclonic seizures and infantile spasms.

One approach to analyzing risks and consequences is shown in the following box.

AFEBRILE SEIZURES
Analysis of Risks and Consequences

Without Treatment

Chance of Recurrence	×	Consequences of Recurrence

With Treatment

Chance of Side effects	×	Consequences of Side effects

+

Chance of Recurrence	×	Consequences of Recurrence

"Should my child begin taking daily medication after her first seizure?"

What are the chances that your child will have another seizure? If her chances of having another seizure were 10 to 15 percent, would you consider this a high chance or a low one? The consequences of a second seizure will depend on the child's age and the type of seizure. The consequences of a seizure could be great for older adolescents or adults if, for example, they are driving a car. The consequences of prohibiting driving are great for this age group. The younger child faces no such consequences. The consequences of everyday activities, therefore, vary with age. The toddler is unlikely to be climbing a tree, while the older child may be climbing when a seizure occurs. Risks and consequences vary dramatically with age, with activities, and also with personality, as well as many other factors. Since the consequences will happen to you and your child, you (and sometimes your child) will have to be the one to evaluate their significance.

Medication is usually started to decrease the chance of another seizure. But does medication do this? It is widely believed that medication is effective in preventing seizures, and indeed, it is clearly effective in people who have frequent seizures. It is not as clear that it prevents a second seizure in a child who has had only one. A number of studies suggest that the risk of a second seizure is just as great for the child who is placed on medication after a first generalized tonic-clonic seizure as for the child who is not. Therefore, whether medication is effective in this situation remains a matter of debate.

Outcome after a FIRST tonic-clonic seizure

With immediate Rx	With delayed Rx
24% recurrence	42% recurrence
87% no seizures 1 year	83% no seizures 1 year
67% no seizures 2 years	60% no seizures 2 years

The child has virtually the same probability of being seizure-free with or without treatment.

Most first seizures will not recur.

You would probably want to try medicine anyway, *if* it involved no risks or negative consequences. Unfortunately, however, there *are* both risks and consequences to medication. The cost of medication can be significant for some families. Every medication has side effects (risks and consequences). The "cost" in terms of side effects can be substantial. You have to evaluate the costs and benefits for your child. The seizures can *always* be controlled by enough medication to put your child to sleep. Would that be worthwhile? Think about your child's quality of life when evaluating the risks and consequences of medication.

"I don't even know the names of the medicines! How do you expect me to know and evaluate the risks of their side effects?"

Ask your doctor about the medicines. We will discuss the various medications and their side effects in detail later in this book. Here is one example of decision making about one medication commonly used in children, phenobarbital. Phenobarbital is a very safe anticonvulsant, but a frequent and often ignored side effect in children is a negative effect on learning or on behavior. Of young children who take this medicine, 20 to 40 percent will become hyperactive, or incur personality or sleep problems. When carefully evaluated, there may also be some subtle effects on the child's intelligence and ability to learn.

To decide whether or not to start phenobarbital, it would be useful to list the pros and cons of the decision. Such a list might look something like this:

After a first nonfebrile seizure, if you start your child on medication there is

- a 25 percent chance of the child's having another "big" seizure,
- a 10 percent chance of a rash developing that will require discontinuing medication and a small chance of a severe allergic reaction,
- a 20 to 40 percent chance of hyperactivity or behavior problems developing from the medication, and
- an unknown chance of learning problems developing.

If you decide not to start your child on medication there is

- a 42 percent chance of his having another "big" seizure,
- a zero percent chance of a rash or a severe allergic reaction developing, and
- a zero percent chance of hyperactivity or behavioral and learning problems developing.

It appears that, after a single seizure, medication reduces the chance of another seizure but does not affect the long-term outcome, and, indeed, phenobarbital, for one, like other anticonvulsant medications, produces its own risks. Are there benefits associated with starting phenobarbital that outweigh the risks?

There are no clear benefits of this medication to the child; one benefit may be your sense of security—or false sense of security—that he will not now have another seizure. The use of medication after a first seizure is not necessarily responsible for your child's not having another seizure, since most children who have had only one seizure will never have another one *whether or not* they are treated. The use of medication in children who have repeated seizures (epilepsy) can, however, have very different and clear benefits.

Each anticonvulsant medication has its own risks and side effects. Some risks are greater than those of phenobarbital in certain children;

some are less. Whenever a new medication is considered, you must weigh the risks and benefits of that particular medication.

We at Johns Hopkins usually do not recommend starting a child on medication after the first seizure. Other physicians come to different conclusions. Parents may weigh the risks and benefits in different fashions. Every child's situation is unique. Therefore, there is no *single* "correct" answer to the question, "Should we start a child on medication after his first seizure?"

We have discussed the considerations regarding treatment of the child after a first "big" seizure. "Smaller" staring seizures are rarely recognized after only one spell has occurred, and, therefore, they are usually treated when recognized, because we suspect that they are not first seizures but recurrences.

Decisions about Everyday Life

Since you are probably not going to raise your child in a padded cell, you will have to assess the risks and benefits of most of his daily activities with questions like these.

"Can my child still ride his bike?"

To help you assess the answer, we would have to ask, "How old is the child?" "How frequently does he have seizures?" "Does he have a warning of the seizure?" "How reliably would he respond to that warning?" "How much does he ride his bike?" "How important is bike riding to him?"

You would have to assess how great the chances are of his being injured on the bike. There are substantial risks to any child of being injured while bike riding. Are they much greater now that he has had a single seizure? He has only a 50 percent chance of having another seizure—*ever.* Thinking carefully about your answers to these questions will enable you to be protective, but not overprotective. Perhaps you can be appropriately protective by choosing where he can ride and insisting that he wear the helmet that has been sitting in the closet.

"Can my child swim?"

We were recently asked to comment about a lawsuit against a physician who had not prohibited his patient with epilepsy from swimming. The child had drowned, as do a number of children without epilepsy who swim. It was not clear that this child had had a seizure at the time of the drowning. Thinking about whether your child should be allowed to swim involves asking many of the same questions we asked about bike riding. "How old is the child?" "How frequently does she have seizures?" "How important is swimming?" "How well will she be supervised?" *Every* child who swims should be supervised. The child who has seizures should clearly be closely supervised. But, if well supervised, should she be prohibited from swimming? These individualized decisions will be dependent upon your analysis of the risks and benefits.

Similar questions can be asked about allowing your child to go out and play, stay at another child's house, climb a tree, go on trips or go to camp, and drive a car.

We permit normal children to take risks. We do not want to shelter a child who has seizures from *all* risks. Taking risks is part of the growing process. We want simply to shelter that child from the *increased risk* associated with a seizure recurrence. But this sheltering must be accomplished at an acceptable cost.

Remember:
- The *risks* of any activity or decision are the parent's or the child's—they are not the physician's!

- The *benefits* of any decision are the parent's or the child's—they are not the physician's!

Therefore:
The decision should be the parent's or individual's—not the physician's.

Assessing risks and benefits remains a very personal effort. What is a high risk for one person is very acceptable to another. The value that one child puts on being allowed to play, ride, or participate in certain activities may be different from the value placed on these activities by his brother, sister, or friend. Physicians, in their paternalistic fashion, tend to be conservative and overprotective. As long as the risks are yours, or your child's, and do not endanger others, then taking them should be your and your child's decision. The physician, the grandparent, or the friend may be advisors, but they should never be allowed to be the decision makers.

We are frequently asked by parents, "Doctor, what would you do if it were your child? Would you start medication? Would you let her swim? Would you do the surgery?" As we have indicated, each individual gives a different value to the risks and benefits of each decision. "What would you do?" is not a question your physician can or should answer.

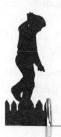

6. What to Do during a Second Big Seizure

"He almost died!" "He stopped breathing and turned blue." "He swallowed his tongue!" "I almost had a heart attack, I was so upset." "I just screamed!" "I called the ambulance, but it took them forever to get here." "I didn't know what to do!"

Remember, more than two-thirds of children (and adults) who have one big seizure *never* have another one. If your child does have another what you should do is stay calm!

"Easy for you to say," you reply. "You've seen a lot of these things. I thought my child was going to die. How can I do nothing? He's my child!"

Certainly, staying calm is the most difficult thing to do. It is easy for the physician or the nurse to recommend, but it's not easy to do, not even for doctors and nurses. Perhaps the most frightening thing about a big seizure is that there is little the observer or parent can do—or should do (see Table 6.1).

The stiffness at the start of a "big," tonic-clonic, seizure is called the tonic phase (see page 28). This is when all of the body's muscles are contracting together. The child arches his back, and since the muscles of the chest are contracted as well, the child is essentially holding his breath. He does turn somewhat blue. In a sense, he *has* stopped breathing. But this phase *will* end! The child will not die; his heart has not stopped; you do *not* need to do CPR. The body has a protective mechanism built in to prevent damage. If the oxygen gets low enough, the

Table 6.1   What to Do for a Person Having a Major Seizure

STAY CALM

During the seizure

- Do *not* put anything in the person's mouth
- Do *not* restrain the person
- Do *not* call an ambulance (unless the jerking continues for more than 5–10 minutes)
- Do try to lay the person on his side
- Do put something soft (coat, pillow) under his head
- Do loosen tight clothing around his neck
- Do remove sharp objects—chair, table, etc.—from the immediate area

After the seizure

- Do stay with him until he is awake and alert
- Do be comforting and reassuring
- Do allow him to go back to his activities if he's all right

body will usually stop the seizure long before the decreased oxygen can permanently damage brain cells.

There is nothing you can do during this tonic phase to get rid of the stiffness or to make your child breathe. Mouth-to-mouth resuscitation will not work, because the patient's chest will not expand.

What Should You *Not* Do?

- *Do not* try to put anything in your child's mouth. During the tonic (stiffening) phase of a seizure the teeth are clenched. If you try to pry them open, you may break a tooth. Once it was thought that a child might swallow his tongue. Now we know that that cannot happen, since the tongue is attached to the back of the throat.
- *Do not* try to restrain your child. You cannot stop the rhythmic jerking of the clonic phase. You can place something soft under the child's head to prevent its hitting a hard surface.
- *Do not* call the ambulance—unless the tonic-clonic jerking lasts five to ten minutes by the clock. Generalized tonic-clonic seizures only *seem* to last a long time. Almost all end—by themselves—in three to four minutes.

What *Should* You Do?

• *You should* turn the child on his side so that the secretions in the mouth, the saliva, can run out rather than running back into the windpipe.
• *You should* loosen clothing around the neck so that it does not further impair the child's breathing.
• *You should* clear things from around him, so that during the clonic, jerking, phase of the seizure, the child does not bang himself against a chair leg or sharp edges of a table.
• *You should,* if possible, put a soft object, such as a pillow, jacket, or shirt, under his head so that his head does not bang against the floor.

The tonic phase seems to last a long time, but in reality it rarely lasts more than thirty seconds to a minute or so. The second phase of a big seizure, the clonic phase, in which the muscles jerk rhythmically, is the violent phase. Restraining the child does not help, because the jerks continue anyway. Unless the patient is jerking against some sort of hard object, he will not hurt himself. *You can* gently support the child on the floor, but you cannot stop the jerking. The jerking is not hurting the child; he will not remember it. But it is very frustrating for the observer, particularly a parent, to stand by and just watch.

The jerking phase of the seizure usually will last up to several minutes. In an unusual seizure, this clonic phase may last five or (rarely) ten minutes—though it may seem like a lifetime.

When Should You Call for Help or an Ambulance?

❏ Jack was six and had not had any tonic-clonic seizures for almost a year. His folks had gone out for the evening for the first time in over a year. Wouldn't you know? Shortly after they left, Jack vomited, felt warm, and started to jerk all over. The babysitter knew that Jack had once had seizures, but she had never seen one. Her first reaction was that he was going to swallow his tongue—if he didn't die first. She called 911. By the time the ambulance arrived, Jack had stopped jerking and was asleep. The emergency medical team listened to his heart, took his blood pressure, and inserted an IV. Within five minutes he was on his way to the emergency room.

When told Jack had had a seizure, seeing him still unresponsive, the emergency room physician ordered a CT scan. His examination was negative, but they did not want him to seize in the scanner so they gave him some diazepam (Valium). His CT scan was normal. The blood chemistries showed a little acidosis; he was breathing shallowly and so they decided to admit him to the intensive care unit and put him on a respirator. Jack fought the intubation and had to be paralyzed. By the next morning, Jack was fine. His family physician saw him and moved him from the intensive care unit, and the following day he was discharged from the hospital.

The sad part about this story is that it happens very frequently. The emergency medical technicians (EMTs) in ambulances are trained to take care of emergencies. A child who has a seizure and is unconscious *might* be an emergency. It is their job to transport that child to the emergency room as quickly and safely as possible. The emergency room physicians are also trained to take care of emergencies. They do not know Jack's prior history and do not necessarily have the time to evaluate the child adequately. A CT scan, while unnecessary in a child who has had a recurrent seizure, could be of value if that child was unconscious for some other reason, like a head injury. Therefore, they ordered the CT scan. The sedation needed to keep a patient quiet during the scan often changes the breathing pattern and, therefore, the blood chemistries. One thing leads to another and before you know it this cascade of events lands Jack in the intensive care unit on a respirator.

If anyone had had the time and the inclination to find out the facts, Jack probably did not need an IV, certainly did not need a CT scan, and would not have been intubated or in the hospital at all.

There is no point at which that cascade of events can easily be stopped once 911 is called. This is why we tell parents that unless the jerking is lasting more than five to ten minutes by the clock, there is no need to call 911. Most seizures seem to last forever, but it is a rare seizure that lasts more than five minutes, and even then there is virtually no evidence that such a seizure does any damage to the brain.

Only if the clonic, jerking, phase lasts ten minutes is it advisable to call an ambulance. Virtually *all* seizures will have ceased before this time, well before the ambulance arrives. The jerking stops by gradually slowing down. Eventually the child relaxes. He often lets out a deep breath and then goes into a very deep sleep. The seizure is over. The brain is "resting." At that point, there is nothing the ambulance crew, physicians, or emergency room personnel need to do.

Only if the clonic phase lasts five to ten minutes is it reasonable to call an ambulance. Why call then? Because *if* the clonic seizure *is* still continuing when the ambulance finally arrives, *then* the ambulance personnel should take the child to the emergency room. It takes a few minutes to get the child on the stretcher and five to ten minutes to transport him to the emergency room. *If the child is still having a clonic seizure when he reaches the hospital, then the emergency room staff may want to give an injection to stop the seizure.* Approximately thirty minutes or more will have elapsed from the start of the seizure. That is the time when medical intervention to stop the seizure *is* desirable.

The timing discussed above assumes that you live in an urban setting, near an ambulance and a hospital. If you live in a more rural or inaccessible setting, it is desirable to reach a physician's office in about that same time.

A generalized tonic-clonic seizure lasting more than thirty minutes is defined as *status epilepticus* (and will be discussed at greater length in Chapter 10). Such a seizure *begins* to cause changes in the brain that look as if they *might* cause permanent brain damage should the seizure and these changes continue. More recent information suggests that even prolonged seizures rarely damage the brain. Rather, these studies show, it is the *cause* of the seizure—the meningitis, low blood sugar level, head trauma—which is the real cause of the permanent damage, not the seizure itself. However, we still recommend that a child with a long seizure be taken to a hospital emergency room to make sure that the seizure stops in a reasonable period of time.

As noted, as the seizure stops, the child usually lets out a deep sigh and goes into a deep sleep, the postictal period. It is as if the brain is resting from its overexertion. The length of this postictal sleep will vary, depending on the duration of the seizure. It may last anywhere from ten to fifteen minutes up to an hour or two. After a short period of time, the child can be aroused but often is confused and prefers to go back to sleep. There is no reason not to let him sleep. This sleep is a healthy recovery phase.

On rare occasions, the patient may have a second seizure while still in this sleepy, postictal state. Serial seizures (one after the other without the patient waking up in between) are also termed status epilepticus. When this pattern occurs, the patient should also be taken to the emergency room so that these serial seizures can be stopped. They indicate that the brain is very irritable and may require medication to decrease this irritability.

"Is there anything else I could do during the seizure? Shouldn't I put something in my child's mouth to keep him from biting his tongue?"

The answer is, "No, you should not." Unfortunately, in many generalized seizures, the patient may bite his tongue. But putting something in the mouth is difficult. Prying the mouth open to put in a spoon or a stick is more likely to break a tooth. If, by chance, someone does have his mouth open early in the seizure, you could put a handkerchief or a shirt sleeve or something soft between the teeth to prevent biting of the tongue. Unfortunately, most people clench their teeth at the start of the seizure.

Never put your finger in the person's mouth, because it can be badly bitten.

"What about mouth-to-mouth resuscitation. Will this help?"

No! When the seizure stops, the patient will breathe on his or her own. During the seizure, your mouth-to-mouth resuscitation cannot get air into the lungs.

It is hard to watch somebody have a seizure and frustrating not to be able to intervene, to stop this terrible thing, not to be able to help. But the best thing you can do is to remain calm. By staying calm, you inspire others around you to remain calm; and when your child wakes up, often confused, he will be surrounded by a less hysterical, more supportive environment.

"What about the child who doesn't have tonic-clonic seizures, but has seizures where he wanders around confused, picking at things, and could injure himself? What should I do during one of those?"

During this type of seizure, what is called a "complex partial seizure," the patient *is* confused and not really aware of what he is doing or of his environment. He is likely to misunderstand and misinterpret things during this foggy state. If the child is wandering around, try to be protective. The myths about people being aggressive during these seizures come from the child's misunderstanding and misinterpretation of what is happening and what is being done to him. If people try to restrain a child who is in this confused state, he may misunderstand the motivation and fight back. Rather, you should be protective, reassuring, and try to direct him away from dangerous objects or from hurting himself. This is perhaps all you can do. Confused ictal and postictal states may last several minutes; occasionally the postictal confusion lasts five to ten or even fifteen minutes. Again, only if this state lasts for a long period of time, more than fifteen minutes, is it necessary to bring the child to the emergency room or a physician's office, where, if it continues, the physician might want to use an injection to stop the spell.

In conclusion, what should you do? In most cases, don't call the ambulance. *It's not needed and won't be of any help. And yet when a child, even one who has had previous seizures, has a seizure in school, the ambulance often is called. Discourage this. It is not only expensive but usually useless. Educating the teachers, school nurses, camp directors, and others who might come in contact with your child that the seizure will be over shortly and that your child will be all right is perhaps the best thing you can do both for yourself and for your child. It is as effective and far cheaper than calling the ambulance.*

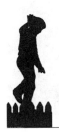

7. Understanding Your Child's Tests: EEG, CT, and MRI

The physician's diagnosis of seizures or epilepsy is made *only* by reviewing the history of the episode or by seeing an episode. There is *no* test for epilepsy.

Certain tests, such as the electroencephalogram (EEG) or video-monitoring can be very helpful in determining the type of seizure and in assisting the physician to decide the type of medication to use. Scans of the brain, such as the CT scan or the MRI, can, at times, be useful in localizing an abnormality that may be causing the seizures. Since most children with epilepsy will have these tests on one or more occasions, it is helpful for you as a parent to understand their utility and their limitations. First, the most common of such tests, the EEG.

The Electroencephalogram (EEG)

We know that the firing of neurons in the brain is carefully modulated by the balance of excitation and inhibition of cells and that groups of cells work together, interacting by exciting or inhibiting one another. The electroencephalogram measures the electricity given off by the brain cells as they interact. The tiny amounts of electricity generated by the brain cells can be detected on the scalp and if amplified many hundreds of times, can be transformed by the EEG machine and recorded (see Figures 7.1 and 7.2).

In most children without epilepsy, EEG recordings resemble wiggly lines, the tiny waves varying slightly in height (see Figure 7.4 and the

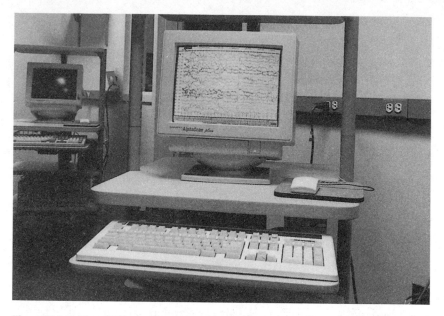

Figure 7.1 Modern EEG machine utilizing digitalized data collection. This allows for great flexibility in reading the records and ease in making the tracing available to multiple physicians.

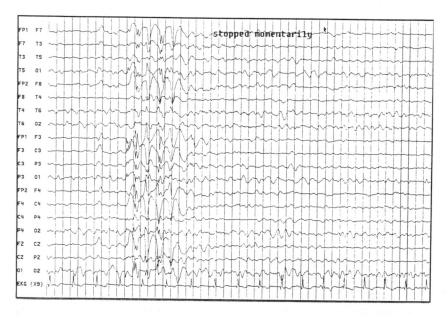

Figure 7.2 Print-out of digital EEG. This record shows a spike-wave burst while a child was hyperventilating.

discussion of EEGs later in this chapter). In most people *with* epilepsy, abnormalities can be seen on the EEG. These are little bursts of electrical activity, called "sharp waves" or "spikes," that interrupt normal rhythm. These bursts are the result of the electrical discharge of a somewhat larger population of cells all firing simultaneously, actually minuscule electrical seizures within very tiny areas of the brain. They are not clinically detectable seizures, because the spikes and sharp waves do not represent *enough* cells firing simultaneously to alter the function or behavior of the person.

When to Do an EEG

The first question to ask is, "Is this EEG really necessary?"

• Some EEGs are done to "rule out seizures." As discussed later in this chapter, EEGs do *not* rule out seizures, nor do they diagnose seizures.
• Some EEGs are done every few months, "to see how the child is doing," "to see if the medications are working," "to see if she is 'getting better.'" These are *not* good reasons for repeating the EEG if the child has not been having seizures.
• Some EEGs are repeated because the child's seizures are getting worse, breaking through the medication, or changing in character. These *are* good reasons to repeat the EEG.
• Sometimes the clinical picture of the child's seizures suggests that they come from one area of the brain. Documentation that there is a focal abnormality on the EEG is helpful to the physician in deciding what medication to use or whether to look for a focal abnormality.
• Certain patterns of abnormality of the EEG (spike and wave, focal or generalized slowing) may assist the physician in searching for a diagnosis or in choosing the best medication for the child's seizures. Looking for patterns is rarely a reason for frequent repetition of the EEG.

Performing an EEG

The EEG is best done with the child relaxed, sleepy, and still. The state of alertness may affect the EEG. Thus, crying, irritability, and restlessness may mask underlying abnormalities on the EEG and make the EEG uninterpretable.

In the past we sedated many younger children for their EEGs, to avoid the movement and its artifacts. New testing protocols have made this more difficult, but we now know that the effects of sedation can be mimicked if a few simple procedures are followed.

For the younger child

- Tell the child what is going to happen: that the technician will be putting some things in her hair, and that *it will not hurt.*
- Keep the child up late the night before the test and awaken him early. Do not let him sleep on the way to the test.
- Bring his favorite blanket or stuffed toy so he can hold it and feel comfortable.
- The EEG laboratory should be quiet and the technician calm, comfortable with children, and reassuring. If this is not the situation, you might consider asking if you can come back another time.
- The electrodes can often be pasted on while the child is in the parent's lap, and the EEG also may often be done with the child in your lap. This option may or may not be offered to you, depending on the practice of the laboratory you go to.
- We prefer that EEGs be done with the child both asleep and awake. This, too, however, is a matter of the specific doctor's preference or the specific laboratory's practice.

Older children usually need nothing more than an explanation of what is going to happen. The worst part of an EEG for them is getting the "gook" out of their hair after it is over.

Sedation for an EEG

Some young children are too anxious or too fidgety for the technician to obtain an EEG without putting them to sleep. When your child will not lie still or go to sleep for an EEG and techniques for helping the child be relaxed and sleepy for the EEG don't work, sedation must then be used. Chloral hydrate is a safe and effective oral sedative for children. A single dose of 55 mg/kilogram (not more than 1-2 grams for a child) given a half-hour before the child arrives at the lab will usually make it possible for the child to go to sleep. Occasionally a second dose of 25 mg/kilogram is used.

Regulators are concerned that any medication which puts a child to sleep could put the child into "too deep a sleep," and that the child might not breathe adequately. They recommend that sedation "only be used under the supervision of a specially trained individual, who is competent to resuscitate the child." We believe that this adds considerable expense to the procedure, with little gain.

Usually you may stay with your child to provide reassurance, but only if you also are quiet and still. Any movement and any touching or patting your child may cause electrical disturbances that show up on this very sensitive machine and will confuse the EEG tracing. A child's muscle movements—crying, squirming, squeezing the eyes shut, or clenching the teeth—can cause the EEG machine to "go crazy" as it picks up the electricity from the muscles. Relaxation and quiet for both parent and child are crucial to a good recording.

Normalities and Abnormalities on the EEG

Most of the pen movements on any EEG are common and normal (Figure 7.3A–D). When muscles twitch or contract, they produce electricity, and this electricity is picked up on the EEG. When people blink their eyes ("eye movement artifact"), this movement also is seen on the EEG. *Artifact* means that the electrical impulse is not coming from the brain, so it doesn't count. (Eye movement artifact is shown in Figure 7.4A.) "Muscle artifacts" can be seen when the child clenches his teeth, for instance (Figure 7.4B). Even during the process of falling asleep, changes are produced in the rhythm of the EEG (Figure 7.3D) that look like bursts of abnormal electrical activity. None of these changes in rate or rhythm on the EEG is abnormal, so don't worry.

Only three abnormalities on the EEG are of importance in the diagnosis and management of seizures: spikes, slowing, and evidence of seizures. Each of these may be either focal (local) or generalized. Each has a different meaning.

Remember, a seizure is an electrical discharge from the brain *that causes a change in movement or behavior*. If there is *no* change in behavior or movement, this is not a *clinical* seizure. Some abnormalities on the EEG may be called *electrical* seizures, but electrical seizures are rarely treated.

The EEG may

• show electrical changes that indicate either an electrical abnormality in one area of the brain or electrical abnormalities in many areas of the brain;

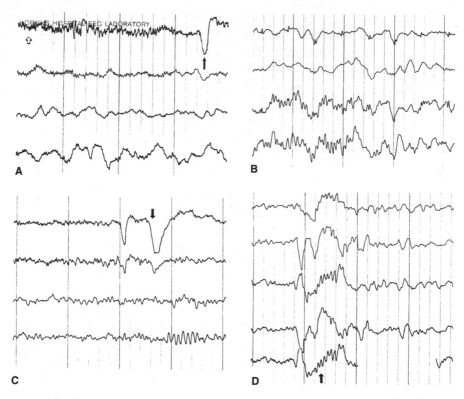

Figure 7.3 EEGs of normal infant and teenager. Record A, of an awake infant, shows blinking (*solid arrow*) and muscle artifact (*open arrow*), both in the first line, or channel. Much normal slowing is seen throughout the record. In B, the bottom two channels show the rhythmical fast activity, called spindles, of the infant when asleep; the two upper channels show a normal amount of slow activity that resembles in many respects the awake record. In the EEG of an awake teenager (C), when the eyes close (*arrow*), very rhythmical activity, known as the basic rhythm, appears in the bottom line; a sleep recording in the same teenager (D) shows a burst of activity (*arrow*) that is normal in sleep.

• indicate to your physician that there is a specific area of the brain involved;
• help your physician to determine the type of seizure your child had; or
• indicate which medication is likely to be most effective for controlling that type of seizure.

Diagnosis of seizures or epilepsy depends on an accurate interpretation of the events that have occurred. The diagnosis of a seizure or of

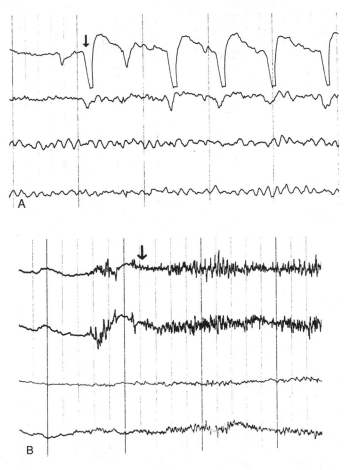

Figure 7.4 Normal EEG with eye movement and muscle artifacts. With the patient blinking (A), the top channel of the EEG record shows the eye movement (*arrow*). In B, the top two channels show muscle activity when the patient bites down or chews.

epilepsy is *not* made by the EEG alone. Furthermore, an EEG does not diagnose or rule out epilepsy. Some people with abnormal EEGs never have seizures. Some people with seizures have normal EEGs.

Spikes

Since a clinical seizure requires that a sufficient number of brain cells fire together to cause the alteration in movement or behavior, one would expect this "firing" to cause a change in the electrical activity recorded on the EEG. That is exactly what does happen. The normal EEG (Fig-

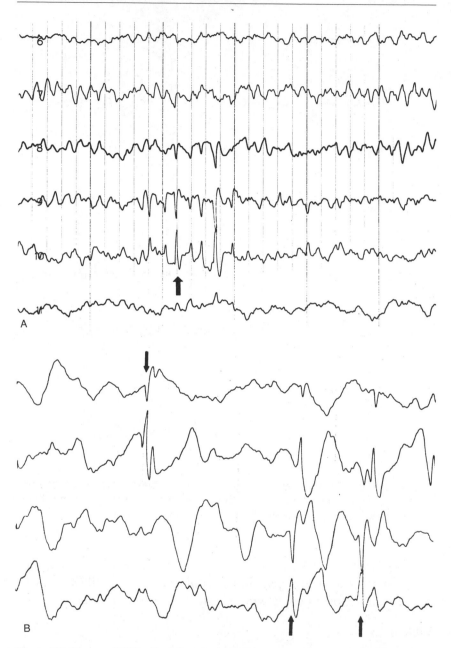

Figure 7.5 Abnormal EEGs. Each line, or channel, on the EEG represents a different area of the brain. In A, since the pointed spikes (*arrow*) shown in channels 9 and 10 do not appear in the other channels, the abnormality is partial (focal) in that specific area of the brain. In B, the multifocal spikes (*arrows*), appearing in several channels, show that they arise in several different areas of the brain and that there are multifocal abnormali-

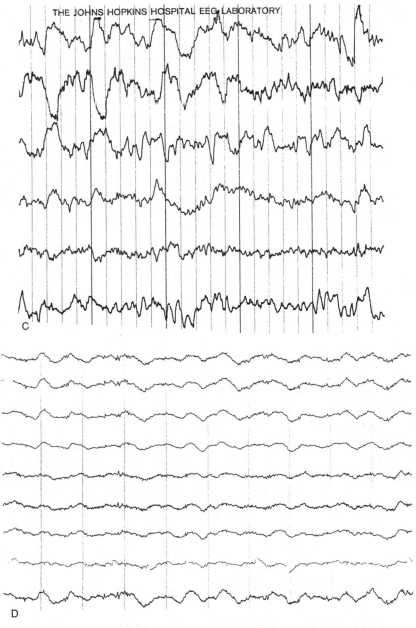

THE JOHNS HOPKINS HOSPITAL EEG LABORATORY

C

D

ties of the brain. In C, the top three channels (from left side of head) show high amplitude with slow waves, as compared to electrical activity from the right side of the head (*bottom three lines*). In D, all channels show low-voltage slow activity, as might be seen in a child in a coma.

ures 7.3 and 7.4) represents an almost random firing of brain cells; when the cells fire simultaneously they produce an electrical abnormality in the EEG called a "spike" (Figure 7.5A).

A spike is a tiny *electrical* seizure. Only if that electrical disturbance spreads to involve more cells (a sufficient number to change behavior) would a true *clinical* seizure occur. Thus, repeated spikes coming from a particular area represent the local response to a provocation there, an epileptic focus or scar. In a child (or adult) who has had a focal seizure, spikes may indicate the area of the brain where the seizure started (Figure 7.5A). Multifocal spikes (Figure 7.5B), by comparison, suggest that there are many abnormal areas of the brain.

Spikes are not of significance unless they are found consistently in one area.

Slowing

The rhythm of the normal EEG varies with the child's age and differs depending on whether the child is awake, drowsy, or asleep. There are well-established limits for these normal variations in rate and rhythm. Slowing may be either focal (Figure 7.5C) or generalized (Figure 7.5D).

A common cause of slowing is postictal, occurring after a seizure, due to inhibition of the firing of cells. It may last several hours. Postictal slowing is best diagnosed by its disappearance soon after the seizure. If slowing lasts for days after a seizure, further evaluation is necessary.

Focal slowing should always be of concern and requires careful evaluation, because it may occur in association with a local disturbance of the brain, such as a concussion, a stroke, or a tumor. In a child who has had a seizure, focal slowing on an EEG (unlike focal spikes) may, therefore, require further studies and appropriate treatment.

Slowing all over the brain—generalized slowing—signifies disturbed brain function caused by acute disturbances of whole brain function—for example, chemical disturbances, lack of oxygen, infection, or severe head injury with loss of consciousness. Generalized slowing may also be seen in children with longstanding chronic brain dysfunction.

EEG Abnormalities Related to Certain Seizure-Types

While the EEG does not diagnose seizures, certain abnormalities on the EEG are commonly associated with certain seizure-types and can help your physician determine your child's treatment and the probable outcome. Thus, just as classification of seizures is useful, so classification of EEGs is useful also.

❑ Roger is in the third grade and has been a very good student. But in the second half of the year the teacher sends you a note that Roger is not working up to his ability. He is not paying attention in class; he often daydreams. Sometimes, when he's asked a question, he claims that he didn't hear the question or that he has forgotten the answer. What's happening to Roger? Is he bored and daydreaming? Is he not smart enough to understand the new work and, consequently, confused? Is he upset or depressed by events at home or school? Is he having staring spells (absence seizures)?

Absence Seizures

The EEG in a child with simple absence (petit mal) seizures often shows brief bursts of spike and wave abnormalities (Figure 7.6). In between these abnormalities the basic rhythm is quite normal. Sometimes spontaneously, but usually with hyperventilation, the EEG demonstrates runs of spikes and waves, with a typical rate of three times a second. This type of "electrical storm," if it lasts more than one second, interferes with the child's alertness or awareness. He will stare into space for a few seconds, then may say, "What? What did you say?" He returns to his normal state just as quickly as he lost awareness. The EEG also abruptly returns to normal.

If Roger has typical staring spells during hyperventilation and has a typical spike and wave pattern on his EEG, the physician will be able to tell his mother that these spells will be outgrown, that he is unlikely to develop other types of seizures, and that his seizures should respond easily to medication.

Atypical Absence Seizures

Atypical absence seizures are often difficult to differentiate from complex partial seizures. The smaller the number of spells per day, the earlier the age of onset, and, most particularly, what manifestations are associated with the seizure, such as lip smacking, picking at clothes, and confusion, may help to identify the type of seizure. The EEG will often help distinguish between them, showing the classical three-per-second spike-wave of simple absence seizures and the somewhat slower spike-wave of atypical absence seizures.

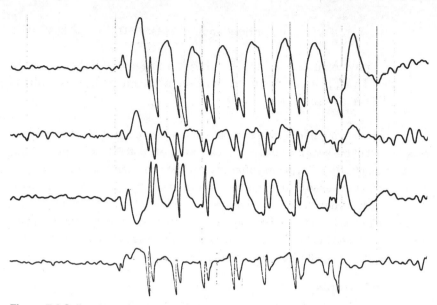

Figure 7.6 Spike-wave abnormality. These brief bursts of spike-wave activity, preceded and followed by normal activity, are often associated with absence seizures.

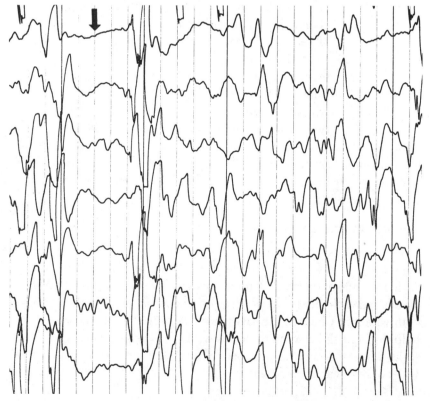

Figure 7.7 Hypsarrhythmic EEG, a chaotic, high-amplitude EEG with multifocal spikes, with a brief voltage suppression (*arrow*), usually seen in association with infantile spasms.

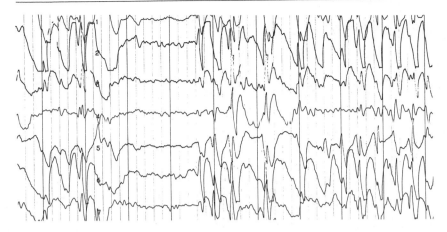

Figure 7.8 The Lennox-Gastaut pattern. Bursts of high amplitude spikes and slow waves are less regular and well-organized than the spike-wave activity of absence seizures.

Other Special Patterns

"Hypsarrhythmia," a very chaotic, high-voltage EEG pattern of spikes, poly-spikes, and slow waves seen in some children of six months to three years (Figure 7.7), is almost always associated with the severe seizure disorder infantile spasms (see Chapter 8). The Lennox-Gastaut pattern is also a chaotic pattern of slow spike-wave and poly-spikes (Figure 7.8), a pattern seen in some children and young adults who have a mixed seizure disorder. The term is used to describe the EEG and also the seizure syndrome (see Chapter 8).

Other types of epilepsy that can be diagnosed by a combination of the clinical pattern of the seizures and the EEG include benign rolandic seizures, which have midtemporal or parietal spikes, and juvenile myoclonic epilepsy of Janz (see Chapter 8).

Special EEG Procedures

Three special procedures that may be part of the routine EEG—sleep induction, hyperventilation, and photic stimulation—are called "activation" procedures, because they can activate patterns of abnormalities on the EEG. Such procedures should be routine with children.

"Why do they do the test both awake and asleep?"

The EEG looks quite different depending on whether the patient is awake or asleep (Figure 7.9A and B). Some abnormalities, spikes for

long

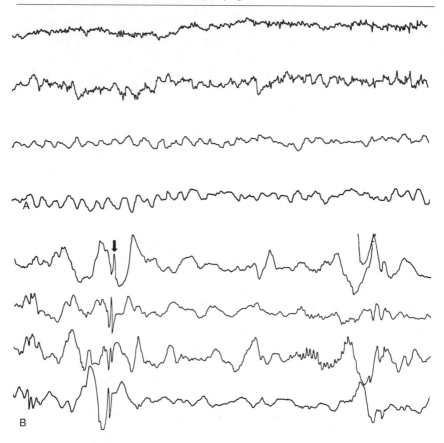

Figure 7.9 (A) Normal awake EEG of three-year-old. (B) The same three-year-old asleep shows spike activity (*arrow*).

example, may be apparent only in a drowsy or sleeping state because sleep changes the organization of brain waves and may allow hidden abnormalities to show up. Some children with epilepsy may have a normal EEG awake and a very abnormal EEG when asleep.

"What is hyperventilation, and why is it done?"

The technician will ask your child to breathe deeply, thus causing changes in the blood carbon dioxide and usually resulting in slowing on the EEG. Such changes as a consequence of hyperventilating are far more pronounced in younger children than in older ones. They can reveal abnormalities on the EEG. In children with absence seizures, over-breathing can even cause a clinical spell and allow the EEG characteristics of this form of epilepsy to become overt.

"What is photic stimulation?"

Flashing lights also may trigger seizures. A special class of seizures is called "photic sensitive seizures." Using a stroboscopic light, which flashes at frequencies from one per second to sixty per second, the EEG technician can observe whether the child is "photic sensitive," that is, that the child's EEG responds to certain frequencies of flashes, with the EEG showing spikes every time the light flashes. Occasionally, "photic driving" can make the brain so active that a real seizure will occur, one similar to episodes that occur under nonlaboratory conditions in a few people. These people are said to have "photic sensitive epilepsy."

"Why Do an EEG Anyway?"

"I still don't understand why one does an EEG," you say. "You've said it doesn't diagnose epilepsy. You've stated that it doesn't rule out epilepsy. It sounds to me like it's useless, one of those boondoggle tests doctors request in order to make more money."

Despite its limitations, the initial EEG is useful.

• Although it does not usually diagnose seizures, the EEG can be helpful in distinguishing between forms of epilepsy. The three-per-second spike-wave pattern of simple absence seizures, the chaotic pattern of hypsarrythmia, or the rolandic spikes of benign rolandic epilepsy (to name a few patterns), when combined with the history of the spell, can identify the type of seizure. The physician can then suggest the best medications for that seizure-type and can often predict the outcome of the seizures.
• A normal EEG, while not ruling out seizures, can be reassuring regarding the severity of the epilepsy, if the child has recurrent spells.
• An abnormal EEG can suggest need for caution and increased awareness of recurrent spells.
• A focally abnormal EEG with either focal spikes or focal slowing can suggest the need for further evaluation with MRI scans.
• The EEG can serve as a baseline, so that if the seizures change in character, or get worse, there is something against which to compare future EEGs.

> Whatever the EEG shows, treatment should be based
> on the whole clinical picture. We do not treat EEGs,
> and we do not treat their abnormalities. We treat patients.

Why Repeat an EEG?

"If that's all they get out of the test, why would they want another one?" you might ask. Others might question, "Will the follow-up EEG really show that the epilepsy is getting better or worse?" The answer to both of these questions is that *an EEG should be repeated only when it will provide useful information.* It should *not* be repeated routinely, say, every three months, every six months, or even every year. If your child's seizures are controlled, you shouldn't care if the EEG is normal or not—that is, until you want to consider stopping medication.

An EEG should be repeated only if

- seizures are continuing despite appropriate medication, or
- seizures are changing in pattern or frequency, or
- seizures that have been well controlled now recur, or
- the child's functioning is changing.

In any of these circumstances, a change in the EEG could provide a clue to the reason for the change. A person who has had a few generalized tonic-clonic seizures, followed by successful control of seizures, might have only an initial EEG and no further EEGs *unless* the physician considers stopping medication, and then a second EEG may provide important information about the possibility of further seizures. A child who has frequent seizures or focal seizures might, by way of comparison, require many EEGs to determine where the seizures are coming from. A child with difficult-to-control seizures might also require many EEGs, or even continuous monitoring of the EEG for days, in order to capture the seizures as they occur and identify their origin in order to plan surgery. But continuous EEG monitoring, either with ambulatory (walking around) equipment or video monitoring, is a special test and should be used only in such special circumstances.

So the answer to the question "Why repeat the EEG?" is that it depends. But if your physician wants a repeat, don't hesitate to ask why. He should be able and willing to tell you.

Intensive EEG Monitoring

For the evaluation of most individuals with epilepsy, no special EEG tests are required. For most such children, the neurological evaluation, one EEG, and in some cases a CT scan or an MRI scan will provide sufficient evaluation. However, in three situations special EEG tests are indicated:

• If the episodes do not seem to fit any particular seizure type, your physician may be concerned that these are not true seizures, but rather are pseudoseizures. Special EEG monitoring may help to separate true seizures from pseudoseizures.

• Special EEG monitoring is always required when surgery is even considered as a possibility. The testing may indicate that the seizures are coming from several different areas of the brain, thus making surgery less likely to be effective. Alternatively, intensive monitoring may indicate that there is sufficient evidence of a focal source for the seizures that it may be worth initiating a series of events and tests that would help in making intelligent decisions about surgery (see Chapter 14).

• Some children with uncontrolled seizures may benefit from intensive monitoring that might identify the type of seizure and indicate alternative medications.

Ambulatory EEG Monitoring

Ambulatory EEG monitoring uses portable EEG equipment to permit long-term constant monitoring of the EEG while a child is out of bed, playing, at home, in school, or on the hospital ward. The advantage of ambulatory EEG monitoring is that it is relatively inexpensive, since it requires neither being in the hospital nor a lot of the supervisory personnel. Thus, it can be performed even when the seizures are of relatively low frequency. The disadvantages are that the physician cannot see the episode and cannot localize its onset. Ambulatory EEG monitoring is useful when:

• the physician needs to determine if the episodes which the child is having are truly seizures. If the EEG does not show the electrical activity usually seen with a seizure, at the time of the episode, that can be evidence that there is some other reason for the episode. The converse may also be true, and episodes thought not to be seizures may indeed have the electrical signature of a seizure.

• there is a need to count the number of seizures the child is having. It is sometimes necessary to check the seizure frequency in order to correctly adjust treatment protocols.

Ambulatory EEG monitoring is not needed for every patient. It is rarely needed to diagnose or confirm epilepsy, and it is often overused. There are various types of portable equipment which can be used for this ambulatory monitoring. All require that the EEG electrodes be glued to the scalp and connected by wires to the recording device; electrodes becoming unglued is the major problem with this form of monitoring. The wires are run to a small device, either a cassette or a minicomputer worn on the belt, which records the electrical activity. Some monitoring systems include a home computer, which can be plugged into the monitor and will store even more information and even recognize seizures. The biggest problem with this monitoring (other than the electrodes coming loose) is that the parents must indicate when the events occur, by pushing a button, and must describe each event on a log sheet. If the parents do not push the button, then even if there is an electrical change on the EEG, the reader of the data record does not know if the child had an event or not. If the parent pushes the button and records what is occurring with the child, then we can see if there was an electrical correlate. Some of the newer computerized recording devices have spike detectors, which detect the electrical activity often associated with seizures. While this permits detection of events that the parents do not see (like brief seizures occurring during the night), it also detects the many artifacts that accompany movement and muscle activity, and this density of information makes the recording more difficult and cumbersome to read.

While ambulatory EEG monitoring permits recognition of major brain abnormalities, such as generalized spike and wave seizures, it is not precise enough for presurgical evaluations. There are additional drawbacks and limitations to ambulatory monitoring, and because the child is monitored at home and it is not uncommon for one or more of the electrodes to become loose without anyone knowing, the monitoring may yield less than accurate reports. It may be impossible to interpret any episodes that occur if not all the electrodes are working. True to Murphy's Law, it is usually the critical electrode that malfunctions.

When used appropriately, however, ambulatory EEG monitors can be exceedingly helpful in selected cases.

Video-EEG Monitoring

The optimal approach to analysis of seizures is to both see and record their onset and their spread. Such an approach is mandatory in situations in which surgery is being considered. When determining if surgery is even an option, it is critical to know the exact area of the brain involved in the origin of the seizures. Video-EEG monitoring allows recording of the EEG from multiple areas of the brain and also simultaneous video recording of the seizures.

Video-EEG monitoring can also be useful when there is a question about what the spells really are. The ability to see a spell that is said to be a seizure *and* to record the EEG at the same time is the definitive way to differentiate seizures from pseudoseizures.

Two examples will illustrate.

❏ Sasha was a fifteen-year-old with a severe behavior disorder and seizures. Despite several years of intensive outpatient psychotherapy, he was once again thrown out of school. His family was exasperated. It was clear to both his neurologist and his psychiatrist that he used his seizures to manipulate his environment. He was taken off medication and these peculiar episodes, which did not sound like seizures, did not increase in frequency. The family was taught to ignore them and Sasha seemed able to control them. But their persistence and his abnormal EEG remained of concern to his psychiatrist.

The only resolution to his problem was to send him to a residential institution where he could be taught better behavioral control. Since the psychiatrist at the institution was uncomfortable dealing with a child with seizures, we brought him into the monitoring unit to see whether all of his spells were pseudoseizures.

Much to our surprise, while most of his episodes were, indeed, pseudoseizures, at night he had genuine tonic-clonic seizures. Placing him back on medication eliminated these true seizures and allowed the psychiatrist at the institution to concentrate on his behavioral problems.

❏ Simon's seizures began when he was two. They would start in his left foot and spread up the left side. At times, he would have a weakness in the left leg that was thought to be postictal paralysis, but at other times the leg was quite normal. Despite intensive attempts with medication, seizures continued to occur several times each day. The EEG showed a focus near the motor strip on the right, and we faced the choice of operating to remove the focus (with the probability of causing paralysis at least of the leg) or of allowing him to continue to have seizures. We decided to wait. After several years, video-EEG monitoring allowed us to see the start of several seizures. The seizures actually began anteriorly in the frontal lobe and then spread into the motor strip. They began in an area that could possibly be removed without damaging his motor ability. Simon was, therefore, put on the list for evaluation with the grid electrodes placed on the surface of his brain (see Chapter 14) and eventually had successful surgery—without experiencing paralysis.

Intensive monitoring allows us to make decisions we were never able to make before. It gives us the opportunity to separate true seizures definitively from pseudoseizures and more successfully to identify children as prospects for surgery. Not everyone needs video-EEG monitoring. Only if an important question must be resolved is the expense warranted. If there is a question regarding surgery, this monitoring should be done at a center capable of doing the surgery. It is difficult, or impossible, for surgical decisions to be made based on tests conducted and interpreted by others.

A number of epilepsy centers are capable of intensive video-EEG monitoring. Video-EEG monitoring is usually carried out in special hospital settings with the patient in bed or sitting in a chair where the video camera and EEG machine can constantly monitor his activities. The EEG and the video are recorded simultaneously in one of several ways which will permit simultaneous analysis of the behavior and the electrical activity. Often these intensive monitoring centers will withdraw medication to precipitate seizures, which can then be recorded.

The principal drawback to this monitoring is its expense. It requires the use of hospital space and the time of nurses or technicians who will monitor the patient and the equipment twenty-four hours a day. Also, analysis of the records (Figure 7.10) is expensive and time consuming. Because seizures must be of sufficient frequency to make their recording feasible, intensive video-EEG monitoring may require many days in the special monitoring unit at enormous cost. Video-EEG monitoring is sometimes used on an outpatient basis for eight to twelve hours. When spells are sufficiently frequent, this abbreviated monitoring may be adequate and is much less expensive.

However, when seizures are sufficiently frequent and disabling to the individual, or when the localization of the onset of seizures is sufficiently important to future decision making about the use of the proper medication or the use of surgery, then intensive monitoring, expensive as it is, is cost-effective. The goals of hospital admission and monitoring must, of course, be carefully defined in advance, in order to make the most efficient use of this complex system.

CT and MRI Scanning

"Dave, I'm so glad you called. I didn't know where to reach you. Joel had a seizure. I thought he was going to die. We had had a good day, he had a friend over and they played nicely. I'd read him a story and put

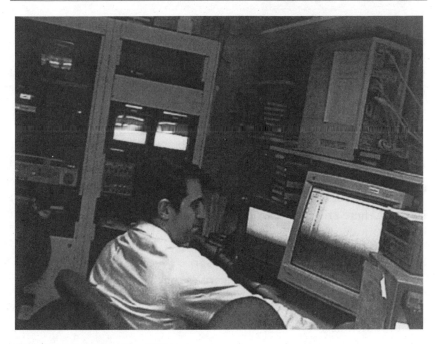

Figure 7.10 Analyzing video-EEG data.

him to sleep in our bed, since you were out of town. I don't know what made me go back and check, maybe I heard a noise. Joel was choking. He was stiff and jerking. I didn't know what to do, I put him on his side and called 911. By the time they arrived the jerking and choking were over and Joel seemed to be sleeping. The EMTs put in an IV and took us to the emergency room. The nurses there took some blood and sent him down for a CT scan, and by the time that was done a doctor had arrived and Joel was awake. The doctor said that Joel had had a seizure but that his blood work looked okay. He said we didn't need to do a spinal tap because he didn't have a fever, and the CT scan was okay, but he wanted an MRI done on Friday. He said it was to rule out a tumor or something causing the seizure. Can you be back home by Friday? I'm scared."

When a child has had a seizure or multiple seizures, the first question parents and physicians ask is, "Why did the seizure occur?" Although more than 70 percent of seizures in children are "idiopathic" (having no known cause) and although most that are "symptomatic" (due to disturbance in the brain) are secondary to something that happened long ago, there is an almost irresistible urge among physicians and families to "take a look," to see if "we can find out why this occurred." Neurologists and neurosurgeons who see adults who have just begun to have frequent seizures, properly consider brain tumors or vascular (blood vessel) problems as a possible cause of these seizures. The causes of seizures in children are different. Tumors and vascular problems are rarely the cause of new onset seizures in children (see Chapter 4).

Modern radiology, through the use of brain scanning, has made it possible to "take a look" relatively easily and at modest expense and without harm to the patient (see Table 7.1).

It is not necessary to do a scan on every child who has had a first seizure. There are good reasons for a physician to request a scan if

- there are repeated focal seizures, or
- there is focal slowing on the EEG, or
- you or your physician are concerned that your child is getting worse.

But remember:

- Most scans are normal in children with epilepsy.
- Most abnormalities found will *not* explain the epilepsy.
- Most abnormalities found will *not* lead to a different approach to treatment.

Just because something abnormal is seen on a scan, it does not mean that this abnormality has caused the seizure or seizures or that it will cause seizures in the future. Only if the abnormality on the scan appears in the proper location of the brain to have caused the seizures can we presume cause and effect.

CT Scanning

CT or CAT scanning (computerized tomography or computerized axial tomography), a procedure introduced in the early 1970s, revolutionized the ability to "see" the brain. Low-dose x-rays are detected and interpreted by a computer, which then generates a picture "just as if we had cut a slice of the brain."

The principal reason for doing a CT scan is to see whether the seizure had a cause that needs to be treated surgically and immediately. Otherwise, an MRI gives far more information.

Why a CT Scan?

The evaluation of a seizure in the emergency room seems always to include blood work and a CT scan. Why? Perhaps to rule out any head trauma as a cause, although a history could usually rule that out. To rule out a tumor, a stroke, or a clot? Again, in a previously healthy child, a seizure is rarely the first sign of such an event.

• Seventy percent of seizures are "idiopathic," of unknown cause.
• In a child who has not had head trauma, an emergency CT is virtually never useful. It is only quickly obtainable and relatively inexpensive.
• An MRI is able to show small and subtle abnormalities that are not seen on the CT scan.
• An MRI is always preferable to a CT scan if any scan is needed. The MRI is usually done after the CT, "to be sure," and the CT is then superfluous, except in the case of suspected head trauma.

MRI Scanning

While CT scanning originally revolutionized our ability to see the brain, magnetic resonance imaging (MRI) has increased our ability to see the brain even more clearly. Unlike CT scanning, MRI does not employ x-rays but rather uses a huge magnet to create an image which is then analyzed by computer in a fashion similar to the CT. It produces pictures of far greater detail.

The advantages and disadvantages of CT and MRI are shown in Table 7.1. The principal disadvantages of the MRI are that, with current equipment, a scan takes a much longer time, during which the child must lie perfectly still in the tunnel-like machine and thus may require sedation. The test is more expensive than computerized tomography. However, when detail of the brain is important, or when subtle changes must be seen, the MRI is indicated. It produces far better pictures of the brain and of most abnormalities than the CT scan does. If it is important to look for an acute abnormality in a sick child who has just had a seizure, the CT scan is faster and cheaper. However, such screening is rarely needed. If the person is having repeated focal seizures, and an abnormality has not been obvious on CT scanning, MRI scanning may show subtle abnormalities causing the seizures.

Table 7.1   Advantages and Disadvantages of Computerized Tomographic (CT) and Magnetic Resonance Imaging (MRI) Scans

Characteristic	CT scan	MRI scan
Speed	10–15 minutes	45 minutes, may need sedation
Ease	Simple, even with sick individuals on life support machines	Difficult with sick patients
		Better for small or subtle changes or problems occurring near bone
Cost	Moderately expensive	Expensive

If your physician wants your child to have an EEG or a CT or an MRI scan, you should feel free to ask him why he wants the test and what he hopes to learn from it. These questions are even more appropriate if he wants to repeat the test.

Other scanning techniques, such as magnetic resonance spectroscopy (MRS), functional MRI (fMRI), single photon emission spectroscopy (SPECT), and proton emission tomography (PET), are specialized techniques that are not part of the initial work-up for a seizure. They are used when seizures are persistent and when the epilepsy team is searching for a single source of origin for the seizures, a source that might be amenable to surgery. These techniques are discussed in Chapter 14, about the surgical evaluation of seizures.

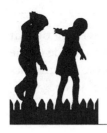

8. The Epilepsies of Childhood: Special Patterns and Causes

Epilepsy and Its Special Forms

Epilepsy is defined as two or more seizures that are not provoked and are not due to an acute disturbance of the brain. Because there are many different types of seizures, epilepsy can take many different forms. There is not, thus, one epilepsy but many. Therefore, if we were to speak properly, we would not speak about "epilepsy" but about "the epilepsies or epilepsy syndromes."

Epilepsy Syndromes

In addition to the many types of seizures discussed in Chapter 2, there are various patterns of recurrent seizures sufficiently distinctive in their course and outcome and in their response to specific medications to warrant distinct names and separate discussions.

Benign Rolandic Epilepsy

Benign rolandic epilepsy is a special form of seizures in children. Often starting after three years of age, it has rather typical clinical manifestations and a typical EEG. It is usually "benign" in that it is outgrown at adolescence whether or not it is treated and in that the children are usually normal before, during, and after this form of epilepsy. In many or most cases, the seizures are infrequent and do not need medication.

Seizures in this form of epilepsy often start with a sensation at the corner of the mouth, which is followed by jerking of that corner. The jerking may spread to one side of the face or cause a twisting of that side. The seizure may, on occasion, spread throughout that side of the body or become a generalized tonic-clonic seizure. These seizures occur more commonly at night and during certain stages of sleep.

The diagnosis of benign rolandic epilepsy is confirmed by an EEG pattern of repetitive spike activity firing predominantly from the midtemporal or parietal areas of the brain near the rolandic (motor) strip—hence the name rolandic epilepsy. Bilateral spike activity on the EEG is not uncommon and interictal activity is more common on the EEG during certain stages of sleep.

The seizures are often so infrequent and benign, occurring only at night, that most children with benign rolandic epilepsy are not treated with medication. If a child's seizures are more frequent or troublesome, treatment can be very effective and may be tapered and discontinued after puberty.

There may be a genetic predisposition to this form of epilepsy.

Juvenile Myoclonic Epilepsy of Janz

Juvenile myoclonic epilepsy (JME) is a syndrome unfamiliar to many physicians. It is easily recognized, if you know what to look for and know what questions to ask of the patient. It is also easily treated.

Epilepsy of Janz starts in late childhood or adolescence, often about the time of puberty. Its hallmark is mild myoclonic jerks, most common as the person is going to sleep or awakening in the morning. An adolescent will describe jerking of the arms or legs, a feeling of being very "jumpy." Some patients have told us that they set their alarm clocks to wake up early and then stay in bed for a half-hour to an hour, until the jumpiness wears off. They say that if they get up more quickly the jerking gets much worse.

If a person has early morning jerkiness, informing your doctor about the jerks may make it easier to diagnosis this particular form of epilepsy.

Occasionally, the jerking increases and becomes sufficiently severe that the person experiences a clonic or a tonic-clonic seizure. In addition, people with juvenile myoclonic epilepsy may experience absence seizures.

The EEG between seizures, in this form of epilepsy, often shows a fast, multiple- or double-spike pattern followed by slow waves, with fast rapid spikes occurring during the jerks. When the diagnosis is suspected, the best way of confirming it is a sleep EEG, continued for ten

or fifteen minutes after the person awakens. It is during this time that
the jerks and the characteristic EEG pattern are most likely to be seen.

Diagnosis is important, because, although this form of epilepsy responds poorly to many medications, it is usually easily controlled with
valproic acid. The seizures often recur when this medication is withdrawn. This type of seizure is *not* outgrown and may require lifelong
medication. A history of epilepsy may occur in as many as 40 percent
of siblings of those with the epilepsy of Janz. Studies of these families
are beginning to provide clues to its genetic basis.

Infantile Spasms (West Syndrome)

Infantile spasms are a special form of epilepsy of infancy readily recognized clinically but initially often mistaken for colic or reflux. In a
typical infantile spasm, the child will suddenly flex his head or his body
at the waist. The arms come up in a startle-like reaction, the knees are
drawn up, and the child may let out a short cry. This spasm lasts just a
second or two, then the child relaxes, but the spasm quickly recurs in
the same form. These spasms continue in a series of five to fifty or more
before the series stops. The child may have many series per day.

Since the mother often thinks that the cry and the flexion represent
cramps or pain, her description may sound to the physician as if the
child has colic, but *colic does not occur in a series of episodes.*

*Infantile spasms are the only type of epilepsy in which seizures occur
in series.*

The series of infantile spasms is most likely to occur when the child
is drowsy, either waking from a nap or going to sleep. A parent might
notice them particularly when the child has been placed in a high-chair
for a meal.

Less frequently, the spasms may be extensor, with the head thrown
back and the body briefly stiffening while the legs are extended; or the
spasm may be unilateral, with one arm coming up, the head turned to
that side and the leg on the same side extended. These brief atypical
spells also occur in series.

Infantile spasms rarely start before two months of age, most commonly beginning between four and eight months. Spells that occur in
series in this age group are usually infantile spasms or one of its vari-
ants. Even untreated, this form of epilepsy gradually disappears during
the second to the fourth year of life. *However,* the child often becomes
developmentally delayed. Shortly after the spasms begin, these children

seem to stop making developmental progress and often lose skills they had previously acquired. A child who had started to sit may stop sitting, may even lose the ability to roll over, may stop babbling, and may function like a much younger child. Because of this deterioration, children with infantile spasms are often thought to have an underlying degeneration of the brain. Only 10 to 20 percent of children with infantile spasms will have normal mental function; the vast majority will have moderate to severe mental retardation. This is the *only* seizure type for which one can predict such a poor outlook (prognosis). The poor prognosis is in part a consequence of the underlying brain pathology, but it may also in some way be a result of the effects of this chaotic electrical activity in the brain. Some people think that the earlier the treatment of these seizures is initiated, the better the outlook. But even infants whose spasms are brought under control with treatment often develop another special form of epilepsy called the Lennox-Gastaut syndrome.

Infantile spasms may occur in the young child who has developmental problems of the brain or with brain damage caused by birth injury, meningitis, or head trauma. Abnormalities of metabolism such as low blood sugar or amino acid problems may also be responsible. All of these are designated as "symptomatic" infantile spasms, since they are caused by the underlying process. A second and smaller group of infantile spasms are called "cryptogenic," since their cause is unknown. Children with cryptogenic infantile spasms appear perfectly normal in development before the seizures begin.

Infantile spasms are virtually always accompanied by an abnormality of the EEG known as "hypsarrhythmia," a wildly chaotic pattern with multiple spikes and slow waves (see page 105). While it may or may not be true, it is useful to think of this EEG pattern as imposing severe "static" on the brain waves so that the brain functions poorly and the child's functioning deteriorates.

A physician evaluating a child with infantile spasms should search for treatable metabolic causes of the spasms and infectious processes. An EEG and a CT or MRI scan should also be requested. Unless a specific treatable condition is found, and one rarely is, treatment for the spasms should begin promptly.

Although ACTH (adrenocorticotropic hormone), a form of steroid given twice a day by intramuscular injection, has been the standard treatment, some physicians use oral steroids, benzodiazepines such as diazepam (Valium) or clonazepam (Klonopin), or valproic acid (Depakote, Depakene), or perhaps vigabatrin. The relative effectiveness of these various medications has not been tested, nor has the duration of treatment been established. Each treatment has side effects, but, as indicated above, there are also substantial risks in not treating this form of epilepsy. Clearly we do not understand the reason for the related retardation or its optimal treatment. Further research is needed. The ketogenic diet (see Chapter 12) may be a new form of therapy.

Lennox-Gastaut Syndrome

The Lennox-Gastaut syndrome, named after the two epileptologists who described its various components, is characterized by two or more types of seizures, one of which is the atonic (falling down) type, by a particular EEG pattern of diffuse spike or poly-spike and slow waves, and by mental retardation.

The syndrome usually begins between the ages of two and six, often in children who previously had infantile spasms. As with infantile spasms, there is no known single cause, but the syndrome commonly arises in children with developmental problems of the brain or acquired brain damage. It is important to search for a degenerative process that may be causing the seizures. Cryptogenic cases, ones for which no cause is found, may have a somewhat better prognosis than cases in children whose seizures are symptomatic of a known disease process.

Children with the Lennox-Gastaut syndrome commonly experience multiple seizure types. In the most disabling seizures the child suddenly falls to the ground, either forward or, less often, backward, frequently injuring himself. Many of these children are forced to wear football helmets with face masks to protect their teeth and faces from trauma. In addition, tonic seizures and atypical absence seizures are common, with occasional tonic-clonic seizures as well.

Children with these multiple, difficult-to-control seizures often are given several simultaneous medications with consequent drug toxicity. The handicapping nature of the seizures, plus the drug toxicity and the continuous electrical abnormalities on the EEG, often reinforce the intrinsic brain dysfunction and produce a severely handicapped child.

Despite this dismal outlook, some children respond well to medications. Some end up with little or no handicap. Some have their seizures controlled with newer medications or with the ketogenic diet. Parents often despair when they hear the term Lennox-Gastaut applied to their child's EEG or to the child's seizures. As with most diagnoses in medicine, there is a range of outcomes. Clearly, as with infantile spasms, the Lennox-Gastaut syndrome is a most frustrating and devastating condition. This group of children make up a large proportion of the intractable seizure population. Research is badly needed to understand their condition and to develop better forms of therapy. The frustration involved in their management and the complexity of treatment lead us to suggest that these children be evaluated and managed under the consultation of sophisticated epilepsy centers with access to newer drugs.

Landau-Kleffner Syndrome and Other Language Impairments

Back in the "old days" we thought we understood a condition called the Landau-Kleffner syndrome. It was a rare malady in which children would usually develop mild seizures and then gradually lose language, first the understanding of language and later speech production. These children always had EEG abnormalities that were often most marked in the speech area over the left temporal regions. It was widely believed that this syndrome was due to "epileptic aphasia" (lack of speech, due to epilepsy). At times the EEG during sleep showed electrical status epilepticus. The natural history of this condition was grim. Many of these children did not recover speech for years. Many of them became mildly to moderately mentally retarded. Various anticonvulsants, steroids, and surgery have been reported to be successful in bringing speech and intelligence back toward normal. No successful treatment has been adequately documented or consistently recommended.

In 1995 a television program featured a child who was reported to have the Landau-Kleffner syndrome. This patient, who had none of the classic characteristics described above, had been retarded and autistic. It was claimed that steroids had returned him to normal. This TV program caused considerable commotion amongst parents whose children are autistic, language delayed or language impaired, or retarded.

As of this writing the confusion remains. If a child who previously had language loses language due to abnormal electrical activity in the speech area, he or she is said to have the Landau-Kleffner syndrome. If the same process were to occur *before* speech was present, presumably speech would not develop and so could not be lost. Would this be Landau-Kleffner-like? Lack of speech can also be due to retardation and to developmental problems of the brain. These problems may be associated with abnormal EEGs and even with seizures. Developmental delays, impairment of speech production, and varying degrees of intellectual impairment are often associated with the syndrome termed *autism*. Thus *autism,* some forms of *retardation,* and the *Landau-Kleffner syndrome* have become intertwined and confused. Until such time as there is specific therapy for any of these entities, the terminology is not important. It is no longer clear that any of these entities is a result of epilepsy. Nor is it clear that normalizing the EEG with medications or even surgery will correct the language delay.

Neonatal Seizures

Seizures in a newborn are often the consequence of lack of oxygen to the fetus during labor, due to metabolic disorders, infections, or developmental disorders. Seizures in a newborn that are due to trauma or difficulties with delivery will often subside over the first days of life and may not lead to epilepsy. Therefore, they may not require long-term treatment.

Other forms of seizures in newborns include:

• Pyridoxine (vitamin B_6)–dependent seizures, often characterized by seizures in utero, which the mother often describes as hiccups, and seizures starting immediately after birth. If 100 mg of pyridoxine is given during the EEG, the change in EEG can be seen, and seizures usually stop almost immediately.
• Benign neonatal seizures often start within the first few days of life in a child who had a normal birth and delivery. The child looks well, and the seizures are outgrown in infancy with or without treatment.
• Familial neonatal seizures, like benign neonatal seizures, are benign, and are outgrown. There is often a family history, and a genetic marker has been found.

Special Conditions That Cause Epilepsy

Most children who have epilepsy do not have mental retardation, cerebral palsy, or other problems. Most children who do have mental retardation or cerebral palsy do not have epilepsy. However, sometimes brain damage due to lack of oxygen, strokes, head trauma, or problems of brain development may lead to both epilepsy and mental retardation or cerebral palsy.

Strokes

Surprising as it may seem, strokes are not uncommon in the newborn period. Thrombosis (blockage) of one middle cerebral artery may occur in the days before or after birth. Often such strokes are difficult to detect, because most of the movements of the infant are not willful, cortical movements. Occasionally the strokes are heralded by seizures in the newborn, but often the only sign of a stroke is that the child displays left-handedness or right-handedness at an age when children should not have a dominant side. The infant splashing in the bath may use only one arm. As the infant begins to sit, she may not use one arm to prop herself up. Walking may be delayed because of the weakness or spasticity of one leg. Even the handedness may go unnoticed for many months. Only when the infant has a seizure and is carefully examined, or has a CT scan because of the seizure, is the stroke diagnosed. The scan shows an absence of brain tissue in the area to which the blood supply was blocked; immature brain tissue does not form scars but is reabsorbed.

These children are usually of normal intelligence. Some, but not all, develop seizures which are on the weak side of the body. If the seizures are difficult to control with medication, and if the child is already paralyzed on that side, a hemispherectomy (removal of that side of the brain—see Chapter 14) may help the child to become seizure free and medication free and to lead a normal life.

Strokes need not always affect a major artery but may sometimes affect only small branches of an artery, and the result is local scarring, which may cause epilepsy. Small abnormalities of blood vessels called *arteriovenus malformations* may have similar effects.

Developmental Abnormalities of the Brain

For reasons that are presently unclear, abnormalities in brain development can result in seizures. The development of the brain includes a series of events in which cells move and interconnections are established in a process so complex that it amazes and awes physicians. Many different abnormalities can occur during this development; the cells may be too large, misconnected, or malformed, or they may not move to the proper place in the brain.

Abnormalities in brain development often involve the entire brain; they tend to be accompanied by mental retardation and cerebral palsy. On occasion, these abnormalities may be focal and produce focal seizures or focal motor deficits. Such abnormalities may be surgically treated if that area of the brain can be safely removed. Less commonly, these developmental abnormalities may involve only one half of the brain, resulting in paralysis of one side of the body and unilateral seizures. If with such abnormalities a child has uncontrollable seizures, removal of that abnormal half of the brain (hemispherectomy) may be a life saving and seizure-curing procedure (Chapter 14).

There are many different developmental abnormalities of the brain, but except for the few patterns of abnormalities (syndromes) discussed below, the details of the developmental abnormalities are not important. What is important is that developmental brain abnormalities *can* be focal and sometimes can be cured by surgery. Although these abnormalities are often difficult to detect early in life, a good MRI with thin "cuts" and special studies are the tests most likely to document these often subtle but important problems.

Tuberous Sclerosis

Tuberous sclerosis is an inherited condition in which children may have white birthmarks on their skin and other skin lesions, mental retardation, and epilepsy. This is an abnormality of cell development affecting many organs of the body. In the brain, cells may be abnormal and may form small tumors. The cellular abnormalities and tumors may in turn cause epilepsy, either focal or generalized. The most common forms of epilepsy in children with tuberous sclerosis are infantile spasms and the Lennox-Gastaut syndrome, discussed above. A diagnosis of tuberous sclerosis is indicated if multiple white spots appear on the skin (see Figure 8.1). Older children may develop acne-like changes on their faces. The CT or MRI scan may show the tumors or areas of calcification.

The outcome of children with tuberous sclerosis varies, as does the epilepsy. Some individuals may be of normal intelligence with no significant problems. Others may have substantial mental retardation and difficult-to-control seizures.

Although there are usually many tuberous lesions within the brain, sometimes only one of them is causing the seizures. Therefore, if a child with tuberous sclerosis has difficult-to-control seizures, it may be worth seeing a pediatric epileptologist at an epilepsy center that does sophisticated epilepsy monitoring and surgery, to assess if the child might be a candidate for surgery.

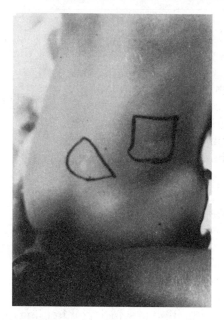

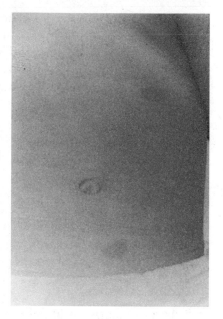

Figure 8.1 Tuberous sclerosis. Multiple white spots, subtle and ash-leaf shaped, are symptomatic.

Figure 8.2 Neurofibromatosis. Café-au-lait brownish and multiple other spots are symptomatic.

Tuberous sclerosis often affects the kidneys, the heart, and the skin. Since tuberous sclerosis may be inherited, if your child has this condition, it is important to talk with your physician about the possibility that your other children may be affected.

Sturge-Weber Syndrome

Sturge-Weber syndrome (SWS) is a neurocutaneous disorder (involving the brain and the skin). Children almost always have a "port-wine stain" (see Figure 8.3), also called an *angioma*. This angioma always involves the forehead and the area around an eye (first division of the facial nerve) but may involve the rest of the face on one or both sides. *Angiomas (or birthmarks) which do not involve the forehead are almost never associated with neurologic problems.* In addition to the facial birthmark, children with SWS may have seizures, a progressive hemiparesis (weakness on one side of the body), developmental delay, and glaucoma (increased pressure in the eye, which may lead to blindness). Sturge-Weber syndrome is not genetic but is a developmental ab-

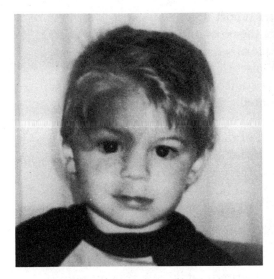

A

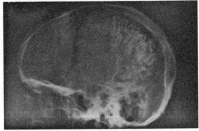

B

Figure 8.3 Sturge-Weber syndrome. Note the birthmark over the child's right forehead, eye, and lip (A); x-ray of the skull of a child with Sturge-Weber syndrome (B), with calcifications of the brain in a classic railroad-track pattern.

normality of the blood vessels to the face and the developing brain. A port-wine stain may occur on other parts of the body. The vascular abnormality involves the coverings of the brain as well as the face and results in seizures in 80 percent of cases and in a paralysis of the opposite side of the body in 65 percent.

Port-wine stain

The port-wine stain can produce a cosmetic handicap, and the child should be seen by a dermatologist in early infancy. Laser technology has enabled the removal of most traces of the stain with minimal scarring. Results are better with earlier treatment.

Glaucoma

Glaucoma occurs in more than half of children with SWS and usually starts in the first year of life. It is treatable. All children with SWS should be seen by an ophthalmologist and followed periodically throughout their life.

Seizures

Seizures occur in more than 80 percent of children with SWS, the majority beginning during the first year of life. One-quarter of the children achieve full seizure control with medication, one-half achieve partial seizure control, and one-quarter report no seizure control with medication. Early onset seizures are the most difficult to control. There is also a correlation between the age of seizure onset and motor development and IQ. Children whose onset of seizures occur within the first year and whose seizures are not controlled have a higher risk of subnormal development. Normal intelligence was found in 44 percent of all individuals with SWS and in 33 percent of those with seizures.

Hemispherectomy or removal of the affected part of the brain has been done in infants and children with SWS whose seizures were difficult to control; the timing of the surgery remains a matter of debate. Aspirin has been given to prevent thrombosis of the blood vessels, but its effectiveness remains unclear. The ketogenic diet is of no use. Headaches may be a substantial problem.

Neurofibromatosis

Neurofibromatosis is also an inherited condition involving many organ systems and with skin abnormalities, in this case consisting of multiple brown birthmarks ("café-au-lait spots") (see Figure 8.2). As with tuberous sclerosis, abnormalities of cell development within the brain may cause mild mental retardation and seizures. Tumors may occur on nerves, creating pressure on the surrounding nervous system tissue and leading to paralysis and other disabling conditions. Your doctor can discuss with you the many forms of this condition, their varying outcomes, as well as the genetic implications.

Chronic Infections

Acute bacterial and viral infections of the brain (meningitis and encephalitis), as we know, may cause acute seizures and may occasionally damage the brain and result in epilepsy. Infections that occur before birth may also damage the brain and lead to epilepsy. The most common infection of the brain worldwide is cysticercosis; in some countries this may be the most common cause of epilepsy, but in the United States it is a rare cause of seizures. A doctor will suspect this diagnosis when single or multiple areas of typical calcification, the result of cysts within the brain, are spotted on the CT. Surgical removal of these cysts may cure the child's epilepsy.

Another brain infection is toxoplasmosis, an infection spread by cats. If a pregnant woman acquires this infection, it may be transmitted to her baby and cause scarring in the brain. Infection, often undetectable in the newborn, may first be manifested as mental retardation or as seizures. A CT scan can detect scars within the brain and aid diagnosis. Also, small scars on the retina in the back of the eye may be noted by your physician and suggest a diagnosis. In addition, blood tests can confirm what the observations suggest. Suspected toxoplasmosis is often treated in an attempt to prevent further damage. The treatment of seizures in affected children is similar to the treatment for those in other forms of epilepsy.

Herpes Virus

Herpes simplex virus is a common human infection. It takes two forms. One is the cold sore which occurs around the mouth. This form (herpes type I) rarely affects the brain. Herpes type II affects the genital region. A baby born to a woman whose cervix is actively infected may, in turn, acquire the virus, which may devastate the child's brain, producing severe retardation, cerebral palsy, and epilepsy. In addition, a brain infection caused by the herpes simplex type II virus may be acquired at any age and produce complex partial seizures and an overwhelming encephalitis. Early detection may enable treatment to be more effective. Children who survive have variable degrees of brain damage and epilepsy.

HIV Infections (AIDS)

AIDS is a continuing problem for infants born to mothers infected with the human immunodeficiency virus (HIV) who acquire AIDS from transfusion, drug abuse, or sexual activity. Infection of the infant may be preventable by treating the mother prior to or at the time of delivery. The virus affects the brain and may produce seizures. The multiple infections that are by-products of the immunosuppression due to HIV infection may also affect the brain and cause seizures. Secondary infections require specific treatment, but the seizures often are treated with standard anticonvulsant medication.

Rasmussen's Syndrome

A rare form of progressive unilateral seizures, usually associated with a progressive hemiparesis (weakness of one side of the body), has been termed Rasmussen's syndrome after the Canadian neurosurgeon who first described it. The sudden onset of intense, constant focal seizures may indicate the presence of Rasmussen's syndrome, a focal, unilateral encephalitis-like condition. While sometimes beginning with either a generalized or a unilateral tonic-clonic seizure, this condition frequently evolves into a state called epilepsia partialis continua (continuous focal epilepsy). The hand, face, or foot may jerk continuously. This condition is uniformly progressive, spreading as if in concentric circles from the initial site. Although Rasmussen's syndrome was originally thought to be viral in origin, recent studies suggest that it is autoimmune in nature. This means that by some mechanism as yet undetermined, the body becomes "allergic" to some of its own brain cells on one side of the brain, and as it destroys them they become intensely epileptic. The seizures do not respond to any current anticonvulsant medications. Steroids have sometimes had a transient beneficial effect, as has plasmapharesis (washing the blood plasma to remove the antibodies) or the administration of large doses of intravenous gamma globulin. All of these therapies at best give transient relief from the inexorable progression of this condition.

Until some more effective form of immunotherapy becomes available, the only effective treatment is hemispherectomy (removal of the affected side of the brain). Removal of only portions of the affected side always results in recurrence of the seizures in the remaining portions. This peculiar condition is limited to one half of the brain. Therefore, removal of the affected half, if done early in the course of the disease, results in cessation of the seizures and permits normal intellectual development. After surgery there will be paralysis of one side of the body and loss of vision to that side, but these children walk, run, and go to school. Without surgery the outcomes are worse. (See Chapter 14.)

Degenerative Diseases

A number of progressive, degenerative diseases of the brain affect children. Epilepsy is commonly seen in most of them. One group is called storage diseases, because the proteins and fats that are normally broken down to waste products (metabolized) and eliminated from the body cannot be broken down in these rare inherited metabolic conditions. These products accumulate within nerve cells and affect their function, leading to epilepsy and mental retardation. These progressive conditions are usually fatal, but the duration of the illness may be quite variable. The names attached to these storage diseases reflect the individuals who described the conditions or the material stored. Different conditions begin at different ages. Among these conditions are Tay-

Sachs disease (GM_2 gangliosidosis), Batten's disease (ceroid lipofusci-nosis), and the various leukodystrophies. In the leukodystrophies, epilepsy is likely to appear later in the course of the progressive disease.

Many other diseases affect metabolism of brain cells and result in epilepsy as well as deterioration of intellect and/or motor function. Each of these has its own age of onset, its own course, and its own out-come. It is beyond the scope of this book to discuss them individually.

Although many of the epilepsy syndromes and some of these infec-tions sound very frightening and can be devastating to both the child and the family, fortunately these conditions are uncommon, as are the degenerative diseases. Most children with epilepsy do not have these conditions and their seizures are controlled. Most children with epilepsy do very well.

Part Three

Treating Seizures and Epilepsy

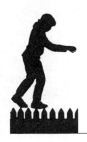

9. Medical Treatment of Seizures

Philosophy of Treatment

Although once it was believed that all seizures should be treated, just because they were there, now it is generally believed that no judgment can cover every individual. Decisions about treatment should be made by the patient (or parent) *and* the physician, acting in partnership. The decision should be based on risk-benefit analysis.

- The risks and consequences of each medication vary with the medicine, with the dose, with the individual's reaction to the medicine, with the age of the child, and with the length of time the child takes the medicine.
- The risk of further seizures varies markedly with the type of seizure, the frequency of seizures, and even the time of day in which they occur. A child who has only occasional tonic-clonic seizures at night will face very different risks from a child whose seizures occur during the day. A child with occasional complex partial seizures has different risks from the child with tonic-clonic seizures or the child with frequent absence seizures.

Most people's seizures can be controlled with a single medicine used in a proper dose to achieve a proper blood level for that individual. *There is no correct dose of a given medication.* The "proper" dose of medication is the dose that completely controls the seizures without causing significant side effects. *There is not a "correct" medication as such. Some medicines work better for some types of seizures than for others. The correct medicine is the one that works.*

The treatment of epilepsy is empirical. This means that the treatment of each person's seizures is a trial or search to find the appropriate dose of the best medicine for that individual. This "experimentation" is often frustrating to parents, since they are used to physicians' knowing, for example, the right antibiotic and dose to use for a child's ear infection. For antibiotics, we know the function, the proper dose, and the side effects. We know how much is necessary to kill the bacteria causing the infection. We can test the drug's effectiveness in the laboratory. We also know, for example, how "heart drugs" work and their side effects; we can use the electrocardiogram (EKG) to see if they are working or if they are producing toxicity. But, since we do not fully understand how anticonvulsant drugs work, and since we do not understand the factors that permit a seizure to occur at a specific time, each child must be his own laboratory as a doctor attempts to find the proper dose of the best anticonvulsant. Side effects will vary with each child's metabolism and his individual reaction to the drug.

How Anticonvulsant Drugs Work in Epilepsy

In an ideal world, we would understand the chemistry and the physiologic mechanisms causing epilepsy—how cells interact, fire, and misfire. Then we would design drugs that interact with the brain and prevent the misfiring—the seizures—without affecting the brain's normal function. As we have previously indicated, we do not know how or why a seizure occurs. While we have many drugs that are effective in treating and preventing seizures, we do not know how they work.

Because epilepsy is a result of complex interactions in the brain, and since these interactions cannot be accurately simulated in a test tube or by a computer, animal experimentation has been necessary for us to understand epilepsy and learn how to control it. Most anticonvulsants were discovered by experimenting with substances to see if they would work in animals that had seizures caused by certain drugs. Such animal seizures, although not the same as epilepsy, have many similarities. Such research has been highly useful, and it must continue.

Although we know little about how these drugs prevent seizures from recurring, we do know a lot about how they are absorbed and metabolized in the body and about their side effects. This knowledge enables us to use them properly, to calculate a dose, and to predict effects and side effects. This knowledge is called the pharmacology of the drugs; your physician will use this knowledge in treating your child and controlling her seizures.

Terms You Need to Know

Drug levels. The term *drug level* refers to the amount of a medication in the blood—to be more precise, the serum levels, since the drug is in the liquid portion of your blood (serum) rather than in the red blood cells. To be still more precise, we should refer to the amount of "free" drug in the serum, since virtually all of a drug is tightly bound to the proteins in the serum and cannot get into the brain to exert its effect; only the tiny "free" (unbound) portion can enter the brain to affect the seizures. When we measure drug levels or blood levels, we usually measure the total amount of a drug in the serum. In most cases this is sufficient, but we can, when necessary, measure the free portion as well, although it is a somewhat more expensive test. In general, when we talk about drug levels in this chapter, we are referring to serum levels.

Toxicity. The term *toxicity* covers a multitude of things. *Toxicity,* in general, refers to all of the adverse (bad) effects of a medication. There are two major forms of such toxicity, allergic and dose-related.

Allergic reactions are "idiosyncratic," which means that each person is different and may react in an unusual fashion to the medication. While anyone may have an allergic reaction to any drug, some drugs are more likely to produce reactions than others. Allergic reactions may be mild (a slight rash) or severe (if the rash continues to spread and involves the membranes of the mouth). Such a severe reaction, termed the "Stevens-Johnson syndrome," may even be fatal. Allergic rashes to anticonvulsants usually occur within the first three to four weeks after starting the medication. We warn every patient starting a new medicine:

Notify your physician immediately if a rash appears, and stop taking the drug until you are seen by the physician.

Most of the rashes are the result of viruses, bites, or allergies to something else, but it is always better to be safe.

Other types of allergic or idiosyncratic reactions can involve the liver, pancreas, bone marrow, or blood cells. They may be mild or severe or even fatal. Some physicians obtain blood chemistries and liver function tests before starting a new medication as a baseline against which to measure any changes that may occur. They repeat the tests periodically. Others feel that these reactions are very rare and tell the families that if the child is tired, weak, jaundiced (has yellowness of the eyes), loses appetite, or begins to bruise easily or to bleed, these could be signs of reactions to the medications. The physician should be notified if any of these symptoms appears, and the medication should be stopped until the cause is found. Whether one of these approaches is more successful than the other at recognizing the early signs of systemic reactions and at preventing serious consequences is unclear.

Dose-related toxicity depends on the amount of the medication in the brain. It may display itself as sedation (sleepiness), ataxia (unsteadiness), tremor, or even increasing problems with learning. Hallucinations and psychologic changes may be signs of dose-related toxicity. Dose-related toxicities are important to recognize, and when recognized are seldom serious, because they are reversible by decreasing or discontinuing the drug.

Half-life. This is the amount of time it takes for one half of the drug in the body to be metabolized (broken down) or to be excreted. Therefore, if a dose of a medicine reaches a level of 10 in your body, that drug's half-life is the amount of time it takes until the blood level decreases to 5. This is important to you because the half-life for some drugs is only a few hours but for others it may be days. A drug's half-life will determine how often your child must take his medicine—one, two, or, rarely, four times per day. The half-life varies with each drug and with the age of the child.

Here is an example: We start your child on drug A, which has a half-life of twelve hours. We tell you to give the two daily doses twelve hours apart. If your child's drug level was 20 one hour after a dose, it would fall to 10 just before the next dose. If 10 were too low to control your child's seizures, she might have a seizure before the evening dose. If we gave the same dose, but told you to give the medicine every eight hours, then eight hours after a dose the level might be 14, and that might be sufficient to prevent a seizure (Figure 9.1).

Steady state. In general, it takes five half-lives to achieve a steady state, a relatively consistent blood level of a drug between doses (Figure 9.2). After one dose of a medicine, let's say that the blood level is 8. One half-life later the level has decreased. If a second dose is then given, the blood level rises. You can see that the blood level is slowly creeping

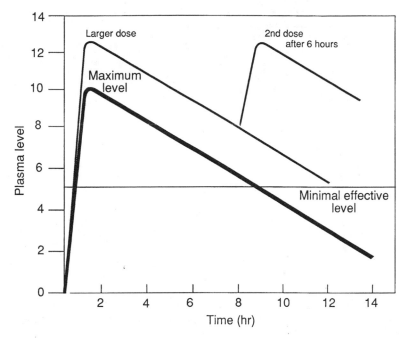

Figure 9.1 Half-life of a drug. Drugs are absorbed at different rates. As shown in the figure, the drug taken by mouth takes approximately an hour to reach its maximum blood (plasma) level of 10, then is slowly metabolized and excreted. The amount in the blood falls to half of its maximum level (5) eight hours later; thus, the half-life of this drug is eight hours. If a second dose were to be given six hours after the first, the body would be absorbing new medicine and the blood level would never fall below the minimum effective level for preventing seizures.

up. If you continue this process, then after five half-lives there is insignificant change in the blood level between doses.

We must allow each new medication sufficient time to achieve a steady state before we know if it is going to work. For example, since phenobarbital has a half-life of three days, it will take at least two weeks to achieve its steady state. If your child has a seizure five days after starting phenobarbital, or after increasing the dose, it may not mean that the drug will not work. It may mean rather that there hasn't been enough time to test that dose of the drug. You have to be patient.

After a first steady state or new steady state is achieved, you will have to allow sufficient time to know if that level will control seizures. As a

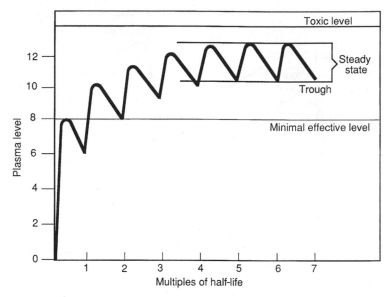

Figure 9.2 Steady state. Steady state is reached at the point when there is relatively little fluctuation in the level of a drug in the body; in general, it takes five half-lives to reach the steady state.

general rule, each new drug and each new dose of a drug should be given a trial of at least seven to fourteen days before a change is considered.

An exception to this rule may occur when the child is having seizures daily or several times each day. Then you may not want to wait two weeks or even one before changing the dose. In this situation, your physician can "load" the child with the drug. This means if she wishes to achieve a high, consistent blood level more rapidly, she can give more of the drug, usually two to three times as much as usual. This will produce an initially high level and may cause substantial temporary side effects.

The side effects of medication are related to both the level of medication in the blood and to the brain's individual reaction. The brain will often become accustomed to a drug. Many people feel sleepy when first started on a medication, but after several weeks, they may become "used" to it and be normally alert.

A second application of the concept of half-life is this: Let's say your child is taking phenytoin (Dilantin) and accidentally took too many pills. You become concerned when you find him very unsteady, acting as if he were drunk. When you discover the overdose and call your physician, she is likely to say, "Don't worry, it will wear off. We have to let it clear out of his system. If he took the extra pills last night, we don't want to give him his usual dose this morning. We want to wait twenty-four hours, the half-life of phenytoin. By evening, he should be feeling better and he can go back to taking his usual dose of medication. If he is still unsteady, then only give him half of the regular dose until he is back to normal. He will become normal over the next twenty-four hours or so."

The physician can predict the time course of the disappearance of the toxicity because she knows the half-life of the drug. She could do it even more precisely if she knew the level of the drug in the blood.

"My child has failed four medications in the past three weeks. What do we do now?"

You will need to start over again. None of the medications was given a sufficient trial to declare them a failure. None had sufficient time to reach a steady state, to determine if they could be effective. Trying to achieve seizure control quickly is the most frequent mistake we see. Individuals are given too many medications in too short a period of time. Patience on the part of the parent and the physician will, in the long run, pay off, and you will not discard medicines that might have worked. Each medication should be given approximately two weeks to reach steady state and several weeks to demonstrate effectiveness. If it then seems not to be working, the medication should be gradually increased to effectiveness or to toxicity before declaring it a failure and starting a new one. It may take two or three months before you can determine if medicine is effective.

"Sam takes his medicine four times each day, but often forgets to take his after-school dose. What can I do about it?"

Change his medication schedule. Most patients at least occasionally forget to take a dose of medication, and the more frequent the doses are the more likely one is to forget.

• Individuals taking medicine once a day have been found to miss 10 percent of the doses. They may remember and take it late, but they usually remember.
• Individuals taking medicine twice a day on average miss 20 percent of the doses. Again missed doses may be taken late.

• Individuals taking medicine three times a day forget 40 percent of the doses, and those taking medication four times a day miss even more.

There is virtually no reason to take medicine more than twice a day. Independent of the half-life, the steady state will almost always provide enough safety to permit twice-a-day dosing. Few medicines have such a small margin that they have dose-related toxicity when given twice a day.

• *If* the medication is given twice a day, *and* the patient has seizures before the second dose, *then* you may want to give the medication three times a day, or try another drug.
• *If* the medication is given twice a day, *and* the patient has signs of drug-related toxicity one to two hours after the dose, *then* his blood level at that time may be too high and the physician may either reduce the dose, spread it out to three times each day, or change to another medicine.

Some medications are now made in a slow-release form. They are slowly absorbed and achieve a more steady state with fewer peaks and valleys. Evidence that they have less toxicity or greater efficacy is not strong.

"Elspeth often falls asleep at seven o'clock, and I'm supposed to give her second dose at 9 p.m. like they did in the hospital. Should I wake her up for it?"

Medications do not need to be given precisely on time. The principles of half-life and steady state mean that there should be little variation from hour to hour, so one or two hours earlier or later should usually make little difference in the blood level or in the child's seizure control. Children are often started on medication in the hospital and medications are given on the nurses' schedule. Parents may not realize that the medication can be given on a more convenient schedule. Discuss the dosing schedule with your physician.

"What will happen if I forget to take a dose of medication? What should I do?"

Again, your steady state blood level should be sufficiently consistent that if you forget a single dose it should make little difference. Take the missed dose when you remember. Missing repeated doses is a different matter; that may affect your seizure control. It is often difficult to remember whether you actually took your medicine or if you only thought that you took it. A daily pillbox (some with several sections for separate doses) allows you to check to see if the pills have been consumed or if they are still in the box.

Blood Levels of Anticonvulsants and the Therapeutic Range

One of the principal advances in our ability to control seizures came when we learned how to measure the amount (level) of an anticonvulsant in the blood and so assess the amount of the drug actually reaching the brain. This advance is only several decades old.

Even now many physicians do not fully understand the use of blood levels and the concept of the "therapeutic range" of a given drug. Parents (and physicians) often believe that these levels ensure control of the seizures or guarantee the absence of side effects, misbeliefs that often lead to misuse of blood level information. Also, some of the new anticonvulsants act by mechanisms unrelated to the serum levels and therefore do not have established therapeutic ranges.

As mentioned above, blood levels are measured in the serum (liquid portion) of the blood, which may be taken by needle stick from a vein or by pricking the finger. (There are several different methods of measuring the drug level, but those techniques are not important here.) The test must be requested and interpreted by your physician, and should always be done with proper quality control.

The level of the drug in the blood will vary, to some extent, depending on how long after the previous dose the blood is drawn (see discussion about a drug's half-life, above). The level of the drug in the blood will be highest one to two hours after a dose, when most of the drug has been absorbed. The level will be lowest just before the next dose. How much variation there will be between those two will depend on the half-life of the drug and the time between the doses (see Figure 9.1). If you or your physician wants to know if the dose of the drug needs to be increased, you should obtain a blood level at the trough (the lowest point). The trough will occur early in the morning, before the child gets her morning dose, or in the afternoon, at the farthest possible time after the morning dose. If the child is complaining about dizziness or fogginess after a dose, you may want to obtain a peak level one or two hours after a dose. It may be equally important to measure the blood level at a time when the child is having seizures to see if the level is low and to measure it when the child is sleepy, dizzy, or having other unexplained symptoms in order to ensure that the level is not too high.

What is the correct blood level for your child? The correct blood level is the amount of the drug that controls the seizures. It is not a specific amount. The optimal level is the lowest level that works without causing toxicity. It will vary from one child to another.

This brings us to the concept of the *therapeutic range,* a concept often misunderstood. Therapeutic ranges for the commonly used anticonvulsants are shown in Table 9.1. It may be useful to understand how the therapeutic ranges for these drugs have been established. A small

Table 9.1   Pharmacological Facts for Selected Antiepileptic Drugs

Drug	Daily dosage range (mg/kg/day)	Serum therapeutic range (mg/l)	Half-life (hrs)	Time to reach stable levels (wks)
Carbamazepine (Tegretol)	10–40	5–14	10–30	1
Clonazepam (Klonopin)	0.05–0.3		24–36	1–2
Ethosuximide (Zarontin)	10–40	40–100	24–42	1–2
Gabapentin (Neurontin)	15–45		5–7	0.5
Lamotrigine (Lamictal)	1–5 (on valproic acid) 5–15 (off valproic acid)		15–60	1–3
Phenobarbital	2–8	10–25	48–100	2–3
Phenytoin (Dilantin)	4–12	10–20	6–30	1–2
Primidone (Mysoline)	10–20	6–12	6–12	2–3
Valproic acid (Depakene, Depakote)	10–70	50–100	6–18	0.5–1

Note: Names of drugs that appear in parentheses are brand names; others are generic names.

number of adults (or children) were carefully studied using a single drug. The lower end of the therapeutic range was then determined by the level at which seizures began to be controlled in a majority of these individuals. The upper end of the range was the point at which some individuals began to show signs of toxicity. Thus, the therapeutic range is the drug level at which most individuals are likely to have their seizures controlled without toxicity. Your child is not an average but an individual. Thus he or she may require a higher-than-average level or a lower-than-average level to control the seizures. He may be able to tolerate more or less than average levels before showing signs of toxicity. Therefore, finding the correct dose of a given drug for your child requires a trial to determine what is "enough" and what is "too much" for *your* child.

The therapeutic range is commonly believed to be the "gold standard" that will guarantee seizure control and avoid toxicity and side effects. It does neither. Yet many physicians misinterpret the therapeutic range as the range where they should keep the blood level, decreasing the dose of the medicine if the blood level is above the range and increasing it if the level is below the range.

To repeat, the correct blood level for your child is enough—enough to control the seizures and not enough to cause toxicity. The therapeutic range is a guide, nothing more.

Common Questions about Blood Levels

Physicians and parents have become enamored of tests and often give them greater importance than is proper. Despite scientific advances, the proper use of anticonvulsants remains an art, not a science. We are often asked such questions as these by both physicians and parents:

"My doctor says that my child's blood level is slightly low and wants to increase his dose. What should I do?"

If you ask us this, we would ask if your child is still having seizures. If he is, then the dose should be increased. If he is not, then we would leave the dose alone; the current level appears to be sufficient to control his seizures. The question of increasing a dose often comes up in a child whose seizures are controlled. As the child grows and increases in size, the blood level will, of course, decrease if your doctor doesn't increase the dose. But we suggest keeping the dose the same as the child grows and gains weight, unless he begins to have seizures again. If the dose is kept the same, then the blood level gradually falls over the months or years. If the child does not have another seizure, it will be easier and safer to take him off his medicine when he has been free of seizures for two years. If he has a seizure, then you know that he needs to stay on the medication longer and that the dose may need to be increased.

"My daughter's blood level is at the upper end of 'normal,' and she is still having seizures. My doctor wants to try another drug. Is that the proper thing to do?"

We would suggest first that he try increasing the dose even further, but slowly, since your daughter is close to the point where many people show toxicity. Sometimes seizures will be controlled with a little more drug without any toxic problems. The upper level of the therapeutic range is like a sign post, "WARNING"; it suggests that you and your physician should be watchful for signs of toxicity.

"Rachel's blood level is 'high,' and my doctor wants to lower the dose. I think that she is doing just fine, and she hasn't had any seizures since that last increase in dosage. What should we do?"

We would recommend that you leave the dose alone. If Rachel isn't having any seizures and has no signs of toxicity, then perhaps this is the level she requires. However, since the level is above the usual range, we would suggest that you keep a close eye on her and on her school performance, to be sure that the drug is not interfering, and that you stay alert for other signs of toxicity.

"Billy's blood level is right in the middle of the 'range.' Is that good?"

The answer to this question is, "It depends." If Billy is not having any seizures and shows no signs of toxicity, then that level is fine and should not be changed. If he is still having seizures, then the level is too low for him, and he needs more medication. If he is too sleepy, too irritable, or having problems in school, then it is important to find out why. There are many causes for problems such as these. Obviously, you should be sure that he is not having seizures. If the level is not high, then the drug is a less likely cause. However, if you can't find another cause, then lowering or discontinuing the drug may be worth trying. If the problem disappears, then it may have been due to the drug.

To summarize, the therapeutic range is a guide and nothing more. It will suggest to you and your physician when it may be appropriate to in-

crease the drug and when to look more closely for signs of toxicity. The range does not tell you when the child is taking too much or too little. Control of seizures and signs of toxicity are the only indicators of that.

Drug Interactions

"Trudy has been on phenobarbital but is continuing to have seizures. Our doctor started her on valproic acid, but several days later she is very sleepy and unsteady. Why?"

You and your physician might assume that she is toxic from the new medicine, but you would probably be wrong. A blood level might show you that the valproate level was actually low but that the phenobarbital level had now increased to the toxic range, and that phenobarbital was the true offender. This effect is due to what we call "drug interactions"—one drug interfering with the breakdown or metabolism of another. Drug interactions are common; some decrease the level of the other drug; some, like the valproate, increase the level of another. The only way you can be sure is by measuring each drug's blood level. Other medications, such as antibiotics or ulcer medications, to name a few, may also interact with anticonvulsants and alter levels. The most common drug interaction we encounter is between Tegretol and its newer forms and erythromycin. Erythromycin may cause the Tegretol level to double, producing severe toxicity. If your child is on Tegretol and your physician wants to start an antibiotic, ask your pharmacist or physician if there are any drug interactions.

While we talk about blood levels of a drug as if they were very important for control of seizures, *it is not the drug in the blood that is important, but rather the amount of the drug in the brain,* which is where these drugs work. However, we cannot easily measure the level of the drug in the brain, so we use the blood (serum) level as an approximation.

Drugs are bound to the proteins in the blood; this is the way they are carried around the body. They cannot get into the brain when they are bound up. Only the small amount of any drug which is not bound to protein (the "free" drug) enters the brain and is actually active. Usually when we measure the blood level, the test measures all of the drug in the blood, both bound and unbound. However, in special circumstances, such as a low serum protein level, when certain other drugs are present, or when there is severe kidney disease, more of the drug may be unbound and thus active. It is possible, and sometimes useful, to measure the "unbound" fraction, but most of the time we do not measure the unbound fraction of the drug, because it requires a somewhat more difficult and, therefore, more expensive procedure.

"How frequently does my child need to have his blood chemistries measured?"

There are two possible answers to this question.

Many physicians evaluate the blood count and the liver chemistries before starting a new medication. As we've said earlier in this chapter, this allows them to have a baseline in case the medication causes an allergic reaction affecting the blood, pancreas, or liver. They might then repeat these chemistries in one month and then every three or four months thereafter. Those physicians are being very cautious, since allergic types of reactions are very rare.

The second group of physicians would respond, "I would recheck blood chemistries only if your child is having problems." *If your child's eyes start turning yellow (indicating jaundice), if your child is bruising easily, develops sores in his mouth, complains of repeated abdominal pain and is vomiting, you should see your physician immediately. These could be the signs of a serious allergic reaction, but such reactions are very uncommon.* If your child is fine and has none of these symptoms, this group of physicians would check the chemistries once a year, or less. Drawing blood for serum chemistries hurts, the tests are expensive, and there is no evidence either that frequent checks allow early detection or that early detection of problems allows better treatment and outcome.

We belong to the second group of physicians, but many physicians belong to the first group.

"How frequently must she have her blood levels of the anticonvulsant checked? She is really afraid of needles."

Since the correct blood level of the anticonvulsant is "enough" but "not too much," we use clinical signs and symptoms rather than blood levels. *Enough* is the amount required to control the child's seizures. *Too much* is the amount that produces side effects such as sleepiness, unsteadiness, learning problems, or behavior problems. If the seizures are under control, the child has enough drug in his system, whatever the blood level. If he has evidence of toxicity, he may have too much, for him, whatever the blood level. Blood levels of the drug may help the physician decide if the sleepiness could be due to the medication or if it is due to one of the many other conditions that can cause sleepiness or behavior problems. If your child's seizures are not under control despite a good dose of medication, we may just increase the dose, or we may get a blood level to make certain that the child is taking the medicine, that he is absorbing it properly, and that he is not metabolizing it too fast. The blood levels do not tell you that he has enough, but they may guide your decisions when you want to give more or less. We do not do blood levels either frequently or routinely.

Your child does not need a blood level test every time he visits the doctor!

"My child's blood level of his medication is low. Why?"

There are several possible reasons. Perhaps the most common is that the child is not on a high enough dose; a second is that she is not taking the medicine or not taking enough. Noncompliance, failure to follow treatment instructions, is a common reason for a low blood level, particularly among adolescents. Also, occasionally an individual absorbs medicine poorly and must take more to achieve the same blood level. Rarely, an individual metabolizes the drug more rapidly than average and, therefore, has a low level. Whatever the reason, increasing the dose should help to determine the answer. If the person is taking the drug erratically or not at all, then prescribing more will usually have little or no effect. If the dose prescribed is too low, a higher dose should correct the problem, as it will do if the patient absorbs poorly or metabolizes rapidly.

"Sally had several grand mal seizures and was placed on a medicine. She has had no more seizures since age three, but she has grown and gained weight. Her physician finds that Sally's blood level has slipped below the therapeutic range. What should he do?"

This question of maintaining the level over time also needs to be addressed. In Sally's case there are two alternatives. The physician could increase the dose, and thus the blood level, to keep it in the therapeutic range, giving her greater protection against another seizure. Or he could leave the dose alone, letting it continue to decrease gradually as she grows. There is not, however, necessarily a correct thing to do. Children who have been free of seizures for two years can discontinue medication with a high probability of remaining seizure free. That chance is better if the blood levels are low at the time the medicine is stopped. Allowing the level to drop slowly is a form of testing. If Sally passes the test, her chance of having a seizure when we stop the medicine is low. If she fails the test and has another seizure, we believe that it is better for this to happen at a younger age. Therefore, our suggestion to this parent and this physician would be not to increase the medicine. We believe that the risks and consequences of another seizure at this age are outweighed by the possible side effects of a higher dose on Sally's learning capacity. Other physicians (and other parents) may believe differently.

Choosing the Best Medication

All drugs do not work equally well for every seizure-type. Therefore it is necessary to classify the child's seizure. For each seizure-type there are several drugs that are usually equally effective. The choice between the drugs is then made on the basis of the drug's side effects, its cost, the child's age, and any previous drug allergies. Some medications are more effective for partial and tonic-clonic seizures, others for absence seizures. We will discuss them in those groupings and in the order in which they were discovered.

Many anticonvulsant medications are available. The following are those most commonly used.

Common Older, "First-Line" Drugs for Partial Seizures and Tonic-Clonic Seizures

Phenobarbital

Phenobarbital is one of the oldest, cheapest, and safest of the anticonvulsants. Since phenobarbital is slowly metabolized by the body (has a long half-life), it usually can be taken only once per day. As with any drug, it can occasionally lead to allergic reactions.

Phenobarbital, like its two close barbiturate cousins, mephobarbital (Mebaral) and primidone (Mysoline), is effective in partial and generalized tonic-clonic seizures but ineffective in absence seizures (and, indeed, may even cause them to increase).

Reactions to phenobarbital and other barbiturate drugs

A skin rash may be the first sign of an allergic reaction to phenobarbital (or to any other drug). A child who develops a skin rash during the first two to three weeks of treatment with any anticonvulsant should immediately be seen by his physician. While most such rashes are *not* caused by the drug, continuing the drug in a child who is allergic to it may lead to severe and even fatal consequences termed the "Stevens-Johnson syndrome."

Side effects that are dose-related are seen in certain children. The most important side effects of phenobarbital in children are its impacts on learning and behavior. While these side effects can occur in any child if the blood level is sufficiently high, certain individuals may react adversely even at "normal" blood levels.

Phenobarbital can also cause sedation (sleepiness). Many children become tolerant of this tired feeling. In others, the tired feeling continues and they do not tolerate the drug. Giving phenobarbital at bedtime may help to minimize this problem. Disturbances of sleep also can occur from use of the drug.

Hyperactivity, a behavioral side effect, may occur in 20 to 40 percent of young children taking phenobarbital. Hyperactivity is more common in children who were quite active to begin with. In one study, more than half of the children had to be taken off this drug because of the side effects of irritability and behavior problems.

Effects of phenobarbital on a child's *learning ability* may be its most disturbing side effect. These symptoms may be subtle and difficult to recognize and may account for some of the learning problems previously attributed to epilepsy itself. Most, perhaps all of these side effects are thought to disappear when phenobarbital is discontinued. Recent studies have also found an increased incidence of depression in adolescents who take phenobarbital, perhaps more frequent when there is a family history of depression. In some children, a depression thought to be caused by an emotional reaction to having epilepsy disappears when another medication is substituted for phenobarbital.

We prefer, for all these reasons, not to use phenobarbital when alternative drugs are available, especially because of our concern about its effects on learning and behavior in the vulnerable young child. When we do use it, we carefully monitor the child's behavior and school performance.

Mephobarbital (Mebaral)

Mephobarbital is said to cause less hyperactivity than phenobarbital, but its effectiveness as an anticonvulsant and its effects on learning have been less well studied.

Primidone (Mysoline)

Primidone is an effective anticonvulsant that is metabolized by the body into phenobarbital. Although the drug has not been well studied in children, hyperactivity and behavior problems have been observed. As with phenobarbital, a child on primidone should be carefully monitored for learning and behavior problems. Primidone must be started at a low dose and increased slowly over several weeks to avoid major problems with sedation and personality change.

Phenytoin (Dilantin)

Phenytoin, the generic (non-brand) name for Dilantin, an excellent anticonvulsant that has been used for many years, is particularly effective for partial and generalized tonic-clonic seizures. Phenytoin also produces side effects, both allergic and dose-related.

Allergic reactions

As with phenobarbital, a skin rash may be the first sign of an allergic reaction to phenytoin. *A child who develops a skin rash during the first two to three weeks after starting phenytoin should be seen by his physician immediately.* Other, more severe reactions to phenytoin may affect the liver or the bone marrow, although these reactions are rare.

Dose-related reactions

The earliest sign of a high blood level of phenytoin is nystagmus (jerky movements of the eyes), a sign of no consequence, since it does not interfere with vision or function and, therefore, does not require lowering the dose of the drug. Noticing it may be useful to your physician, however, because it indicates that the drug is in a "good" therapeutic range. If, with the onset of an even higher blood level, the child begins to be unsteady on his feet and awkward with his hands, to act drunk, you should notify your physician. He will usually reduce the dose. Sleepiness or exaggeration of the "drunkenness" follow if the blood level goes even higher. Vomiting may also occur. All of these signs disappear over several days (several half-lives) if the dose is reduced.

Because phenytoin has an unusual metabolism, when its level in the blood is in the therapeutic range, small increases in dosage can cause large increases in the blood level and, thus, in toxicity. Therefore, when the blood level is in the therapeutic range but the dose must be increased to control seizures, increases should be introduced slowly and by small increments or the child may become toxic.

Other side effects

Phenytoin also affects behavior and learning. The child's mood may change, and she may seem to have less energy. The child's motor abilities and her alacrity in performing tasks may also be affected. Hyperactivity is less common than with phenobarbital, however, and the effects on learning may be less severe than with phenobarbital.

Some of the dose-related side effects of phenytoin are cosmetic, that is, they affect the appearance of the child. Gum hyperplasia (overgrowth of the gums) occurs in almost one-half of the children who have therapeutic blood levels. The overgrowth is made much worse by poor dental hygiene; thus, when children are wearing braces, gum overgrowth becomes an even more severe problem. *Children taking phenytoin should be taught good tooth-brushing techniques, and young children should have their teeth brushed by their parents. Good hygiene will diminish the gum swelling but not necessarily prevent it entirely.* Overgrown gums can be cut back by the dentist. Overgrowth of the gums may make secondary teeth come in with wide spaces, and the child may later require extensive orthodontic care.

Children who have been on high doses of phenytoin for long periods of time often develop coarse facial features and more extensive body hair. The hair does not disappear when the drug is discontinued, although it may decrease. Such a side effect may become a cosmetic problem, especially for young women. *Although phenytoin is an excellent anticonvulsant, we prefer not to use it as our* initial *drug in young children because of its cosmetic side effects.* The cosmetic effects seem to be a lesser problem in adolescent and adult patients.

Carbamazepine (Tegretol)

Carbamazepine is an excellent anticonvulsant medication for partial and generalized tonic-clonic seizures and is our initial choice for children with these seizures, because of its apparent lower incidence of effects on learning and behavior and its lack of cosmetic side effects. Earlier concerns about carbamazepine's effect on the blood and bone marrow seem to have been greatly overstated, especially for children.

Carbamazepine is a seemingly very safe and effective anticonvulsant.

We start it slowly, however. If we were to begin with the amount of medication needed to control the seizures, the child would become toxic, because carbamazepine "induces its own metabolism." The half-life is longer when the medication is first introduced into the body; the body's metabolism hasn't been induced, or "turned on," and the drug accumulates. Therefore, when starting carbamazepine, the drug should be begun at a low dose and increased each week for the first several weeks to reach and maintain the appropriate blood level.

Side effects of carbamazepine

The side effect of carbamazepine that worries most parents (and physicians) is a decrease in the white blood cells, which are responsible for fighting infection. The normal white blood cell count is in the range of 5000–8000 cells. Children (or adults) who are taking carbamazepine often have lower white cell counts, perhaps 3000–5000. In one in ten such children, this lowering of the white count is temporary; it persists in only 2 percent. Usually this persistent low white cell count is of no consequence, since the child is able to fight infections just as well as anyone else.

If your child has a low white count while on carbamazepine, don't panic. Sometimes your child's white count may be low from a viral infection. Your physician may want to repeat the count in five to seven days. If it has come back toward normal, the carbamazepine can be continued. If it has dropped further, the drug may need to be stopped temporarily. Stopping the drug suddenly may cause seizures to recur, so it should be tapered.

Aplastic anemia, in which the bone marrow stops producing blood cells, is a *very* rare but serious complication. We are aware of only a few reported cases in children. There appears to be no way to predict if a child will develop this condition. Frequent blood counts are expensive and painful and, besides, we have not found them useful.

Allergic side effects

As with other anticonvulsants, a *rash occurring within the first two to three weeks after starting carbamazepine may indicate a potentially serious situation and should always be checked out promptly by your physician,* who can then decide whether to discontinue the drug. Rare effects on the liver, bone marrow, and blood clotting cells (platelets) have also been reported.

Dose-related side effects

The signs of dose-related toxicity from carbamazepine are important, because they are briefly experienced by almost everyone who uses the drug. The first sign of mild toxicity is double vision, sometimes accompanied by blurred vision or dizziness, most likely to occur one to two hours after a dose, when the amount of the drug in the blood is at its highest. Such symptoms last one to two hours, until the blood level decreases, and do not constitute a serious side effect. If the symptoms are persistent and bothersome, your physician may want either to lower the dose or to spread out the medicine in more frequent, smaller doses.

More significant toxicity is displayed in unsteadiness, ataxia, sleepiness, or foggy thinking. These symptoms should be brought to the attention of your physician, who will want to check the blood level of the drug and perhaps change your child's dose. All of these symptoms disappear when the dosage is decreased or the drug is discontinued.

Because of carbamazepine's short half-life, physicians often recommend that it be taken three or even four times each day. We, and most patients, find that taking a drug this often is cumbersome and that doses are often forgotten. We prescribe the drug to be taken only twice a day. We tell the patient (or the parent) to observe carefully if seizures occur before the next dose. If they do, then we assume that the blood level dropped too low or that the time between doses is too long, and we change the schedule to three or, infrequently, four times a day.

The other reason why we may decide to give the drug more often than twice a day is a patient's experience of signs or symptoms of toxicity shortly after taking a dose. This indicates that we have given too much at one time, and again we will instruct the patient to take a smaller dose of the drug three times a day. We have found that the seizures of most children can be controlled if they take carbamazepine only twice a day. A new, slow-release formulation of carbamazepine, designed to be taken twice a day, has recently become available.

In children taking carbamazepine who are given erythromycin (an antibiotic often used in place of penicillin) for infection, high levels of carbamazepine and toxicity often develop. If your physician prescribes erythromycin, he may need to lower the dose of carbamazepine temporarily.

Valproic Acid (Depakene, Depakote)

Although useful in treating partial seizures and tonic-clonic seizures, valproic acid is particularly useful for treating absence seizures and partial complex seizures and, therefore, is discussed below.

Drugs for Absence and Other Generalized Seizures

Ethosuximide (Zarontin)

Ethosuximide is very effective in treating simple absence seizures but has no effect on partial seizures or on generalized tonic-clonic seizures.

Allergic side effects to ethosuximide include rashes, blood problems, and liver disease, but such complications are *very* infrequent. Dose-related toxicity is also uncommon, and the drug dose may be increased even when the blood level is well beyond the usual therapeutic range. Occasionally, hyperactivity and effects on learning have been noted at high blood levels, but the data are, so far, inadequate.

In general, ethosuximide seems to be well tolerated, safe, and effective, and it is our drug of choice for simple absence seizures.

Valproic Acid (Depakene, Depakote)

Valproic acid, a major anticonvulsant medication with a uniquely broad range of actions, is effective in tonic-clonic seizures as well as in absence seizures, complex partial seizures, and myoclonic seizures.

There is no universal agreement about how this drug should be used. Some physicians note that valproic acid has a very short half-life, and they therefore recommend using it three or four times a day. These same physicians recommend keeping the blood level above 90–100 micrograms/ml. We, and others, find this drug very different from the other anticonvulsants and believe that its effectiveness has little to do with the blood level. We find that it works better after the child has taken it for several weeks and that it continues to work for several weeks after the drug is stopped. If necessary for seizure control, we recommend increasing the dose up to a fixed amount based on the child's weight (30–60 mg/kg), virtually ignoring the blood level but watching for toxicity. Which of these two approaches is correct remains to be determined.

Allergic side effects of valproic acid

The most severe allergic reaction to valproic acid is a severe, sometimes fatal liver failure. Such a reaction, which usually occurs only in children, happens in one out of 800 children younger than two years of age, in one out of 7,000 children ages two to ten, and in fewer than one in 100,000 children older than ten. The risk is lower when valproic acid is the only drug used.

While valproic acid is, in general, a safe anticonvulsant drug, it should be used with great caution in children younger than two years of age, and then preferably as the only drug.

Valproic acid may also cause severe, persistent abdominal pain, accompanied by nausea and vomiting (pancreatitis). It may cause a decrease in the blood's clotting cells (platelets) and thus in the body's ability to form blood clots. Because frequent tests of blood counts, bloodclotting, and of liver function are expensive and painful and, in addition, will not predict whether your child will incur one of these problems tomorrow or next week, we do not perform them on a frequent or routine basis.

In general, we counsel parents that if their child is taking valproic acid and is ill for several days or has changes in behavior or school performance, they should ask their doctor if this could be due to the anticonvulsant.

We caution parents that if their child who is taking valproic acid has persistent vomiting, yellow skin (jaundice), darkened urine, easy bruising, or a tendency to bleed from cuts, they should contact their physician immediately.

In some children, valproic acid may cause an increase in the blood level of ammonia, leading to sleepiness, headache, nausea, or vomiting. Children with these symptoms should have a blood ammonia level test, and if the ammonia level is found to be elevated, the valproic acid dose should be decreased or the medication stopped.

Valproic acid itself rarely affects learning or behavior negatively. It seldom causes sleepiness. If these symptoms occur when the drug is started, they usually are a consequence of an increase in the level of some other drug the child is taking, particularly phenobarbital. Valproic acid increases the blood level of phenobarbital by 30 percent; thus, the dose of phenobarbital must be decreased by one-third when valproate is begun.

Depakene may be irritating to the stomach and cause nausea, vomiting, and a decrease in appetite. These symptoms decrease if the drug is taken along with meals. Depakote, a slightly different form of the drug, is said to have fewer effects on the stomach.

Weight gain, loss of appetite, and temporary loss of hair may also occur in some individuals who are taking valproic acid.

Although the list of side effects of valproate seems long, we repeat that it is an excellent anticonvulsant drug, and, if used properly, it is also very safe.

The Benzodiazepines (Diazepam, Clonazepam, Clorazepate, and Lorazepam)

Benzodiazepines are a class of anticonvulsant that includes a number of individual drugs. Diazepam (Valium) and lorazepam (Ativan) are commonly used to treat status epilepticus; clonazepam (Klonopin), clorazepate (Tranxene), diazepam (Valium), and lorazepam (Ativan) are also frequently used for long-term therapy. All of these drugs may be useful in absence seizures also, but they are most effective in myoclonic seizures, sometimes in drop attacks (atonic seizures), and also in complex partial seizures. Since these drugs generally cause sleepiness, irritability, and hyperactivity in young children, as well as personality changes in all ages, they tend to be used as "add-on drugs," that is, when other medications have not succeeded in controlling the seizures. Also, the brain often becomes tolerant of these drugs, so doses must continually be raised to maintain a beneficial effect.

Allergic and cosmetic side effects of the benzodiazepines are uncommon, but the other side effects greatly limit their usefulness.

"Not Approved for Use in Children"

New medications, and many old medications, are "not approved" for use in children. This does not mean that they do not work in children. It does not mean that they are more toxic in children. It merely means that they have not been tested in children. The Food and Drug Administration (FDA) approves the claims and cautions (printed on the package insert) made for drugs. In order for a drug company to claim usefulness and establish the indications for a particular antiepileptic drug, it must have demonstrated that the drug is effective in controlling seizures, and it must have proved the drug's lack of toxicity. Infants and children may metabolize drugs differently than adults do, and drugs therefore cannot be "approved" for use in children without appropriate testing in children. To establish the effectiveness of a new drug, it is usually tested against one type of seizure, most commonly partial complex seizures. Its effectiveness against other types of seizures, generalized tonic-clonic or myoclonic, is rarely tested before marketing. Therefore, the drug is not "indicated" for other types of seizures. In reality, a new anticonvulsant's toxicity and effectiveness are evaluated as the drug is used in practice. Felbatol, a drug that *was* tested in children and found effective and safe, when used more widely, was found to have major side effects. When your physician wants to use a drug that is "not approved" or "not indicated" for your child, you should ask in detail what is known about its use in children and its effectiveness for your child's seizure-type. Insurance companies and HMOs may not pay for medications that are not prescribed according to FDA indications. For children whose seizures have been difficult to control with current medications, it may be very useful to participate in one of the many studies of new drugs. That way, more drugs will perhaps be studied and approved for children.

New Antiepileptic Medications

In the past decade seven new anticonvulsants have been approved for the treatment of epilepsy. Some but not all have been studied in children. Extensive experience with these new medications will come only with extensive use. Past experience has taught us that "the latest, newest, safest" drug may have serious side effects. Although many drugs have been studied in children, and many of those drugs have been "approved" by the FDA for specific uses in children, their role in the treatment of the childhood epilepsies remains to be determined. Many children and adults with difficult-to-control seizures have benefited from these new medications, however.

Felbamate

USE WITH GREAT CAUTION

Felbamate was introduced in 1993 with great fanfare. It was the first new anticonvulsant in more than a decade and had been shown to be effective in a wide range of seizure-types, including partial seizures and the Lennox-Gastaut syndrome. It was heralded as a medication with few side effects. Nausea, weight loss, insomnia, and changes in behavior were occasionally sufficiently severe to discontinue the drug. One year later, reports of aplastic anemia and liver failure appeared, and most patients on the drug were taken off. This withdrawal was unfortunate, because the drug was of great benefit to some patients. At present, few patients are started on Felbamate.

Reports of the usefulness of Felbamate in treating the Lennox-Gastaut syndrome, partial complex seizures in children, juvenile myoclonic epilepsy (JME), and infantile spasms remain unconfirmed, because of the reported side effects. Aplsastic anemia appears to occur in one patient out of every 4,000 to 5,000 patients, and liver failure in less than half that number. Aplastic anemia has *not* been reported in children under fourteen years and seems to be more common in adults, in women, in those with autoimmune diseases, and in those with prior hematologic problems.

Blood counts and liver function tests should be monitored carefully.

Gabapentin (Neurontin)

Gabapentin is metabolized by the kidneys and excreted largely unchanged into the urine; it does not, therefore, affect the metabolism of other medications that are metabolized largely in the liver. Its advantage seems to be that it may be effective in partial seizures and that it does not interfere with other medications. The drug should be increased slowly (daily) to the maximum for your child's weight. Withdrawal of the medication should be done slowly, because of the risk of withdrawal seizures. Hyperactivity may occur and seems more common in children with prior behavioral problems.

The role of gabapentin in difficult-to-control seizures in children is unclear. Its mechanisms of action are unknown.

Lamotrigine (Lamictal)

Lamotrigine appears to be effective in the Lennox-Gastaut syndrome, and may be effective in treating many other types of seizures, as well. Its spectrum of usefulness seems to parallel that of valproate (valproic acid). Lamotrigine has been used primarily as an add-on drug, but it may be useful alone. Its major side effect is a rash, which occurs in up to 10 percent of individuals. The rash may proceed to the Stevens-Johnson syndrome (see p. 137). This rash appears most commonly when lamotrigine is added to Depakene or Depakote. A child who is receiving valproate must start lamotrigine very slowly; valproic acid markedly slows the metabolism of lamotrigine.

The drug should be stopped immediately if a rash appears!

Adverse effects include rash, ataxia, dizziness, diplopia (double vision), and hyperactivity. Apart from the rash and the need for a very slow increase in dosages to effective levels, this appears to be a useful new drug.

Topiramate (Topamax)

Topamax may be useful for difficult-to-treat partial and generalized seizures. It may be useful in the Lennox-Gastaut syndrome and in infantile spasms. Its mechanisms of action are unclear.

Side effects include headache, sleepiness, behavioral problems, psychomotor slowness, confusion, and weight loss. Kidney stones can be a problem.

Tiagabine (Gabitril)

Tiagabine selectively blocks the brain from scooping up GABA. GABA is a brain chemical that inhibits transmission of impulses between nerve cells and may decrease seizures (see Figure 1.2). Tiagabine therefore theoretically increases the GABA in the brain. It neither inhibits nor enhances the metabolism of other anticonvulsants.

Dosing in children starts low and is gradually adjusted upward depending on the clinical effect. There are several studies of tiagabine's effect on partial seizures in adult patients. There are currently no published studies of its effectiveness in children.

Side effects include dizziness, difficulty thinking, sleepiness, depression, and nervousness. Most were mild. Limited studies and the newness of the drug prohibit comments about its potential role in childhood epilepsy.

Levetiracetam (Keppra)

Levetiracetam was approved by the FDA in 2000 and, while widely used, it has not yet been approved for children. Its mechanism of action is unknown but appears different from that of other anticonvulsants. Side effects include sleepiness, irritability, and other behavioral changes. Interactions with other drugs appear limited.

Vigabatrin (Sabril)

Vigabatrin has not been released in the United States, nor is it approved for use in children. It is a novel drug which works by preventing the breakdown of GABA. The drug seems to have limited pharmacologic interactions. Its effects seem to last for several days. In adults it is effective against partial seizures, but it has little documented efficacy against other seizure-types. In children it is said to be very effective against infantile spasms, and it may have particular efficacy in children with infantile spasms due to tuberous sclerosis.

Loss of peripheral visual fields, optic atrophy, and peripheral retinal atrophy have been reported in 25–50 percent of adults. An opthalmologic exam should be conducted every three months in adults. The visual deficits do *not* disappear when the drug is discontinued.

The use of vigabatrin in young children with infantile spasms must be carefully monitored.

Tegretol Analogues (Carbatrol, Tegretol-XR, Oxycarbazepine [Trileptal])

Carbatrol and Tegretol-XR are new and different formulations of carbamazepine created to change the absorptive characteristics. The advantage of all of these new Tegretol analogues over Tegretol is said to be the ability to give the medication twice a day instead of more frequently. Since we usually give Tegretol twice each day, the advantage of the new medications is unclear. Their cost is equivalent to Tegretol's. Trileptal may have slightly different actions and side effects than carbamazepine.

Zonisamide (Zonegran)

Zonisamide was approved by the FDA in 2000 but has been used in Japan since 1989. It has multiple mechanisms of action and works against many seizure-types, some that are very difficult to control. Zonisamide is currently available only as a 100-mg capsule that is somewhat difficult to dissolve in water. Dosing is gradually adjusted upward. Side effects include drowsiness and nausea, and studies have reported psychosis, kidney stones, and decreased sweating.

How to Choose among the Many New Medications

We don't know how to choose among the many new medications, nor how to choose between the old, "first-line" medications and the newer drugs. We haven't had enough experience with the new drugs yet. It sometimes takes months or years to find the side effects of new medications. We prefer not to find them in our patients. As a team we tend to be very conservative, and we are third or fourth in line to try the new drugs in our children. When faced with a child with difficult-to-control seizures who has been tried on and failed most of the older medications, we choose the new medication which has been reported to have been effective in that type of seizure *and* has been seen to have the least-serious side effects.

Therefore we have little personal experience with: tiagabine (Gabitril), gabapentin (Neurontin), oxycarbazepine (Trileptal), and zonisamide (Zonegran), and virtually no experience with vigabatrin (Sabril).

A recent statistical analysis of the newer anticonvulsants by Dr. David Chadwick found that no one drug was superior to another in reducing seizures by 50 percent. He also found no significant difference in tolerability or side effects between them. Children and patients with generalized epilepsies were excluded from his analysis.

"Sylvia has failed every medication we've tried, or else she's had side effects—she's been too sleepy, or irritable. I thought that it was time to get another opinion from an epilepsy center. Can you help us?"

This story is so common that we would be remiss if we didn't put it in this book. Our response is, "Let's look at the problem carefully. We often find that the seizures started just two months ago. One medication was started and Sylvia became irritable and the physician, responding to the parent's complaint, discontinued the first drug and began a second. Three days later, while the first drug was at too low a level and the second had not yet achieved a therapeutic level, Sylvia had another seizure. Therefore the second drug was deemed a failure and yet a third was tried. We could go on with the story, but you get the idea.

What was wrong? Too many drugs used too rapidly. This was partially because the parent wanted "IT" fixed, pronto! And it was partly because the physician did not explain the proper use of the medications to the parent and acquiesced to the parent's demands.

Patience!! The most important ingredient in treating seizures is patience. Patience on the part of the parents and on the part of the physician.

It takes a week or sometimes longer to achieve stable blood levels with a new medication. If the medication must be increased slowly, then it may take even longer. It takes the body time to adjust to the medication and sometimes to change the metabolism of the drug. It then takes a week or longer, depending on the frequency of the seizures, to assess whether the drug is achieving seizure control. Therefore if you change drugs every two weeks, you never know if the medication was working or if you had even achieved a therapeutic level.

Medications should rarely be changed before two weeks and preferably not until a month has passed, unless there is a rash! Medications should be slowly increased to effectiveness (preferably until there are no seizures) or to toxicity, before adding another medication. Then, if possible, the first medication should be slowly withdrawn to allow the child to be on only one medication.

The most common mistake we see made by parents and by physicians is too many medications used in too low a dose and changed too rapidly.

Remember:

• One medication is always preferable to two. Multiple medications can increase the chance of cognitive side effects and can decrease the effectiveness of each drug.
• Two drugs may be necessary in an attempt to control the seizures of a child with difficult-to-control seizures. However, the physician should strive to discontinue the first medication after adding a second.
• Three simultaneous drugs are rarely necessary and are likely to produce substantial (if unrecognized) cognitive effects.
• Four simultaneous medications are too many!

Generic Drugs or Brand-Name Drugs?

Generic drugs are medications which are no longer under patent protection and so can be made by any manufacturer. Since each medication may be made slightly differently, the rate of absorption and metabolism for the same drug may differ depending on the manufacturer and even among batches from the same manufacturer. Thus, the blood level may vary. In a sensitive individual, small changes in blood level may either allow seizures or cause toxicity. Therefore, we strongly urge that children take the brand-name drug rather than the cheaper generic form, at least until the generic drugs become more standardized and consistent. We strongly urge that you always stick to the form made by the same manufacturer, and this can only be done by using the brand-name drug.

The choice of an antiepileptic drug must be individualized, taking into account the seizure-type and concerns about possible side effects in a particular child. The pharmacology of these medications is important, because it tells us how long we should expect to wait to see the impact of our therapy and how frequently the drug should be administered.

All medications have potential side effects, and parents should be familiar with the ones most commonly associated with the drug their child is taking. It is crucial to monitor the impact of therapy—to know whether seizures have been completely controlled and whether there are any unwanted side effects. It is always the response of the child that is important, not what the blood level is. Understandably, one-drug monotherapy is preferable to multidrug polytherapy, and a concerted attempt at seizure control with a single drug should be made before another drug is added. Most seizures in children can be controlled using this careful approach. After control of the seizures is achieved, the question will be how long the therapy should be continued.

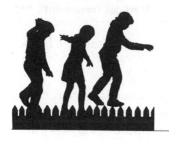

10. Status Epilepticus: A Medical Emergency

"Suppose the seizure lasts more than 30 minutes. Suppose the child has one seizure after another without waking up between them. What do I do then?"

Both long seizures and rapidly recurrent seizures are termed "status epilepticus." *Status epilepticus is a medical emergency!* How long is a long seizure? Some people define a long seizure as one lasting twenty minutes, some thirty minutes, some an hour. We would recommend not being too concerned about a tonic-clonic ("grand mal") seizure that lasts fewer than ten minutes. There is no evidence that even thirty minutes of generalized tonic-clonic movement does damage to the brain. Even an hour of tonic-clonic seizures is unlikely to do damage to the brain, but we would *not* recommend purposely allowing a seizure to continue that long.

There are actually two types of status. One is the status epilepticus that most people think about, *convulsive status,* in which the patient is having tonic-clonic, shaking seizures for this long period of time. A separate type, *nonconvulsive status,* is an episode when a patient has absence spells, staring spells, or periods of confusion lasting a half-hour, an hour, or (rarely) days. This nonconvulsive status is not life-threatening or brain-damaging but should be recognized and treated.

Convulsive Status Epilepticus and Its Treatment

Physicians are taught that a seizure lasting more than thirty minutes can do permanent damage to the brain. The medical literature says that as many as half of the patients with status epilepticus die or are left with permanent brain damage. But sometimes the things we think we know are not true!

Studies show that it is not the seizures but the *cause* of the seizures that does the brain damage. Status epilepticus can be a consequence of infection of the brain, such as meningitis or encephalitis. It can be a consequence of head trauma, brain tumors, or other serious causes. When status epilepticus is "symptomatic"—due to something serious—usually it is the "something serious" that does damage to the brain *and* causes the status epilepticus. It is this *symptomatic* status that may result in death or permanent brain damage. Whether the seizures themselves cause further damage is much less clear.

The first seizure a child experiences may result in status epilepticus and in that case is often the *only* seizure he ever has. Whether the patient's first seizure is status or a brief, generalized, tonic-clonic seizure, most children (70 percent) never have another episode. Although there are many different causes of status epilepticus, *in most children the cause remains unknown.* When status epilepticus is of unknown cause or is part of a seizure disorder, it rarely causes permanent brain damage.

There are many causes of status epilepticus; whatever the cause, it is important to stop the prolonged seizures as promptly as possible. It is also crucial to evaluate each child and each episode of status to identify any underlying cause that may require specific treatment.

The treatment of status epilepticus is a task for skilled physicians, not for parents. But we're sure that you would like to know what the physicians are doing and why. First, they will take your child into a special place in the emergency room to make sure that he is breathing properly. They may give him oxygen by mask, suction saliva out of the throat, and observe him for a few minutes to see the seizures. While they are observing, they will draw some blood to check for infection and to check for the level of blood sugar and other chemicals in the body that could be out of balance and causing seizures. If your child has previously had seizures and is taking medicine, the physicians will want to check the blood for the level of the anticonvulsants. They may also check for any drugs or medications taken accidentally. They will start an intravenous line (IV) to introduce fluids and so that they can give anticonvulsant medications into the vein if necessary. Intravenously is the best way to give medications when a child is continuing to have seizures, because it is the quickest way to get the medicine to the brain to stop the seizures. All of these things should take place in the first several minutes after arrival in the emergency room.

During this time the medical team also will take a brief history, searching for reasons for the status. They will be particularly concerned about any current illness, because meningitis or encephalitis, which could be a cause of the seizures, would require prompt treatment. The medical staff will want to know from you if the child has ever had seizures before, if there possibly has been an injury to the head, and things like that. Anything that you can think of that might have led the child to have a seizure *at this particular time* may be of help to the physicians.

If the seizures have been continuing more than ten minutes, the physicians will want to give medication to stop them. Various medications may be used, but drugs like diazepam (Valium) or lorazepam (Ativan), quick-acting effective anticonvulsants, are used initially. Unfortunately, although they work quickly, they often do not continue to work over a long period of time, and when they wear off—in ten to twenty minutes in the case of diazepam, or longer in the case of lorazepam—another seizure may occur. Therefore, the physician usually will give an additional drug, such as phenytoin (Dilantin), which works less quickly than the other but lasts longer, or phosphenytoin, its less irritating cousin.

If this status epilepticus is the child's first seizure, then the doctors will probably want to do a lumbar puncture (spinal tap) to look for infection. They will study the blood for possible chemical changes and, perhaps, do an EEG then or the next day. They may even do a CT scan.

If the child has had other seizures or has epilepsy, then looking for a cause of the status may be slightly less important.

The most common cause of status epilepticus in a person who has previously had seizures is that the level of medication in the blood is too low. This may be because the child is not taking his medication, or it has been forgotten, or an interaction with some other medication has lowered the level. Substitution of a generic drug that is less well absorbed may also result in status epilepticus.

It appears that children whose first seizure lasts a long time fall into two groups. Three-fourths of first seizures last less than four minutes. The other quarter last an average of more than thirty minutes. It appears that if a seizure lasts longer than ten minutes it should be treated with medication to prevent its going on for the longer time. Children who have had a long seizure the first time are more likely to have a long seizure if they have a second one. Therefore, if your child had a seizure lasting more than ten minutes the first time, it might be advisable to have rectal diazepam (Diastat) available, in case another seizure occurs *and* lasts more than ten minutes. Lorazepam (Ativan) given beneath the tongue is also a good treatment.

In almost all instances, the status epilepticus can be controlled within one-half hour to one hour from the time the child arrives in the emergency room and treatment is started. Only in an unusual situation, when there is an acute process occurring in the brain, such as infection or damage from a head injury, do seizures continue and prove difficult to control. Treatment of severe prolonged status epilepticus can be enormously challenging for the physician, requiring large doses of medication given in an intensive care unit. Sometimes general anesthesia is required to stop the seizures.

The outcome of status epilepticus, even in these severe episodes, depends more on the cause than on the duration of the seizures. Rest assured that most children who experience status epilepticus recover and are just as normal as they were before the seizures. It appears to be very, very rare for children who have status without a known cause to suffer any permanent damage, even from prolonged seizures.

Nonconvulsive Status Epilepticus and Its Treatment

Just as there are many types of seizures, so there are diverse types of status epilepticus. Since these other types do not involve shaking, they are called nonconvulsive status epilepticus.

A child with "petit mal" seizures or absence seizures may just stop and stare and be unaware of his environment for brief episodes, lasting from a few seconds to a minute or two. On *rare* occasions, these absence seizures may continue for a long time—thirty minutes, an hour, occasionally even a day or two. This type of status is much harder to detect, since there is no shaking. The child may seem confused, or dull, or just quite different from his or her usual state. Sometimes there is confusion and the child seems lost, wandering around, unable to answer. On other occasions, a child acts as if his IQ had suddenly decreased twenty or thirty points. He or she may be able to answer you, but not with usual quickness or alertness. The child may appear dull or just different. While there are many possible causes for this change, one cause could be that the child is in nonconvulsive status.

In addition to this suddenly altered state, the child may have brief eye blinks or staring or repetitive movements, but the only thing that may be different is that the child is not his usual self. When this state lasts for hours, when it is clear to you that something has suddenly changed, your physician should be consulted. The change could be due to medication or illness, it could be the effect of other drugs, it could be a different kind of illness, but *it could be nonconvulsive status.* How can you tell? The answer is, you can't. Even the physician can't necessarily tell from just looking at the child.

An EEG done during the episode is the only *certain* way to establish this nonconvulsive status diagnosis. The EEG usually shows constant spike-wave abnormalities that clearly interfere with cortical function, with thinking. If the EEG confirms the "spike-wave stupor" or nonconvulsive status, then the physician can give small amounts of medication (diazepam) in the vein; this will usually stop the brain wave abnormality abruptly and allow the child to return to normal.

❑ **Joanne was a bright, sparkly second grader when we first met her. She was referred because of a "weird" episode the previous week. One day in school, she quite suddenly did not seem herself. She was quiet, wandered about the class, and responded inappropriately to the teacher. Her mother took her home, and after another hour or two, when she still wasn't herself, she had been taken to the hospital. No cause for the sudden change was found, but the next morning an EEG showed slowing, as if she might have previously had a seizure.**

When we saw her the following week, she was fine and back to her usual self. Since she had never had seizures and was otherwise normal, we asked her mother to bring her back during another episode, should one occur.

It was almost a year later when we received a call from Joanne's mother in the middle of the day. "She is doing it again." We didn't remember Joanne, but we told her mother to bring her in immediately. A very attractive, dull ten-year-old came into the office. She could answer questions and count, but seemed to be mildly retarded. If her mother had not insisted that this was not Joanne's usual state, and if our records had not confirmed a previously sparkling young lady, we might have been fooled.

An immediate EEG confirmed "spike-wave stupor," a continuous electrical status on the EEG, and after a small dose of diazepam (Valium), she immediately returned to her usual state. When she was admitted from the EEG lab to the ward,

the resident wanted to know why we were admitting this perfectly normal, charming young lady. With anticonvulsant medication, she has never had another episode.

❑ For two years, Jamil, age four, had had a multitude of seizures of various types, drop attacks, generalized tonic-clonic seizures, and complex partial seizures. None of the multiple medications had been of benefit, and he was developmentally delayed. He was started on the ketogenic diet (see Chapter 12). On the diet his seizures came under complete control, his speech and demeanor improved, and he became a normal five-year-old. After two seizure-free years on the diet, we tapered him off and he continued to do well, having no seizures for the next year. Then his sister first noted some mild staring spells. "I think he's doing it again," she told her parents. When he had two generalized seizures he was brought back to see us, and the EEG showed spike-wave abnormalities. Jamil was restarted on the diet at home and after one day of fasting the parents noted that his speech had improved. Three days later he had more ability to focus. He had no more staring spells or seizures. The EEG returned to normal and the parents stated that they hadn't realized that his speech and behavior had gotten so bad until they saw the dramatic improvement. Jamil had been in nonconvulsive status for months and despite his history of seizures, no one had recognized it until he had two big seizures and an EEG was obtained.

Nonconvulsive status epilepticus can be subtle, long-lasting, and difficult to detect without an EEG. Only a very careful history of an unexplained change in function or behavior can lead the physician to suspect nonconvulsive status and to obtain an EEG. The physician should maintain a high index of suspicion that such changes in behavior could be electrical in nature and thus easily treatable.

There is no evidence that spike-wave stupor causes permanent damage to the brain, even when it goes on for hours or days. However, it clearly disrupts the child's level of function. Spike-wave stupor can easily be treated, but it is far better to prevent these seizures with continued use of an appropriate anticonvulsant medication.

Although many myths and fears still persist about status epilepticus, with early recognition and appropriate treatment, children who have an episode of status should return to their previous function and have no residual effects.

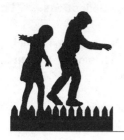

11. The Outlook for the Child with Seizures

Once upon a time it was believed that epilepsy was forever. In those olden days, only twenty to twenty-five years ago, physicians were taught never to discontinue anticonvulsant medicine. They were taught in particular not to discontinue the drugs before puberty, because seizures might increase in frequency at puberty, and you were never sure when puberty might start or when it would end. After puberty came driving, and you wouldn't want to stop medication before that, because the child might never be able to get a driver's license. Then physicians were urged not to discontinue medication because the individual was driving. In those days, it was said: "Eventually people will stop taking medicine on their own. Then, if they have a seizure, it will not be the doctor's fault."

None of those old teachings was true!

Under this old philosophy, many people were kept on medicine for many years, and some are still taking it.

Now we know that

• Seventy-five percent of children who have been seizure-free for four years will remain seizure-free as medication is slowly withdrawn.
• Seventy-five percent of children who have been seizure-free for only two years will remain seizure-free as medication is slowly withdrawn.

• Some children can be taken off medication after only one year seizure-free.
• For most people epilepsy is *not* a lifelong disorder.
• For most children epilepsy is a benign disorder. Most of them will outgrow their epilepsy.

Therefore, your child can probably look forward to being seizure-free and medication-free.

Unfortunately, this is not true for all children. Roughly 70 percent of children who have a single seizure will *never* have another. Roughly 75 percent of children who have two seizures (the definition of epilepsy) will have them controlled with medicine and become seizure-free also. Can we predict which children will have difficult-to-control seizures and which will have "benign" epilepsy? To a large extent we can.

❏ "Ellie had her first seizure last evening, Doctor. It was the worst thing I ever saw. I thought she was going to die, or swallow her tongue. I called 911, and they took her to the emergency room. After a whole bunch of tests the doctors said it was nothing to worry about. They said she didn't even need treatment. They said she might not have any more seizures, but that even if she did have more she would be fine. What do you think, Doctor? You're an epilepsy expert. Shouldn't she be on medication?"

What Is the Outlook after a First Seizure?

Many children who come in with a first generalized tonic-clonic seizure have had seizures before, but they were not recognized as such. Some will have had staring spells that were thought to have been daydreaming, or they will have had jerks early in the morning which were thought to be "normal." Some will have had episodes of jerking of the face which the family thought to be tics. All of these may really have been unrecognized seizures, and the tonic-clonic seizure that brought them to the emergency room was really not their first seizure; it was the first *recognized* seizure. The child has "newly recognized epilepsy," not a first seizure. The distinction may be important and affect the outlook. A careful history is critical to making the distinction.

Risk of Recurrence		

First nonfebrile seizure	Chance of 2nd seizure	Chance of further recurrence
	Within 1 yr. 29%	3rd seizure 72%
	Within 2 yrs. 37%	4th seizure 58%
	Within 5 yrs. 43%	10+ seizures 29%
	Within 10 yrs. 46%	
	In lifetime 50%	

Factors that increase risk

- Neurologic problems (mental retardation, cerebral palsy, autism)
- Abnormal EEG, CT, or MRI
- Prior febrile seizures
- Occurrence during sleep

Other factors

- A long first seizure does not increase the chance of a recurrence, but, if there is a recurrence, then the second seizure may also be prolonged.
- Todd's paralysis increases the likelihood of multiple further seizures.
- Two or more seizures on one day are considered a "flurry" of seizures and count as a single episode.
- Medication decreases the risk of a second or further seizures, but it is not guaranteed to prevent them.

After a true first seizure, 30 percent of people will have a second seizure and half of these will occur within six months of the first. Eighty percent of second seizures will occur within two years of the first. Although a person who has had a seizure has a lower threshold and a higher chance of having another seizure at some time in their life, most will not develop epilepsy.

Children who have neurologic problems such as mental retardation, cerebral palsy, or autism have a higher probability of having more seizures. If the child's EEG is abnormal, or if she has abnormalities on the CT scan or MRI scan, then she has a greater chance of having more seizures. If the first seizure was long, twenty to thirty minutes, the child has no greater chance of having more seizures, but if he does have another it is more likely to be long also. If your child had a long first seizure, you may want to ask your physician about having some medication at home to use if the child has another seizure. Although anticonvulsant medication given after a first seizure *does not prevent* epilepsy, it will decrease the probability of another seizure by approximately 50 percent. However, medication alters only the short-term outlook of a child who has had a single seizure.

Most physicians now do not start a child on medication after a first seizure unless there are very special circumstances.

What Is the Outlook after a Second Seizure?

For most children the outlook (prognosis) is good. Although, as is shown in Figure 11.1, almost three-fourths of children who have two seizures will have a third, only 30 percent of those who have two will have 10 or more seizures. A Todd's paralysis (weakness on one side of the body after a focal seizure) and neurologic deficits are predictors of ten or more seizures.

Roughly 10 percent of children who have two seizures will go on to have intractable epilepsy. *Intractable* seizures (or what we would term "difficult-to-control") are those which fail to respond to two medications and occur more than once per month.

Children with benign rolandic epilepsy, or childhood absence (petit mal) seizures, have a good prognosis. Those whose seizures are symptomatic (associated with pre-existing prior brain damage or dysfunction), or cryptogenic (whose cause is unknown but presumed to be pre-existing), have a worse prognosis than those whose seizures are idiopathic (of unknown cause and occurring in an otherwise normal person).

The factors most predictive of difficult-to-control seizures are:

• symptomatic or cryptogenic seizures
• Early seizure frequency (the greater the frequency, the more difficult to control)
• Focal slowing on the EEG, indicative of a focal brain abnormality

Children with myoclonic seizures, atonic seizures, and neonatal seizures are most likely to develop difficult-to-control epilepsy. Children with a few seizures scattered over a year are likely to come under control, whereas children with the same number of seizures scattered over weeks or a month are more likely to have difficult-to-control epilepsy.

These children whose seizures are more likely to become difficult to control perhaps need even more vigorous treatment with the newer anticonvulsants, with the vagus nerve stimulator, or with the ketogenic diet.

Questions You May Have

"What is the chance of my child coming off medicine and staying seizure-free?"

After being free of seizures, on medication, for two years,

• those children who have had idiopathic seizures, and who have no evidence of neurologic dysfunction, and whose EEG is normal or near normal have a 90 to 95 percent chance of remaining seizure-free without medication;
• those children who have had epilepsy caused by old and nonprogressive brain damage, such as a birth injury or head trauma, have a 40 to 60 percent chance of staying seizure-free off medication, even if their EEGs are moderately abnormal;
• those children whose EEGs are severely abnormal, and, particularly, if their EEGs are worse than when their seizures began, have a 90 to 95 percent chance of having *more* seizures if medicine is discontinued—even if they have been free of seizures for two years on medicine.

These scenarios represent points on a spectrum. How then does someone decide whether or not medication should be discontinued? Here we have to go back to our risk-benefit analysis (see Chapter 5). Remember that the risks are yours and your child's, as are the benefits. Thus, you both have to be full partners with your physician as these decisions are made.

Your child can *gradually* stop taking medicine whenever you both are willing to accept the risks of another seizure. As we said, the risks vary with the cause of the seizures and the normality of the EEG. But also remember the consequences of another seizure. These consequences vary with the age and the ability or disability of the child. A seizure once the child is driving can be both emotionally and physically devastating. If medication can be stopped one year before driving, life becomes much easier.

"What is the worst that can happen if my child continues taking the medication?"

If your child has been free of seizures for two years and is tolerating his medication well, then probably not much will happen if he continues to take medication. However, if he continues to take medicines for a long time, chronic effects can occur that vary with the medicine. In addition, if your child is a girl, eventually she may want to have children. While the risks of any medication on the fetus are small, they are many times greater than if she were taking no medication at all. If a woman doesn't need medication to control seizures, the baby will be better off not being exposed to these drugs. Also, you'll never know how much better your child will function without medication unless your physician discontinues it.

"What is the worst that can happen if we decide to discontinue my child's medicine?"

Medication should never be stopped suddenly, since this could cause status epilepticus. It should only be stopped under your physician's direction. When the medication is decreased slowly over four to six weeks, the worst thing that can happen is that your child will have another seizure. The consequences of another seizure vary with the individual's age and circumstances. You and your child will have to determine how much weight to give this matter. When people's medication is discontinued, they tend to worry about having another seizure. In our experience, this concern diminishes over time and is usually negligible after about a year.

"What is the best that can happen if my child continues taking the medication?"

The best that can happen if medication is continued is that your child will be no worse off than he is now. He may also not be as fearful if he is taking medication, even though he is constantly reminded that another seizure may recur. But, unless he takes medication forever, at some time in his life he will need to face this worry. If the decision is to stop medication, you and he should choose the time at which this concern will have the least impact. For example: you might want to discontinue medication at a convenient time during the summer when school is out.

"What is the best that can happen if my doctor discontinues my child's medication?"

The best that can happen is that your child will remain seizure-free and that there will be an improvement in his learning and behavior. Many adults who have had their seizure medication stopped say, "I'm not so tired any more. I feel so much better. I can think much more clearly." Many parents say, "Mary is a different child. Her school work is better. She's not so irritable and she's not so tired all the time. I never realized the medicine was affecting her in that way." Another benefit is that your child would not have to take medication each day, a reminder of his potential problem. He would no longer have "controlled" epilepsy. Now he would be either "recovered" or "cured" and could get on with his life, unimpeded.

For the normal child who has only a 5 to 10 percent chance of having another seizure, we would recommend discontinuing medication. In general, the consequences, should a seizure recur, will be small. For the child with handicaps who may have a 50 percent chance of another seizure, we would also recommend trying to discontinue medication. The consequences of another seizure for him are also small, but since he may be less able to compensate for the subtle effects of medication on learning and behavior, the benefits of being free of medication may be even greater. Should a seizure recur, and if it is apparent that the child is functioning better off the original medication, it may be possible to substitute a less toxic anticonvulsant.

On balance, we believe that avoiding the chronic effects of medication and their effects on learning and psychological function outweigh the risks of another seizure in most children who have been seizure-free for two years.

"Can't we wait until she's older and less vulnerable to discontinue the drug? She's still just a little girl."

Sure. No problem. But soon she'll be driving, and it will be hard to give that up for a period of time when she discontinues medication.

Won't you be afraid to let her drive after stopping the drugs and before you know that she'll be seizure-free? Then she'll be off to college and not under your watchful eye. Is that a better time to discontinue medicines? You could defer it until she finishes college and gets a job. Or maybe wait until she's married and then her husband can keep an eye on her. You wouldn't want her on medications when she's planning her pregnancy, would you?

In short, there is no good time to discontinue medications, but when a child has been seizure-free and is not yet driving would seem to be the easiest time to try discontinuing medicines. There may be other fringe benefits to discontinuing medications, in terms of cost savings, insurance, and perhaps even in terms of jobs that may be open to your child. But these are less important than trying to put the epilepsy in the past.

"Are there situations in which you would discourage someone from discontinuing medicine?"

Yes. We would recommend continuing medication for the child whose EEG is severely abnormal, where the chance of recurrence is very high, although if the child and parent were determined to try to discontinue medication we would be supportive. In some of the special forms of epilepsy, such as the juvenile myoclonic epilepsy of Janz, or the Lennox-Gastaut syndrome (Chapter 8), where the chance of recurrence of seizures is very high, we would suggest continuing medicine. In each case we would make an individual decision, discuss the risks and benefits of alternative courses of action with the parent and child, and help them to reach a sound decision.

"If we stop the medicine, how long will we have to worry about the seizures coming back?"

Most recurrences happen shortly after the medication is stopped, indeed, many while the medicine is being tapered. One-half of the recurrences happen within six months of stopping medication, 60 to 80 percent occur within one year, and virtually all within two years of stopping the medicine. This is another reason why, if possible, it would be better to discontinue medicine before or during the early teenage years, because the consequence of a seizure would be less severe before the individual has begun to drive or has a job.

In summary, most epilepsy in children is not forever. Therefore, treatment for most children should not be forever. Decisions about discontinuing medication can begin to be made when the child approaches being seizure-free for two years. You should discuss the risks and benefits of continuing medication and of stopping medication with your physician.

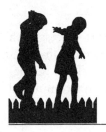

12. The Ketogenic Diet

History of the Diet

The ketogenic diet is one of the oldest forms of treatment for epilepsy. While recommendations for fasting are found in biblical and medieval writings, this special diet was devised in the 1920s when there were few effective treatments for epilepsy. The ketogenic diet is high in fat, adequate in protein, and has negligible amounts of carbohydrate. It was created to simulate some of the metabolic effects of fasting, a state known to decrease seizures in some individuals.

It has been known for centuries that fasting ameliorates seizures. In the early 1900s, a boy in New York who was experiencing uncontrollable seizures was taken by his desperate parents to Hugh Conklin, an osteopath, faith healer, and disciple of the well-known faith healer Bernarr McFadden. Conklin recommended prayer and ten to twenty days of fasting, as well as osteopathic treatments. When they prayed and fasted with this child, his seizures improved. Experience demonstrated that prayer alone was insufficient. Others confirmed the benefits of fasting for seizure control. In order to search for the mechanism by which this improvement occurred, the boy's father, a lawyer, made a generous donation to the newly established Department of Pediatrics at the Johns Hopkins University School of Medicine, which was being directed by his brother, John Howland. At the time, Howland was initiating studies of metabolism in young children. Together with his younger colleague, James Gamble, he began studies of the metabolic effects of fasting in children with epilepsy.

Simultaneously, researchers elsewhere began to report success with fasting as a treatment for epilepsy. Physicians at the Mayo Clinic devised a diet that would "simulate the effects of fasting." This diet derived about 90 percent of its calories from fats; it contained minimal protein and virtually no carbohydrate. This diet remains the basis of today's ketogenic diet.

In the absence of glucose (sugar), muscle protein and fat cannot be completely "burned" and leave a residual "ash" in the body in the form of ketone bodies, which are washed out in the urine. Protein that is burned leaves uric acid, which also appears in the urine. At the time, it was believed, erroneously, that the presence or absence of uric acid held the key to the seizure control. When a fast was broken by eating glucose or protein, the uric acid in the urine disappeared. If the fast was broken by eating fat, the uric acid excretion was maintained. A diet was developed that was high in fat and had just enough protein for growth and as little carbohydrate as possible. This was termed the *ketogenic diet* because it caused a continuous excretion of ketones in the urine. (Ketones also account for the "sweetish" smell of the breath of children who are on the diet.)

Today we know that it is not the uric acid in the urine that accounts for the effectiveness of the diet. However, the ketones in the urine are a good index of the degree of metabolic change that has occurred. But the excretion of ketones, while necessary, is not alone sufficient to document the anticonvulsant effectiveness of the diet. *In 2002 we still do not know how the ketogenic diet works.*

Since the only available effective medications in the early 1900s were phenobarbital and bromides, which failed to control many individuals' seizures and both of which posed major toxicity problems, the ketogenic diet came to be widely used—with substantial success. In a number of reports from the Mayo Clinic, from New York Hospital, and from Johns Hopkins in the 1920s and '30s, it seemed that 20 to 40 percent of children with difficult-to-control seizures had their seizures completely controlled by the diet. An additional 30 percent experienced a substantial decrease in the frequency of their seizures, and 25 to 40 percent did not benefit.

However, even then, physicians looked askance at this highly restrictive diet, which they considered unpalatable. Their most favorable comments were often "Yuk!" or "What normal school-age child would stick to a diet like that?" In 1939 the first highly effective anticonvulsant, Dilantin (phenytoin), was discovered. Clearly it was far easier to take pills than to stick to a rigid diet. Gradually, during the 1940s and '50s, other anticonvulsants were discovered, fewer children were placed on the diet, and the diet was used less and less.

At Johns Hopkins Hospital during the 1940s and 1950s, the diet continued to be used, under the leadership of Dr. Samuel Livingston, one of the pioneers in pediatric epilepsy and one of the doctors who prescribed the diet extensively. The supervising dietician for the diet, Millicent Kelly, remained at Hopkins after Dr. Livingston retired, and the hospital continued to start eight to ten children a year on the diet. It was one of the few institutions using the diet at that time.

In the 1960s a modified form of the diet using medium-chain triglycerides (MCT oil) was developed. It had the alleged advantage of allowing more protein and carbohydrate in the diet and therefore "greater variety" in the meals. Dieticians and physicians used this diet in place of the older, "classic," ketogenic diet. As new anticonvulsants became available, few in the medical profession, and even fewer dieticians, retained or gained experience with either form of the ketogenic diet. Often, those who used the diet miscalculated it, because of their lack of experience, and as a result it was not effective. Therefore, the use of the diet, even at Johns Hopkins, gradually withered away. That is, until October 1994.

In the fall of 1994, Charlie Abrahams, the two-year-old son of a Hollywood producer, was brought to us with intractable seizures. His father, Jim Abrahams, had read about the diet in the first edition of this book and wanted to start Charlie on it. Charlie's seizures were quickly controlled and, freed from medicine and the effects of the seizures, Charlie started to blossom. He is now a normal young man, free of seizures. Mr. Abrahams felt compelled to inform other parents about the diet as an alternative to medication, and so he made a videotape, which is available from the Charlie Foundation (address given below). After a segment about Charlie appeared on a television program, the demand for the ketogenic diet was rekindled!

What Is the Ketogenic Diet?

The ketogenic diet is a carefully calculated diet that should be initiated only under the supervision of a physician familiar with it and a dietician experienced with the calculation of the classic ketogenic diet and with the subtleties of adjustment needed for each individual.

Remember:

• The ketogenic diet is a medical therapy, not a fad diet.
• The ketogenic diet is not something that you can do on your own.

This is not the place to discuss the ketogenic diet in great detail. There are two principal sources of information: First, the videotape for parents, "The Ketogenic Diet," which discusses the diet in parents' own words and those of older children on the diet, can be obtained from the Charlie Foundation, 1223 Wilshire Boulevard, Box 815, Santa Monica, California 90403. Enclose a check for $10 made out to The Charlie Foundation. Second, a book has been written for parents, describing how the diet is done. It is *The Ketogenic Diet: A Treatment for Epilepsy,* by John M. Freeman, Millicent T. Kelly, and Jennifer B. Freeman, and is in its third edition. A copy can be obtained at many bookstores or from Demos Publications, 386 Park Avenue South, New York, New York 10016 (tel. 800-532-8663). Before we begin a child on the diet, we require the parents to watch this videotape and read this book.

Other sources of information include a videotape made for dieticians about how to calculate the diet. This, too, can be obtained from the Charlie Foundation, for a small fee. A physician's prescription is required to obtain the tape.

Choosing and Managing the Diet

The ketogenic diet contains a high ratio of fat to carbohydrate and protein. Most of the calories are provided as fats, using butter and heavy cream. Seizure control is greatest when the diet contains a ratio of fat calories to protein/carbohydrate calories of 3 or 4:1. A typical meal might consist of a very small portion of meat, fish, poultry, or cheese, a slightly larger portion of fruit, additional fat served as butter or mayonnaise, and a serving of heavy (whipping type) cream. It doesn't sound very palatable, does it? It is this perception of the diet as unappealing that has interfered with its more frequent use.

When your child is severely handicapped by seizures and massive amounts of medication, what do you have to lose by trying the diet? Not much! What do you have to gain? If it works, a lot. If it doesn't, you've lost very little other than the time invested in learning how to prepare the diet. If your child is seizure-free and less drugged, then the rigors of the diet are worthwhile. If the child's seizures continue after one to three months on the diet or if the diet is poorly tolerated, then the diet can be discontinued and the child returned to medication.

The diet is initiated with 36 to 48 hours of starvation and limited fluid intake. During this time, the child should be observed closely, in the hospital, for signs of hypoglycemia (low blood sugar)—paleness, sweatiness, unresponsiveness, or seizures. Too much ketosis or acidosis can also occur, characterized by vomiting or heavy breathing. The blood chemistries can confirm this excessive acidosis, and small amounts of orange juice will allow the child to regain balance.

After the two days of fasting the child is given one-third of the diet for 24 hours then two-thirds the next day. We usually give this as an eggnog because it is easier for hospital dieticians to measure and prepare. The eggnog can be diluted and served as a milkshake, it can be frozen and served as ice cream, or it can be microwaved and served as "scrambled eggs." After three meals of the two-thirds diet the last two meals are served as the full diet.

We usually initiate the diet in the hospital so we can carefully observe the child during the starvation and so we can instruct the parent in diet preparation and in how to avoid extraneous carbohydrates. Menus can be created to fit most children's food preferences. It is surprising how much variety a creative and innovative parent can introduce into this restricted diet.

WARNING: The diet should not be attempted on your own. The diet will only work when it, and you, are carefully supervised by a dietician familiar with using the diet. The diet may be dangerous if not done properly.

WARNING: The diet is deficient in vitamins B and C as well as in calcium and these must be given as supplements in a sugar-free form.

Also, remember that today many things like toothpaste, vitamins, and children's antibiotics and cough syrups have added glucose. If your child is on the ketogenic diet, you must read every label carefully and, if in doubt about added sugar, check with your physician, the dietician, or the manufacturer.

Small deviations in the diet can result in loss of ketosis and a seizure. Indeed, if a child has been well controlled on the diet and has a seizure, you can almost be sure that the child has eaten a cookie, a piece of candy, or a bit of dog food. (Yes, small children can get into the dog food!) Should this happen, a day of starvation followed by reinstitution of the diet usually will reachieve control.

The diet is not for all children with epilepsy. Indeed, for most children it is far easier to take a few pills each day. Most children will have their seizures easily controlled with medication. However, when anticonvulsants are ineffective or their side effects are overwhelming, the ketogenic diet can often control seizures with few if any adverse effects on behavior or learning.

You do not have to try all of the new medications before trying the ketogenic diet. Children with difficult-to-control seizures (see Chapter 8) who do not respond to the first medication, properly used, may have only a 10–20 percent chance of responding to any other medication. The ketogenic diet might be considered early in that child's course. This is particularly true of children with the Lennox-Gastaut syndrome.

The diet is cumbersome, particularly at first. It requires careful weighing and measuring of food. It also requires strict compliance: sometimes a few extra nuts or a piece of a cookie can allow seizures to break through. For older children, teens in particular, this may be a very difficult diet to adhere to. There is little experience with the diet in adults. We have prescribed the diet for children under the age of one year, where it can replace breast milk or formula.

At the present time we are willing to try the diet in children who have difficult-to-control seizures and have not responded to at least two anticonvulsant drugs. We have even successfully used the diet in children who would appear to be candidates for focal epilepsy surgery. We do not know what limitations might be put on use of the diet in the future, but these are our current restrictions.

Our success rates in patients who are chosen using these restrictions remain about the same as has been reported from many centers over the past sixty years. Table 12.1 reports outcomes for a group of 150 children placed on the diet at Johns Hopkins.

The 150 children studied at Hopkins averaged 410 seizures per month at the time of initiation of the ketogenic diet. They had, on average, failed to have their seizures controlled by more than six medications. One year later, approximately half of the children were still on the diet. Almost 27 percent had a substantial (greater than 90 percent) decrease in their seizures. Four years later, most of the same children had discontinued the diet. Twenty-seven percent had a greater than 90 percent decrease in their seizures, and most had discontinued medications.

Roughly 30 to 40 percent of patients find that, after giving the diet a good try for one month or more, it is not sufficiently effective to con-

Table 12.1 Outcomes of Children on the Ketogenic Diet

Length of time after starting diet	Number remaining on diet	Seizure status			
		Seizure-free	90–99% improved	50–90% improved	<50% improved
12 months	83 (55%)	11/150 (7%)	30/150 (20%)	33/150 (22%)	9/150 (6%)
More than 48 months	15 (10%)	20/150 (13%) 0 on diet	21/150 (14%) 7 on diet	24/150 (16%) 7 on diet	18/150 (12%) 1 on diet

Notes: N = 150. At initiation of the diet, patients averaged 410 seizures per month.

tinue, and they return to trying medications or surgery. However, even unsuccessful patients are glad that they made the effort.

A few patient stories may help to show the range of children who have tried the diet.

☐ Victor was four years old, the youngest in a large Italian family. His seizures had begun at two. This previously bright-eyed "devil" had become dull and severely handicapped by frequent drop seizures and by tonic seizures. His family finally forced him to use a helmet to avoid injury to his mouth and face. Unresponsive to several medications, Victor was referred to us for further therapy. We recommended the ketogenic diet and started to explain what this meant. His father said, "No way! What would we do on Sunday when the family gathers for dinner? Do you think Victor is going to eat whipped cream while the rest of the kids are digging into their pasta? Grandma would cry if he didn't eat her cookies. Don't you have any other medicines?"

The dialogue continued over the next year as we tried various combinations of medicines and Victor's seizures were unchanged. Finally, having run out of options, the family agreed to try the diet. Victor's seizures were gone within two weeks and his helmet in less than a month. His medications were withdrawn over the next few months. Amazingly, family dinners continued. His grandparents stopped trying to stuff him with pasta and his cousins understood that he was on a "special diet." Everyone was delighted to have Victor back and not to have to worry that he was going to fall and hurt himself.

What do they have to say now about the diet? "No problem, we wish we'd started it earlier!"

For children with drop seizures, the ketogenic diet seems to be the most effective form of therapy. Medications such as valproate, felbamate, lamotrigine, benzodiazepines, and vigabatrine are easier to administer, but they are frequently ineffective and have major side effects. The ketogenic diet may avoid all of those problems.

❑ Sarah had severe developmental abnormalities of her brain. She had trouble breathing at birth and was placed on a respirator. She couldn't swallow and had a tube inserted into her stomach. She was unable to see, hear, or respond to her parents. The only thing she was able to do was seize, and this she did hundreds of times a day. Medicines were of little benefit and seemed to make her irritable. We first met Sarah when she was one year old and hospitalized for one of her periodic aspiration pneumonias. Mom had heard of the ketogenic diet in her local support group and asked if it might be appropriate for Sarah.

We pointed out Sarah's severe brain damage and that we could not make that better but said that perhaps the diet might control her seizures and allow her to be on less medication. Her mom asked us to go ahead with the diet.

Starting the diet for Sarah was easy. We merely switched her tube feeding from a standard formula to a ketogenic formula. Over the next several weeks her seizures began to decrease in frequency. Over the next year she was able to discontinue medications and her seizures were reduced to one or two jerks per day. Sarah's development improved slightly. Her mother says that she now responds when they talk to her; she is less irritable and more fun to be with. It is hard to measure any improvement in Sarah's quality of life, but her mom is delighted with the changes and is confident enough to have started to work outside the home on a part-time basis. She attributes the dramatic change in the family's quality of life to the ketogenic diet.

Sometimes it's not just the decrease in seizures that is the benefit of the diet. Sometimes it may be the decrease in medicines. When dealing with profoundly handicapped, tube-fed children who are further handicapped by seizures, switching to the ketogenic diet may be easy, requiring little effort by the family. It may be worth giving the diet a trial to see if the child (and family) will benefit.

❑ William was seven and had a mixture of partial complex seizures that occasionally generalized. He was on three medications and continued to have one or two generalized seizures per week. The family saw the television program about Charlie Abrahams and got the video tape. They wanted to put William on the diet immediately. After reading the book they still were eager to try the diet. William was admitted, fasted, and started on the diet, which was fine-tuned at home. Despite our best efforts and the hard work of the family, William continued to have one generalized seizure every other week and some brief complex partial seizures. We increased the ratio of fats to protein and carbohydrates and decreased the calories, but nothing made a substantial difference. Finally, we said that perhaps William was going to be one of the 30 percent of children for whom the diet doesn't work. We recommended discontinuing the diet.

"Why do you want to do that?" asked the mother. "William is on less medicine, he's doing better in school and he's a much nicer child. He's not so hyperactive. The diet's no problem and I don't want him to go back on those medicines. Can't we continue?" William agreed: "The diet's no big deal."

Although seizure control is the aim of the diet, in 30 to 40 percent of children we do not achieve substantial control. However, other benefits of the diet include the ability to reduce medications and their toxicity. For some families these changes are sufficient reason to continue the diet. As always, the decision about the benefits and the hardships of a treatment remain with the family and the child.

❏ Doug was fourteen. He'd had seizures since the age of four. Two medications had substantially controlled them and in the past two years he had been averaging one generalized seizure every three to four months. He was passing in school but was unable to participate in sports and after-school activities. "I'm just too tired at the end of the day," he said.

The family was eager to put Doug on the diet so that he could discontinue the medications. Doug was equally eager. We actively discouraged them, since we thought that in this child there would be insufficient benefit to warrant the rigors of the diet. Finally, the family's persistence overcame our resistance and Doug started the diet. In the nine months that he's been on the diet, he's had no seizures, medication has been discontinued, and his school work has improved. Best of all, he now has the energy to participate in Boy Scouts and after-school sports. "We told you the diet would work," say the gloating parents.

Summary: We have not recommended the diet for children who have rare seizures. Often we are asked by parents of children with newly diagnosed epilepsy, "Can't we go on the diet instead of using medications?" Our answer has consistently been, "No. The diet is far more difficult than taking a few pills, and most seizures will easily respond to medication." We have reserved the diet for children whose seizures have failed to be controlled by two or more medications. Perhaps, when the diet is better studied, we may advocate its wider use in children less handicapped by seizures and medications. It should be used earlier for those we predict will have difficult-to-control seizures.

❏ **Stephen is an exceedingly bright nine-year-old who had had intractable seizures despite three medications. We started the diet a year ago, and controlled his seizures and managed to get him off medication. When we told him that we were writing about the ketogenic diet for this book, he asked if he could write something. He e-mailed us the following paragraph.**

"Dr. Freeman, my ketogenic diet helps me get off of my drugs. You can eat cheese, salads, meats, peanut butter, mayonnaise, and macadamia nuts. You will not get to eat ice cream, bread, honey, cake, or brownies. I like it because I can make new recipes like mashed potato turnips. I do not like it when my friends laugh at my food."

Thanks, Stephen.

Parents' Questions about the Diet

"Is my child eligible for this diet?"

The diet appears quite effective in children with myoclonic and atonic (drop) types of seizures, the types most resistant to current medications. However, it can be used in virtually all forms of epilepsy. There is no upper age limit to its use, but children over the age of ten who have normal intelligence may have developed sufficient food preferences and sufficient independence that maintaining the diet can be difficult. We have used it successfully in preteens and adolescents when the individual and family are well motivated. The diet has been used with equal success in small numbers of highly motivated adults.

"Will my child have to remain on this diet for life?"

No. Most children whose seizures are controlled on the diet remain on it for two years. After that time they can gradually be taken off the diet, and the seizures usually do not return, even without additional anticonvulsant drugs.

"That sounds like a miracle. How does the diet work?"

We don't understand how the diet works. The results do not seem to be merely the effects of the dehydration, or of the ketosis, or of the acidosis (increased amount of acid in the blood) that accompany the diet. Research is ongoing to understand the effects of this diet on seizures.

How long will my child have to stay on the diet before we know whether or not it will work?"

Some children with multiple atonic seizures per day will stop having seizures during the starvation phase of the diet. Most for whom the diet will be effective will cease having seizures during the first several weeks. However, since some will respond later, we recommend continuing the diet for three months before giving up.

"When can we stop the anticonvulsants?"

If the child is on barbiturates, we often begin to taper them off during the starvation phase, since the barbiturate level in the blood may increase and make the child sleepy. We continue the other anticonvulsants for several months until it is apparent that the diet is effective in controlling the seizures and that it is tolerated. Then we slowly taper the other anticonvulsants over several months.

"What are the complications of the ketogenic diet?"

During the starvation phase of the diet, the child's blood sugar may drop, with symptoms like weakness, dizziness, paleness, sweating, and sleepiness. If these occur, it is imperative to measure the blood sugar and to give a small amount of glucose before continuing starvation. We have mentioned that supplementary vitamins and calcium are needed to prevent deficiencies. Your child should gain little weight on the diet if it is properly calculated, and growth may be slightly slowed. However, both will catch up when the diet eventually is discontinued. Despite the high fat content, the diet does not appear to cause atherosclerosis. Kidney stones can occur, but may be prevented by appropriate fluid intake.

"Is the diet always a last resort to control seizures?"

This diet has been used mainly as a last resort. However, since it is so effective when nothing else works, it should be used earlier in the course of difficult-to-control epilepsy.

"Isn't there any other alternative to the ketogenic diet?"

There is another form of the diet, called the MCT diet, in which the fats are given in the form of an oil. Although giving fats in this form allows the remainder of the diet to be more flexible, our experience shows that the MCT diet is not as effective as the classic ketogenic diet and that it is less well tolerated. We prefer the standard ketogenic diet.

More detailed information about the ketogenic diet can be found in *The Ketogenic Diet: A Treatment for Epilepsy* (see page 367).

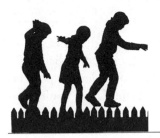

13. Vitamins, Minerals, and Complementary and Alternative Therapies for Epilepsy

Vitamins, Minerals, Other Special Diets

Despite many anecdotes, there is no evidence that food allergies or the elimination diets used to treat them play any role in the cause or treatment of epilepsy. *The only special diet shown to be effective for treatment of epilepsy is the ketogenic diet, discussed in Chapter 12.*

Vitamins

Vitamins are small molecules known to be necessary for certain chemical reactions in the body. Although a balanced diet contains sufficient amounts of vitamins and does not require supplementation, vitamin deficiencies *can* occur when diets are unusual. Deficiencies can also occur, although rarely, when an individual is unable to absorb vitamins from food. There are also rare inherited conditions in which a person's body chemistry requires unusually large amounts of a specific vitamin. In just a few circumstances, a vitamin deficiency can cause seizures.

One example of a deficiency or dependency known to produce epilepsy is deficiency of pyridoxine, vitamin B_6. Lack of B_6 may cause difficult-to-control seizures, usually in a newborn. Since there is no test for the deficiency, the physician may give small doses of the vitamin to see if it controls the seizures in the infant. Occasionally, when older children have difficult-to-control seizures, pyridoxine may be given to see if it will control the seizures.

Except in rare, specific problems, the addition of other vitamin or mineral supplements to a balanced diet is of *no* documented benefit in the treatment of seizures. However, there is also no evidence that vitamins and minerals, *in standard amounts,* do harm. Thus, while vitamins are not considered alternative therapy, they could perhaps be considered complementary therapy. At present, vitamin supplementation and special diets other than the ketogenic diet should not replace anticonvulsant therapy; but they may, if desired, be used in reasonable amounts as supplements to standard therapy.

Megadoses of vitamins can be harmful.

Minerals

Calcium is a very important mineral for the normal functioning of brain cells. Low levels of calcium, a condition called hypocalcemia, can cause seizures. Hypocalcemia can be the result of severe kidney disease, causing too much calcium to escape from the kidney into the urine. It may also, but rarely, be the result of a hormonal problem that has the same effect. Children who are having repeated seizures, especially those who are not responding to medication, should have the level of calcium in their blood tested. If it is low, then the cause should be sought and extra calcium given if necessary.

Magnesium is a mineral which interacts with calcium, and low levels of magnesium may cause symptoms, such as seizures, identical to those of hypocalcemia. Hypomagnesemia may actually produce a low blood calcium level. Although rare, hypomagnesemia is a readily treated cause of difficult-to-control seizures.

The role of any trace elements and of minerals other than calcium and magnesium in the course or treatment of epilepsy is unclear.

Complementary and Alternative Therapies for Epilepsy

The rest of this chapter is intended to give a brief overview of nontraditional therapies (also called alternative therapies and complementary therapies) for epilepsy. The authors do not claim any expertise in these alternative or complementary therapies and therefore do not advocate one alternative therapy over another—nor indeed do we advocate any of these therapies over traditional therapies. Most practitioners of these therapies see them as supplemental to the traditional use of anticonvulsant medications for the treatment of epilepsy. If alternative therapies are used in addition to anticonvulsant treatments, and the seizures are controlled, then, in consultation with your physician, it may be possible to decrease or even eliminate medications.

Despite the many new anticonvulsant medications available, some children continue to have seizures. When two medications have failed to control the seizures, the individual has only a 10 percent chance of having the seizures controlled by any of the newer medicines. The quality of life of children with difficult-to-control seizures is often impaired both by the seizures and by the side effects from multiple medications. One hundred percent of such children will have distraught parents who are frustrated that their physicians cannot bring the seizures under control and who are usually unhappy with the side effects of the multiple medications. The treating physicians are also frustrated by their lack of success in controlling the seizures. Typically, the physician will add the newest medication that has been promised to be "more effective," "safer," and have "fewer side effects." And yet the seizures often continue. The child, now on two, three, or four medications, "is not her old self" or "is always tired." The parents say it was almost better when she was having more seizures.

What children with epilepsy and their parents want is seizure control with no side effects—an improved quality of life. Dissatisfied parents start looking for another physician, for another approach, for anything that will allow their child to be seizure-free, or often even more important, free of the side effects of the medications. They want some reassurance that the future will be brighter than the present, that there is light at the end of the tunnel.

The parents turn to friends who have heard of someone's friend who went to someone who . . . Or they search the Internet and read about a therapy that promises . . . The woman in the chat room said that her child's seizures were due to imbalances in the . . . ; another said that the seizures were due to lack of . . . , or to an excess of. . . . Offered new hope, the frustrated parents of these children turn to alternatives to the medications and turn away from the physicians who seem to have failed them. The alternative therapies promise to redress the imbalances which some say are causing the epilepsy and the side effects.

There are many alternative and complementary therapies and combinations of them: massage therapy, chiropractic, osteopathy, craniosacral manipulation, homeopathy, Chinese herbal medicine, neurotherapy (also known as biofeedback), magnetic stimulation, aroma therapy, and pet therapy—to name a few. Some would even place the ketogenic diet in the category of alternative therapy. Alternative therapies are just that, alternatives to what has been variously termed "traditional medicine," "evidence-based medicine," "Western medicine," "allopathic medicine," or "anticonvulsant drug therapies." We are having trouble even finding the proper term for our current treatment of epilepsy, which is usually scientifically tested and evidence-based but is not always Western in origin. A common term is *allopathic,* which means "producing a different effect." Alternative and complementary therapies are usually used *in addition* to pharmacologic (drug) therapy. When complementary therapies help, the hope is that the multiplicity of drugs and their side effects can be minimized or eliminated.

A list of the traditional and alternative therapies discussed in this chapter appears below. We discuss traditional Chinese medicine first because the theoretical basis behind that therapy helps us in discussing other alternative and complementary therapies.

Herbal therapies
    Traditional Chinese herbal medicine
    Phytotherapy (non-Chinese herbal medicine)
Physical therapies
    Traditional Chinese medicine
    Acupuncture
    Massage therapy
Other alternative therapies
    Homeopathy
    Chiropractic manipulations
    Craniosacral-massage therapy
    Osteopathy
    Hyperbaric oxygen
    Carbon dioxide therapy
    Vagus nerve stimulation
    Cerebellar stimulation
    Transcranial magnetic stimulation
    Biofeedback

Most complementary and alternative therapies have several things in common. They lack allopathic medicine's "scientific" rationale, and they often depend on theories of the causation of seizures which lack evidenced-based support. These therapies usually have not been tested in controlled studies and rely on anecdotal evidence of effectiveness. However, parents and patients trapped in the morass of continued seizures, multiple medications and their side effects, and an uncertain future are desperate for any hope. Parents, afraid of the side effects of medicine, may turn to these "more natural" approaches.

Thirty percent of Americans have visited a practitioner of these treatments, although usually not for seizures. As we have said, we do not advocate any of these treatments as a primary therapy for epilepsy. We *never* encourage alternative treatments instead of pharmacologic treatment of epilepsy. However, in this edition of our book we felt it was important to describe some of these therapies and tell readers where to find out more about them.

We should add that not long ago, the ketogenic diet was considered an alternative therapy. Over the recent years, through studies, the ketogenic diet has been demonstrated to be both safe and effective in controlling difficult-to-control seizures and has taken its place among the standard treatments for seizures in children. It thus has been given its own chapter in this book (Chapter 12). Vagus nerve stimulation, also once considered an alternative therapy, has also taken its place among the accepted therapies for epilepsy (see Chapter 14). We hope that in the future the other alternative and complementary therapies will be subjected to rigorous testing that will—or will not—establish their efficacy.

There is nothing wrong with using one or more of the alternative approaches discussed in this chapter as an adjunct *to traditional anticonvulsant treatment. There are many additional alternative therapies which we have not discussed and about which we know even less. Alternative and complementary therapies should always be used with the knowledge and advice of your treating physician, however. You should be aware that most of the therapies discussed in this chapter are unproven, but when they are used with traditional allopathic therapies, they are rarely harmful.*

It is very important that you tell your neurologist if you wish to use alternative therapies. Although your treating neurologist or primary physician may know very little about these therapies and may very well fail to endorse or approve them, you should inform him or her when you are considering embarking on a course of alternative medicine. Some therapies are incompatible with Western medicine. Most practitioners of alternative medicine will initially use the therapy as an adjunct to the child's current anticonvulsant medications, with the hope that as (or if) the seizures abate, traditional medications can be reduced without an increase in seizures and with a resulting decrease in side effects. But *some herbs are dangerous when combined with anticonvulsants.*

Most complementary and alternative therapies come out of belief systems that are unfamiliar to those of us who have been trained in evidence-based medicine. Many such therapies are based on a holistic concept. *Holistic medicine* is medical treatment that makes a point of dealing with the whole person, not just with his or her physical condition. In this system, disease and dysfunction are understood to be a result of misalignments and imbalances between the environment and the individual as well as among the vital forces inside the individual's body.

The Theoretical Bases for Evidence-Based Therapies for Epilepsy

Before discussing alternative therapies in detail, we review here the theoretical and belief systems that form the basis of evidence-based therapies for epilepsy.

As discussed in Chapter 1, the brain functions properly when there is a balance between the electrical excitation and inhibition of cells termed neurons. The relative excitation and inhibition of these cells (threshold) is influenced by the local (intracellular and extracellular) environment, as well as by the systemic (whole body) environment. We know that many factors—genetics, age, stress, anxiety, lack of sleep, poor nutrition, disposition—influence the predisposition to and the occurrence of seizures.

A seizure is a change in a person's physical state (such as alterations in consciousness, uncontrolled movement or sensation) due to an electrical discharge in the brain. What does Western science know and not know about seizures?

- We know that a seizure is due to excessive discharge of a large number of these electricity-generating neurons. We do not know whether the discharge in an individual seizure is due to excessive excitation or to lack of sufficient inhibition.
- We do not know why some individuals have a predisposition to seizures (low thresholds) and others lack this predisposition.
- We do not know why some children have seizures once a day and others have them once a year. In fact, we do not know why most individuals who have seizures have them at all.

• We know that some individuals have seizures that occur only during the night (nocturnal seizures). Some people have the seizures as they go to sleep, others have them early in the morning before awakening, and still others during the wake-sleep transition. We do not know the reasons for this.

• We know that the type of seizure is determined by the location of its onset in the brain and the direction and speed of its spread, but we do not know the many factors which influence these variables.

• We know that stress, nutrition, family history, and many other factors play a role in an individual's seizures. But we do not know how they exert that influence.

In short, our scientific understanding of the physiology of epilepsy is less advanced than patients and even health care practitioners believe. The question remains: is our understanding more scientifically based than the understanding that emerges from some of the belief systems underlying the alternative therapies?

Despite what we know and don't know about seizures and epilepsy, Western medicine has identified and in some cases synthesized a number of medications and tested them, first in animals and (if effective) then in humans with epilepsy. The effectiveness of these compounds as additions to the individual's other treatment has been evaluated, to see if the compound decreases the number of seizures. These studies are often carried out by comparing the new medication's effectiveness in controlling seizures with the effectiveness of a placebo (a substitute benign substance, often referred to as a "sugar pill"—something that has no specific therapeutic activity for seizures).

The Theoretical Bases for Alternative and Complementary Therapies for Epilepsy

Alternative and complementary therapies take many of these same observations about seizures and epilepsy and create different therapies based on different theoretical bases. Most of these therapies have not been studied in the more rigorous manner of Western medications, but over time they have received enough anecdotal reports of benefit to patients that they have become established treatments.

When expressed in this fashion, the primary difference between the alternative or complementary approach and the allopathic, evidence-based, scientific, Western approach is the type and quality of the evidence of therapeutic effect, not the underlying theories or beliefs. (See www.quackwatch.com for more information about this.)

Traditional Chinese Medicine

Eighty percent of the traditional Chinese medicine treatments used for the management of epilepsy are herbal therapies.

Chinese Herbal Therapies

Traditional Chinese herbal therapy is hundreds of years old. Its aim is to eliminate the causes of disease by correcting the imbalances within the individual and the individual's environment. Since each condition and each individual may have different imbalances, it is important to differentiate (diagnose) the type of imbalance producing the problem. Differentiation (diagnosis) is made by taking a careful history of the nature of the condition, assessing the quality of the pulse, and the color and quality of the tongue. The personality that the person exhibited in the past and the current emotional state are noted, as are the sort of foods ingested and other aspects of the patient's physical condition. Based on this multiplicity of factors, a diagnosis (differentiation) is arrived at, the nature of the imbalance is determined, and its causes—due to excesses, deficiencies, or neither—is diagnosed. The condition may be defined as the "cold type" or the "warm type," which will determine the herbal combinations to be used and will define the specific preparation of each herb.

Words often have very different meanings in traditional Chinese medicine (TCM) than in Western medicine. In TCM the term *heart* refers not only to the organ in your chest but also to the circulation as a whole and includes the brain. The term *liver* refers not only to the organ but to a person's disposition. Thus, for example, in evaluating a headache, the practitioner of traditional Chinese medicine must look not only to the head, but to the heart, the lung, and the liver to find the dysfunctional organ system.

The formulas for treatment of the various conditions and of the various epilepsies are defined in the *Chinese Herbal Materia Medica,* which consists of more than 400 Chinese herbs. These herbs are to be prepared in very specific ways for (or by) the individual. A practitioner of traditional Chinese medicine prescribes the Chinese herbs, in specific combinations calculated for that individual's specific imbalance (dysfunction). To overcome the imbalance, it is critically important for all the herbs to work in the same direction, toward balance. Since the imbalance producing the disease is different in each individual, the combination of herbs and the duration of treatments will be different for each person. This makes the designing of controlled trials impossible.

Acupuncture

In addition to the differentiation of imbalances discussed above, the practitioner of traditional Chinese medicine assesses the Qi (pronounced *chee*), the vital forces of the body. Imbalance is expressed as misalignment of the vital forces (Qi) and the relative balance between the yin and the yang. Yin is the inhibitory side of the body's status, and yang is the excitatory index. These "vital forces" flow throughout the body along meridians (pathways) of body energy. Imbalances or blockages can cause disruptions and symptoms. Acupuncture is used primarily to treat pain and discomforts, but it also can have a role in the treatment of epilepsy.

In this belief system, epilepsy is caused by too much yang (excitation) and/or insufficient yin (inhibition), with the imbalance resulting in seizures. The flow of vital forces can be modified through acupuncture at the appropriate sites (points on the meridians). Acupuncture as a part of the treatment of epilepsy is intended to increase the yin and decrease the yang. Massage and moxibustion (see below) are used when required to further adjust these vital forces. Since each individual's symptoms are due to different imbalances, the combinations of herbs and choice of acupuncture points are tailored to that individual. Elements of the belief in "imbalances" and in "flow of vital forces" also seem to underlie many of the other types of alternative therapies.

Western medicine and traditional Chinese medicine start from different belief systems. Each explains the individual's dysfunction in its own way, and each attempts to correct that perceived dysfunction using modalities suited to its belief system. The Eastern system of beliefs and of therapies has persisted for centuries. As incomprehensible as it is to those of us trained in the evidence-based tradition, people must have derived benefit from these therapies, or they would not have persisted.

Practitioners of TCM say that the treatments have either no side effects or fewer side effects than Western medical treatments. They say that in treating epilepsy, TCM may be combined with Western medicine and, when there is benefit, Western medications may be tapered.

Phytotherapy

Phytotherapy, like Chinese herbal therapy, starts with the belief that the individual has an imbalance and that specific herbs may restore this imbalance. Although TCM utilizes combinations of Chinese herbs prepared in very specific ways, phytotherapy uses individual herbs chosen because of their specific effects. Some herbal therapies may be effective in treating specific problems, but few have been adequately studied.

Herbs are not evaluated by the Food and Drug Administration because they are considered food additives and not drugs. The herbalist cannot claim to cure or prevent disease, and there are no requirements for testing the safety or efficacy of herbal treatments. People often use herbs because they believe that "natural" substances are preferable to, and safer than, synthetic substances such as medicines.

Herbs have a far longer history than Western medicines in the treatment of disease. Some herbs have been shown to be effective. Their active components have been isolated, tested, often synthesized, and then they have become part of standard evidenced-based medicine. Quinine, used to treat malaria, was originally derived from chichona bark; and aspirin developed from willow bark, digitalis from foxglove.

Many herbs are known to produce sedation and to affect the nervous system. Kava, lobelia, valerian, and passion flower have been shown to have effects on the central nervous system. While a few herbs have been shown in laboratory or animal testing to have anticonvulsant effects, there has been little testing in humans of either their safety or their efficacy. Clearly there is a need for further laboratory, animal, and human research on herbs. One source for further information is www.herbs.org.

Homeopathy

Homeopathy is a therapy that attempts to treat symptoms rather than diseases. Homeopathy practitioners believe that the symptoms are the result of the body's attempt to restore itself to health. Homeopathy looks for the one substance that will cause similar symptoms in a healthy person and gives it to the patient in very dilute doses to help the person fight the disease-causing symptoms. The underlying theory is that if a substance given to a healthy person causes similar symptoms, then if given to a sick person in very diluted form it will help to stimulate that person's body to restore itself to health.

The homeopathic claim is that a holistic approach using detailed information about the patient's seizures, including the EEG and the events which precipitate the seizures, and about the patient's mental, emotional, and physical state, will make it possible for the homeopathic practitioner to prescribe the correct remedy. This remedy when diluted to the maximum is intended to be taken with the anticonvulsant medications as a complementary therapy for epilepsy. In general, the more diluted the solution—the less of the substance given—the more powerful the remedy. One drop of the appropriate substance is diluted with 99 drops of alcohol to make a 1:100 solution. This solution is then diluted 100-fold to make a 1:10,000 solution and may be further diluted so that the substance is present in 1 part per million, or less. Homeopaths assert that, although such infinitesimal quantities are considered by some to be no more than placebos, the clinical experience shows that the infinitesimal dose is effective. One source for further information is www.homeopathic.org.

Adjustments, Manipulations, and Massage

We have introduced the concept of Qi (chee—the vital force) and the flow of the yin and yang along meridians in our discussion of the theories underlying Chinese acupuncture. Several other alternative and complementary therapies are based on similar belief systems.

Chiropractic

Chiropractic is the third largest health care profession in the United States. There are eighteen accredited chiropractic colleges, there is regulation and licensing of chiropractors on the books in all states, chiropractors are considered primary health care providers by many health systems, and their services are covered by health insurance. Chiropractors adjust the "flow of fluid" along the spine by manipulations. Visits to chiropractors account for almost half of all visits for alternative therapies. Most visits are for chronic low back pain, neck pain, anxiety, depression, arthritis, and strains and sprains.

In the treatment of epilepsy, spinal adjustments are primarily directed to the upper cervical spine and are meant to correct aberrant bio-mechanics, which practitioners believe cause the seizures, and to allow activation of appropriate neural pathways, resulting in a decrease or cessation of seizure activity. Chiropractors often find "subluxations" (partial dislocations) of the cervical spine, label the dislocation the cause of problems, and claim to correct it by manipulations. *Manipulations of the upper cervical spine may be dangerous and result in damage to the vertebral blood vessels and in strokes. Manipulations of children's spines may be particularly dangerous.*

Chiropractic should *not* be used instead of pharmacologic care in the treatment of epilepsy. Some individuals believe that it may be given a brief (several weeks) trial, to see if it will enhance the pharmacologic treatment of the seizures. For more information, see www.chirobase.org.

Craniosacral Therapy

Craniosacral therapy, like acupuncture, is based on the concept of the flow of vital forces. The spinal fluid, which bathes the brain, is said to have hydraulic pulsations that aid in neurotransmission. The well-trained therapist can detect the subtle imbalances affecting the flow of an individual's cerebral spinal fluid over the surfaces of the brain, down through the spinal canal, and even through the membrane that covers the brain and spine canal and the tissue that covers the muscles. The therapy is said to be "experiential" and uses very gentle pressure over the sutures of the head or along the spine and fascia to readjust the asymmetries and blockages which result from the subtle imbalances and impair the individual's sense of well-being. This very gentle pressure is said to be able to realign the pulsations and allow the body to respond and self-correct.

This therapy is often a part of a holistic approach that might also involve homeopathy, naturopathy, and hydrotherapy. The treatments are said to allow the body to be "detoxified." There have been no attempts to validate either the theory underlying this therapy or this therapy's role in treating epilepsy. Nevertheless, some parents have said that, when used in addition to pharmacotherapy, this therapy has helped their child.

Osteopathy

Osteopathy believes that the patient is a "dynamic system," and that the pulsations of the brain and cerebrospinal fluid affect the movement and alignment of the bones of the skull. Epilepsy is one manifestation of "impaired" skull-bone movement or alignment. For example, it is said that the compression of the head during the birth process may result in impairments of the bony alignment of the child's skull and cause seizures. The trained hands of the osteopath can detect the misalignment of the skull bones and readjust them. There is little support for the theory of osteopathy and little evidence to support its efficacy in the treatment of epilepsy.

Massage

Massage therapy has many different forms, each directed toward relaxation and reduction of anxiety and stress. Reduction of anxiety and stress may also decrease the propensity for seizures. There are no studies of the role of massage in the specific treatment of epilepsy, but just as anxiety and stress can be precipitating factors in seizures, massage may be beneficial as a supplement to the pharmacologic therapy of seizures. Although sensory input such as pain, application of heat, cold, or other stimulation, or the pressure of massage has been known to stop the spread of Jacksonian seizures, the relevance of this finding to massage therapy is unclear. Massage can do no harm.

Oxygen, Hyperbaric Oxygen, and Carbon Dioxide Therapies

The brain needs oxygen to survive and function. Oxygen gets to the brain via the circulatory system. Lack of oxygen or lack of circulation to the brain for more than several minutes may cause the death or dysfunction of neurons and may result in seizures.

During a seizure, the increased rate of firing of the neurons uses more oxygen, and the blood flow to the brain or to the firing part of the brain increases. During a generalized tonic-clonic seizure, just as there is stiffening of the muscles of the body, there may be stiffening of the muscles of the chest and therefore a lack of air exchange. The seizing individual's lips may turn blue, and the body's oxygen saturation may decrease.

There is a widespread misperception by both the medical profession and by families that this lack of oxygen during a seizure may do damage to the brain. There is little evidence to support this. Children and adults recover from seizures and are back to their old selves. Even prolonged seizures (status epilepticus), when due to fever or drug withdrawal, does not damage the brain. Lack of oxygen or lack of circulation after a *stroke can* cause acute seizures and *can* damage the brain, causing chronic epilepsy. This does *not* suggest that giving extra oxygen can treat or prevent epilepsy. It does not indicate that increasing oxygen or circulation can improve brain function.

Why do emergency medical technicians and nurses give oxygen when a child is having a seizure? Because it gives them something innocuous to do while they are waiting for the seizure to end. There is no evidence that oxygen needs to be given or that oxygen given by mask during a seizure even gets to the brain.

Hyperbaric oxygen is oxygen delivered under increased atmospheric pressure within a special high-pressure chamber. This procedure can slightly increase the amount of oxygen saturated in the blood, and thus it has been used to increase brain oxygenation. Since there is no evidence of oxygen deficiency in the brains of children with seizures or those with brain damage and developmental delay, there can be no benefit to them of hyperbaric oxygen therapy. Since the increase in saturation occurs only during the time a person is in the pressure chamber, there can be no lasting benefit. Hyperbaric oxygen treatments are a very expensive way to obtain unneeded extra oxygen with no therapeutic or even theoretical benefit.

Carbon dioxide (CO_2) enhances oxygen delivery to the brain by dilating the brain's blood vessels and therefore increasing the flow of blood. Carbon dioxide levels can be increased by having the individual rebreathe into a paper bag. Again, there is no evidence that the brain of an individual with epilepsy, with or without evidence of other brain damage, is deficient in either blood flow or oxygen, and there is no evidence that increasing either blood flow or oxygen affects seizures. Therefore there is no reason to believe that increasing brain oxygen is beneficial to children with brain dysfunction or epilepsy. In addition, when the individual stops breathing into the bag, the CO_2 quickly returns to normal, as does the dilation of blood vessels.

Other New Alternative Therapies

Since epilepsy is a balance between electrical excitation and inhibition in the brain, other types of electrical stimulations may affect that balance.

Cerebellar Stimulation

This particular treatment method is no longer in vogue. In cerebellar stimulation, electrodes were placed on various parts of the cerebellum and stimulated episodically. While effective, the operation to place the electrodes was substantial, and the parameters of stimulation and the placement of the electrodes were never established. However, the principle of electrical stimulation to increase inhibitory inputs to the brain is sound and led to the development of vagus nerve stimulation.

Vagus Nerve Stimulation

Vagus nerve stimulation (VNS) has been shown to be effective in decreasing seizures (see page 241). This technique, now approved, is no longer considered an alternative therapy. Electric stimulation of the vagus nerve with precise inputs can increase inhibition in the cortex and therefore decrease seizures.

Transcranial Magnetic Stimulation

Electricity creates a magnetic field. It appears that stimulation of specific areas over the cortex can create an electric field which may be either excitatory or inhibitory, depending on the interval. This stimulation can have widespread influences on the local blood flow. The role of this form of stimulation in the management of epilepsy remains to be determined.

Biofeedback

The EEGs of some individuals with epilepsy have abnormal sensory-motor rhythms (SMR), which are detected using brain mapping. These rhythms can be altered by biofeedback. It is said that altering the SMR in some individuals may decrease the frequency of seizures. Controlled studies of this time-intensive and expensive technique remain to be performed.

Conclusion

One theme underlies many of the alternative and complementary therapies, and that is that epilepsy is a multifactorial disease: stress, lack of sleep, nutrition, and disease may all affect the individual's propensity to seizures. Even in allopathic medicine these factors are recognized, although often not given the attention they deserve. It takes time to listen to the patient and to become aware of the multiple factors involved in their quality of life. Treatment of seizures is—or should be— more than the adjustment of medications to diminish the seizures.

Many of these complementary and alternative therapies place emphasis on relaxation and stress reduction, doubtless always a good thing in the treatment of seizures. Some portions of these therapies may be useful; we need to find out which ones. Vagus nerve stimulation and the ketogenic diet were, until recently, considered alternative therapies. Now they have been adequately studied.

Until these other therapies are adequately studied, they should not be used as alternatives to pharmacologic therapies but may, if desired, be used as complementary to standard treatment, with the knowledge of your physician.

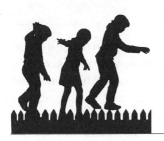

14. Surgical Approaches to Epilepsy

❏ Wendy had her first complex partial seizure when she was thirteen. Her initial evaluation, including a CT scan, MRI, and EEG, revealed no cause, and medication was prescribed. Phenobarbital made her sleepy, and phenytoin (Dilantin) only slightly reduced the frequency of her seizures, now occurring three to four times a week. Carbamazepine (Tegretol) was added, and then valproic acid (Depakote), and the seizures became less frequent. However, Wendy's school work began to suffer while she was taking several medications, and she became depressed. At sixteen she couldn't drive and because of embarrassment she became less social and more isolated. When she was eighteen, other medications became available, but despite attempts to adjust medication, her physicians were unable to completely control her seizures. By this time, Wendy's school work had suffered and she had been turned down by the colleges of her choice. She was about to enter the local junior college.

When we first saw Wendy, she was a highly motivated young lady, depressed about the seizures and about her future. She had received psychological counseling, which had helped some, but the seizures—during which she would suddenly stop what she was doing, stare, then wander about the room picking at her clothes, and remain in a confused state for ten to fifteen minutes—were still occurring several times each week despite good levels of medication.

Our evaluation suggested that the seizures came from the right temporal lobe. Surgery was discussed, but Wendy, now twenty-two, was afraid. She was away from home, finishing college and about to begin a master's program in psychology. We worked with her, long distance, to adjust the medications, but she had problems either with drug toxicity or with seizure control. Finally she decided she was willing to have the surgery. Repeat evaluation suggested that the focus was in the anterior right temporal lobe. This was removed surgically and revealed mesial temporal sclerosis, an old scar that had not been visible on the scans.

Wendy has had no seizures in the past ten years, has finished her Ph.D. in psychology, and says that life and her work are both much easier now without seizures and without any medication. "I only wish that we had done the surgery much earlier," she says. "It would have made growing up so much easier."

❑ Ted had his first tonic-clonic seizure at fourteen. The initial CT scan showed a small abnormality in the anterior left temporal lobe, probably caused by bleeding from abnormal blood vessels. The doctor decided to wait and see what would happen. Six months later Ted began to have complex partial seizures and he was referred to us. We began administration of carbamazepine (Tegretol) and discussed the option of surgical removal of the malformation, both for the control of seizures and because the malformation might bleed again.

The lesion was removed when Ted was fifteen, one year after his first seizure. He is now completing high school. He's on the basketball team, and he lives without seizures and without medication.

When we recently asked Ted how he felt about all that had gone on, he replied, "It wasn't any big deal. I didn't like having my beautiful hair shaved off, but that's all behind me now."

These two examples of temporal lobe surgery involved small, focal lesions in the anterior temporal lobe, an area which is easily removed at surgery with very little risk. They are often used as examples of epilepsy surgery, but these are the easy ones. The decisions are not difficult, the surgery is not hard, and temporal lobectomy can be done by many neurosurgeons when the lesion is clear. The patients are out of the hospital in a few days and quickly back to work or school. In cases such as these, surgery should be done far earlier than it was in the past, and the disability associated with continued seizures and medication can be avoided. This type of temporal lobe surgery is often done in adults and is being done increasingly in children. Other types of epilepsy surgery for focal and for unilateral seizures are discussed later in this chapter.

Even within the focal surgeries there are two major types, temporal lobe surgery and extratemporal surgery. As we have discussed (Chapter 2), complex partial seizures with staring, lip smacking, picking at the clothes, and brief alterations of consciousness, with or without a secondary generalized tonic-clonic seizure, often arise in the temporal lobe but could be of frontal lobe origin.

• If an individual is experiencing complex partial seizures *and* he has an EEG showing temporal lobe abnormalities, even without MRI findings, he may be a candidate for temporal lobe surgery. This is by far the most common type of epilepsy surgery performed, and it is done mostly in adults. It is very successful in eliminating seizures and should be done early in the course if several drugs (or perhaps only one drug), properly used, have failed to control the seizures.

• If the MRI shows scarring and shrinkage (sclerosis) in the mesial temporal lobe, that is additional evidence that the seizures may prove difficult to control and additional evidence of the site of the problem. Unfortunately, although those seizures often start in childhood, the mesial sclerosis is not commonly seen until late adolescence, and these children are not easily identified.

Adults with partial complex seizures and mesial temporal sclerosis whose seizures are not controlled by one or two medications should seriously consider a surgical evaluation.

Thinking about Surgery

No one wants to think about surgery on the brain—except as a very last resort. This is often true of physicians as well as patients and parents. Surgery is often left as the last alternative. *Surgery should not be the last alternative, it should be among the first things thought about. Thinking about surgery for epilepsy is* NOT *the same as doing epilepsy surgery.*

• *If* the seizures come from one area *and* that area can be easily removed without causing problems, surgery should be done, and earlier rather than later.

• *If* the epilepsy is caused by a lesion, a developmental problem, a cyst, or a tumor, then the seizures may be less likely to respond to medication. You and your physician should know whether surgery is or is not an option early in the course and at least think about surgery as an alternative.

Contemplating surgery is overwhelming. Except in the rare instance of a rapidly growing brain tumor, this surgery is not an emergency. Epilepsy surgery should never be placed "on the fast track." It should be done only after careful consideration of its potential risks and benefits. As discussed later in this chapter, the risks and potential benefits may not be known until all of the noninvasive and invasive evaluations discussed in this chapter have occurred.

We believe that decisions about surgery require working through a series of questions.

1. Is the child (or the adult) having seizures?
2. Are the seizures recurrent and difficult to control?
3. Are the seizures coming from one location?
4. Can the source of the seizures be easily removed?

If the answer to these four questions is yes, then the next step is to obtain more information. What are the *risks* of the operation? Is there a risk of losing some motor function, language function, vision, or intellect? What are the potential *benefits* of the surgery? Is it likely to get rid of the seizures? Is it likely to allow the child to be free of medication? Will it improve the child's quality of life? How much? In what way?

These are only some of the thoughts and concerns you should discuss with your physician as you progress toward making decisions about a surgical treatment.

If your child has seizures that are recurrent and difficult to control, your physician will want to establish if they are coming from a single location in the brain. If your physician has done an MRI, EEG, and perhaps several days of monitoring and feels that your child may benefit from a surgical intervention, then it is time for you to get involved in the decision. If your child is not being seen at a hospital that does epilepsy surgery, you should feel free to explain to your physician that before making such a monumental decision you would like a second opinion.

The epilepsy community, and particularly the pediatric epilepsy community, is fairly small, and your physician should be able to give you the names of several centers specializing in epilepsy and epilepsy surgery. Most physicians will be very understanding if you seek a second opinion, and will provide you with your child's records. In addition, you can begin doing research yourself. Go on the Internet (see page 366), call the Epilepsy Foundation, talk with other parents. These are just some of the ways you can get the names of epilepsy centers. You should call the center and ask pertinent questions about their programs: How frequently they do epilepsy surgery? In what age ranges? With what success rates? You will find that most centers will want to do their own monitoring, even though it may have been done recently elsewhere. This is perfectly reasonable, since it is on the basis of the interpretation of the monitoring that the center will be able to decide how to proceed. Centers such as ours review all of the child's records prior to making an appointment to see the child, so that we can have the most cost-effective visit with the parent and child.

We have written elsewhere in this book about the work-up for epilepsy surgery, about the various scanning processes, about the initial video-monitoring. After all of that work-up has been completed, and if it confirms that your child is a candidate for surgery, then think very seriously if this is the avenue you want to pursue. Your physicians will explain to you just what surgical procedure they are recommending and just what it entails. They should explain—until they are sure you understand—the potential risks and benefits of the procedure, and the risks and benefits of not doing surgery.

Epilepsy surgery is never an emergency. You should not approach this as an emergency or allow anyone to intimidate you into making a quick decision. There is plenty of time to decide if you want the surgery done and where you want the surgery done, as well as to carefully consider the alternatives. Epilepsy surgery is an irreversible procedure.

Take the time to talk with other parents whose children have had the surgical procedure, to obtain their perspective. Only another family who has been there can tell you what the decision-making process was like, how they weighed the choices, and about the hospitalization and the recovery process. Other parents can provide wonderful tips for dealing with life in the hospital and after the patient goes home. (Tips from one parent are appended at the end of this chapter.) We also encourage older children to talk with other kids who have been through the surgery, because peer interactions are really important. If another family lives close by, we encourage a visit, so that you can ask questions and hear of problems and outcomes. This is of particular importance if you are considering a hemispherectomy, for no one can imagine how well a child can do with only one-half of a brain. It has to be seen to be believed. Many families tell us that the best thing we provide is a family network.

Finding the right place to do the surgery can be complicated. Different centers perform different surgeries, and there is often a waiting list for all of them. Remember, this isn't an emergency. Do not make the mistake of choosing a center on the basis of who can do the operation soonest. *There is not just one center for epilepsy surgery in the United States, nor just one surgeon.*

Unfortunately, in this era of managed care, not all patients are able to go to the center of their choice, because of the constraints of insurance. (Insurance issues are discussed in Chapter 26.) It is important to recognize that epilepsy surgery, and all of the preliminary evaluation and follow-up care, is *very* expensive. Out-of-network costs can escalate rapidly, leaving a family with a mountain of bills that is overwhelming. No one should have to sell their home, move to another city, or go to extremes to be able to have surgery for their child. Most epilepsy programs can recommend a center for the surgery that is within your network. The evaluation for epilepsy surgery is a long and tedious process. If traveling great distances is a limiting factor, a center can be found near where you live. Most centers are willing to help you find the place that will be able to meet your needs and those of your child.

Tumor Surgery and Epilepsy Surgery

There are two categories of brain surgery in a patient with seizures. One we call "tumor surgery," the other "epilepsy surgery." A tumor in the brain may cause seizures. (We are using the word *tumor* in its original sense of a swelling or mass.) We are talking about not only abnormal growths and cancer but also abnormal blood vessels, areas of prior bleeding, and cysts, which may press on the surrounding brain, causing seizures. These tumors can usually be seen on brain scans. The surgeon or neurologist may recommend removal of the tumor, and as an additional benefit, the seizures may be controlled. Removal of such abnormalities is called tumor surgery, and its purpose is different from epilepsy surgery. The sole purpose is to remove the tumor.

Epilepsy surgery is primarily intended to eliminate the seizures, whether or not a tumor is present. Abnormalities of the brain causing seizures may be subtle, local abnormalities of cells or local scarring, with nothing pressing on the surrounding brain. In these cases, separating normal tissue from abnormal ("epileptic") tissue may be difficult. Removal of these "epileptic" and electrically abnormal areas to control seizures is defined as epilepsy surgery. Sometimes scars, tumors, or blood vessel abnormalities are removed incidentally while removing the abnormal tissue causing the seizures. As we continue our discussion of surgery, we are focusing on epilepsy surgery rather than tumor surgery.

While surgery should *always* be considered for an individual with a focal seizure disorder when there is a *clear* focal lesion on the MRI scan, unless that lesion is thought to be a growing tumor, medication is usually the first treatment option. However, with a focal lesion arising from a safe area of the brain, as was true with Ted (discussed earlier in this chapter), surgery may be a better option than having the patient take two or three medications and suffer their side effects. *Surgery should be performed only after careful evaluation in an epilepsy center with full capabilities for both evaluation and for surgery, and then only after full consideration of risks, benefits, and alternatives.* Decision making about the timing, the risks, and the benefits of evaluating for surgery and doing surgery is discussed later in this chapter.

There are many different types of epilepsy surgery. Most epilepsy surgery is "focal excisional surgery"—surgery to remove a focus. Larger excisions, or "resections," like removal of lobes of the brain or even a whole hemisphere (one-half of the brain), can be done when large areas of the brain are functionally and electrically abnormal. Resections of areas of the cortex can also be performed. In rare occasions, sectioning (cutting) of the corpus callosum (the tissue connecting the two hemispheres) can be done to minimize the spread of seizures, when the foci of the epilepsy cannot be removed.

Each procedure must be carefully designed for the individual. Each procedure is appropriate only for specific seizure problems, and each has its own risks and benefits.

Surgery for Partial (Focal) Seizures

General Considerations for Focal Surgery

Partial (focal) seizures and partial seizures that secondarily generalize (Chapter 2) are, by definition, always focal (local) in origin. Any child with partial seizures deserves some evaluation to find the source of the focal abnormality. If the EEG shows focal slowing or if the child has had several seizures that seem to start from the same area of the brain, then he should have an MRI scan, to search for a focal, structural problem that might be cured by surgery. Surgery is rarely considered for the child who has had only a few seizures, unless there is a tumor or vascular abnormality or obvious scarring—*rare* causes of seizures in children—and then the surgery done is tumor surgery. Ted, whom we discussed above, had a structural problem. Surgery early in the course of his epilepsy cured him of seizures.

In the absence of a tumor, vascular abnormality, or scarring, a reasonable trial of medication is indicated to try to control focal seizures.

Consideration of surgery proceeds step by step. The process can be stopped at any step if evidence suggests that the individual is not a good candidate for surgery or if the risks and negative consequences of the surgery seem too great.

Is Your Child a Candidate for Surgery?

• As we've said, if there is no tumor growing in the brain, epilepsy surgery is never an emergency.
• Surgery should always be a carefully considered alternative to medications.
• Surgery should only be done after careful consideration of its risks and benefits.

We start with the case of a young woman who should *not* have been a candidate for surgery, but who underwent the operation anyway. Candice's experience lets us see where decisions can go wrong.

❏ **Candice was seventeen years old, a ballet dancer on her way to a promising career with a New York group. She had just finished high school and was to enter the conservatory that fall. On a summer camping trip with her friends she had a generalized tonic-clonic seizure. She was taken to the local emergency room and had recovered before she arrived. The CT scan performed there showed a lesion high in the right parietal lobe. The physician showed her the scan and the "tumor" and suggested that she be transferred to the teaching hospital fifty miles away. She called her parents and, with their permission, was sent to Northern State Medical Center. The MRI done the next morning again showed the lesion.**

"It looks to me like a small tangle of blood vessels, an angioma," said the

chief of neurosurgery. "I'd advise that you start on Dilantin to prevent another seizure and go back home. There are several excellent medical centers there, and I'd recommend that you make an appointment with one of their neurosurgeons."

Candice went home and talked with her parents. Her brother, Charles, was a resident in neurology in another part of the country, so she had access to other advice as well. Candice wanted the thing taken out *now*! "I don't want to take Dilantin. It will affect my balance and my dancing. Suppose I had another one of those things during a performance, what would that do to my career? And besides, I want to have children in the future, and Charles says that Dilantin could affect my children. When I have a child, I don't want to take any chances."

The local neurosurgeon looked at the MRI that Candice had brought with her and said that the lesion was close to the surface and the surgery should not be any problem. He said it should take about two hours. The surgery was scheduled for the following week.

Before we go on with this story, let's pause and see what is wrong with this picture.

- Candice has had only one seizure. Will she ever have a second one? We don't know.
- Candice has a lesion in her brain. Was that what caused her seizure? We don't know.
- The lesion hasn't caused any problems other than perhaps the seizure. Is it growing? How long has it been there: a month, a year, a lifetime? We don't know.
- Will Dilantin control her seizures? Will it cause side effects? Could another medication control the seizures without side effects? We don't know.

The decision to do surgery in this case has been made far too rapidly—by the surgeon and by the patient—with inadequate consideration of the risks and benefits of the surgery and of the alternatives.

❏ Charles flew home to be with his sister on the day of the surgery. After about six hours in the operating room, the surgeon came out to say that he hadn't been able to find the lesion. "It just wasn't obvious at surgery. We should have repeated our own MRI and localized it better. We'll give her a week to recover and do another scan with our new 3-D equipment and operate again then," he said.

When Charles asked the surgeon if he was sure that he could remove it all, the surgeon's response was, "There are never any guarantees with this kind of surgery." When asked if he could be certain that she would not have any seizures after the surgery, he responded, "We can't be certain. The surgery is to remove the lesion, and hopefully the seizures as well." After a long discussion of the risks and possible benefits of another surgery, the surgeon changed his mind. "You're right," he told Charles. "Maybe we shouldn't re-operate." The re-operation was canceled.

Five years later Candice has continued to dance. She has a beautiful baby. She takes her Dilantin daily and has had only one further seizure in all of those years. More careful consideration of the risks and benefits of the surgery and of the risks and benefits of not doing the surgery might have prevented the first operation. Fortunately, the outcome was good anyway. There was never any reason to rush the decision.

We find that evaluating the pattern of the seizures—their frequency and behavior—is most helpful in the initial screening of a potential candidate for surgery. Your child must have a sufficient number of seizures in order to establish a reliable and consistent pattern that can be evaluated. This will take time. If your child's seizures always follow the same pattern (for example, with the seizure always starting in the right hand, or with the head and eyes always turning to the left), this would suggest that the seizures may start in a particular location in the brain. The advantage of knowing such details is why careful observation is critically important. Repeated EEGs may also be required to document a consistent area of abnormality. (The location of the various areas in the brain is shown in Chapter 2.)

Routine EEGs may, or may not, show a focal abnormality, so special EEGs or video monitoring may be necessary. If your doctor finds multiple abnormal areas on the EEG, then your child is probably *not* a candidate for surgery.

The next question at this stage is whether the focal abnormality, if present, is in an area which can safely be removed. The anterior portions of the frontal lobe and temporal lobe are the portions of the brain that can be removed without causing neurologic problems. Therefore, children whose seizures repeatedly appear to come from these areas should be considered good candidates for evaluation for *possible* surgery early in the course of their epilepsy. If, on the other hand, the seizures appear to come from near the motor or speech area, the likelihood that surgery will cause neurological problems is higher; in such a case, surgery requires a more careful evaluation.

If your child has had repeated focal seizures, your physician will probably have some thoughts about whether or not your child might be a candidate for surgery. If he has not brought up the subject, it might be appropriate for you to ask him. After your physician has found answers to the two preliminary questions noted above, *and* if your child does seem to be a good candidate, *and* if the seizures are difficult to control with medicines, *then* it is the appropriate time for you and your physician to discuss the possible risks and benefits of surgery. If your child is a good candidate for surgery and you are interested in considering surgery, then the next step in the evaluation can take place.

Getting your child an evaluation for surgery enables you and your physician to assess the potential risks and benefits of surgery. *It is not a commitment to do surgery.*

Confirming that Your Child Is a Candidate for Surgery

The second step in the process of evaluating your child for surgery should take place in an epilepsy center capable of carrying out the full evaluation *and* the surgery.

If the center does not know your child, they will want to review his records carefully and may want to repeat EEGs and scans before deciding if further evaluation is in order. The center might also think that further trials of medication might be useful before considering further evaluation. Sometimes we find that patients referred to us have pseudoseizures, not true electrical seizures (see Chapter 3). Sometimes a diagnosis of pseudoseizures requires video monitoring. Other children have multiple areas of abnormality and thus are not candidates for surgery. However, if, after the initial review, the child is still considered a possible candidate, then the next step is to document that there is indeed a single seizure focus and that it is in an operable location. This will usually require video-EEG recording.

Video-EEG monitoring (see Chapter 7) is the use of continuous monitoring of the EEG with simultaneous video recording to document both the clinical and the electrical onset of the seizures. It is essential to appropriate evaluation for surgery. The duration of this monitoring will depend on the center and on the frequency of the seizures. In general, we schedule one week in the monitoring unit, although for an individual with frequent seizures, a few days is often sufficient to analyze enough spells and determine if there is a consistent focus. If the seizures are less frequent, or if they subside in the hospital setting, as they often do, then we may withdraw one or more of the medications to permit seizures to be recorded. Since this drug withdrawal is done in the hospital setting, with trained personnel readily available should status epilepticus occur, the risk of abrupt withdrawal is minimized.

If, after careful analysis of the recorded seizures, a focus is identified, then consideration of surgery can proceed. If the abnormal area is situated far forward in the temporal lobe or frontal lobe, areas that can be removed safely, then it may be possible to proceed directly to surgery. Surgery should never proceed, of course, until you and the surgeon have fully discussed the risks to your child, the chances of controlling the seizures, and any other questions you or your child may have.

Risk-Benefit Discussion with Your Physicians

Discussion of the possibility of surgery and its risks and benefits should be an ongoing process. When a focus and its location have been identified, surgery can become a more serious consideration, and a more detailed discussion of its risks and benefits is then possible. The risks will depend on the area to be removed. Surgery is most often performed to remove a focus from the frontal or temporal lobes of the brain, areas from which large amounts of tissue can usually be removed without major complications.

As with any operation, there is, of course, a risk of the patient's dying or suffering major complications of anesthesia. While the consequences of anesthetic complication can be great, the chances of a major anesthetic complication's occurring are in the range of less than one per one thousand. Infection also is always a risk; so is bleeding or clotting of a blood vessel. All these are potentially serious and capable of causing additional brain damage. Fortunately, these complications occur infrequently.

Generally, as noted, frontal and temporal lobe removals are considered by neurologists and neurosurgeons to be "safe" procedures, but as with any decision-making process, the risks and their magnitude must be weighed against the possible benefits and the chances that those benefits will occur.

What are the benefits of the focal operations? The maximum benefit would be freedom from seizures, freedom from taking anticonvulsant medicine, and freedom from neurologic deficit due to the surgery.

This is everyone's goal. What are the chances that the goal will be achieved? Surprisingly, it is difficult to give numerical answers to this question. Surgical centers often quote 60–75 percent "good outcomes." This means that perhaps 50 percent of those undergoing an operation will be cured of their seizures, another 10–25 percent will have substantial decrease in the frequency of their seizures, and about 25 percent—one in four—will not be helped.

You cannot, however, apply these statistical figures to your child. Your child's chance of success will depend on the cause of the seizures and the exact location of the focus. The figures quoted also depend on how specific centers select patients for surgery. If they only select "ideal" candidates their success rate will be higher. If they take some of the more difficult patients, they may be less "successful," statistically. Your child is unique and, therefore, the discussion and the chances of success are unique. Recent advances in evaluation techniques may have made your child's chances of having a successful outcome better than the published statistics.

In calculating the statistical chances of successful surgery, it is important to differentiate between surgery to remove a lesion (or tumor) and surgery to remove an "epileptic region." Epilepsy usually comes from the area immediately surrounding a lesion, and a lesion is more easily identified and removed. An epileptic region is more subtle and has less identifiable margins and, therefore, is more difficult to remove completely. The success rate for surgery to remove lesions causing epilepsy is far higher than that for surgery to remove epileptic regions. In general, the latter surgery is more successful when more tissue is removed.

Whether the risks of surgery are worth the possible benefits is a very personal decision. The possibility of being totally free of seizures will have different value to different people. The risks each individual and family are willing to take to achieve that condition are also very personal. However, it is our belief that, in general, physicians and surgeons have been far too conservative in recommending surgery. Temporal lobe removal may be preferable to taking medication for a lifetime, even if the medication is controlling the seizures with minimal side effects. The anterior part of the temporal lobe on either side, as noted, may be removed without causing neurologic problems. Much of the frontal lobe on either side can also be safely removed, although frontal lobe surgery is less successful.

Because language function is usually in the more posterior part of the left frontal and temporal lobes, surgery that might involve that area requires very careful evaluation, in order to weigh the possible risks and benefits. Similarly, since motor function is in the posterior frontal lobe, consideration of surgery near that area also requires careful thought.

When making decisions about surgery, it is your responsibility to look for an epilepsy center that is equipped to evaluate your child properly. Such an epilepsy center should have not only the proper equipment but also the proper team and the proper experience. The best way to find out how capable a center's staff are is to ask them questions. They should not mind your inquiries; in fact, they should encourage you to ask questions.

- Feel free to ask how many children with your child's type of seizures they have evaluated.
- Does the center have a team approach? Do the epileptologists work together with the surgeons in deciding about the surgery and its boundaries? Is there an epilepsy nurse or social worker who can help you and your child prepare for the evaluation?
- Ask about the surgeon's experience. How many similar cases has he or she handled? What were the outcomes?
- Are there other children who have undergone the evaluation? Have they had the surgery? Can you and your child meet them? Can you talk with them about what it was like?

Surgery on the brain is scary. You and your child should enter the decision-making process as partners with your physicians, and you and your child should be well informed and comfortable with your decisions and with your epilepsy team.

Evaluation of Language

Speech is usually located on the left side of the brain, in the posterior frontal and temporal lobes (see Chapter 2). However, in 10 to 15 percent of left-handed people speech is on the right side. It is vital to know where it is before proceeding with surgery.

The Wada test, named after the neurosurgeon Juhn Wada, is designed to localize speech and memory. A catheter is threaded from the groin of the awake patient up to the internal carotid artery, the main artery supplying one side of the brain. After a small injection of a dye, which can be seen on x-ray, a small amount of barbiturate is injected and that side of the brain is briefly "put to sleep."

As the test begins, the patient is asked to hold his arms up in the air and to count. If the injection is done on the left side of the brain, the right arm becomes weak as the left side of the brain goes "to sleep." If speech is on that same side, the patient will simultaneously, but briefly, lose the ability to speak or count. Memory is also tested at this time, by showing the patient objects and pictures. When the medication wears off, the patient will be asked to recall the objects he has seen. Speech and memory, if interrupted during the test, quickly return when the drug wears off. In this crude fashion the laterality (side) of speech is determined. The same procedure may also be carried out on the other side of the brain, because occasionally speech is located on *both* sides.

If testing on the right side produces no change in speech or memory, then it can be assumed that operating on that side will not threaten those skills. If speech is on the left and the surgery is to be done near that area, then a far more careful evaluation of speech, language, and the extent of the epileptic region must precede a decision to operate.

Young children cannot provide the cooperation necessary for a Wada test. However, in young children it is less important, because the brain mechanisms for speech, if damaged at surgery, *will* transfer to the other hemisphere of the brain. In children there is little risk in doing a Wada test. In adults there is a very small chance of a stroke.

Detailed neuropsychologic testing may be performed prior to surgery to assess the patient's intellectual function and personality. Some physicians use these very detailed neuropsychologic tests to assess specific brain functions and to predict their function after the surgery.

Newer scanning and imaging techniques may, in the near future, provide more precise localization of language and speech than is currently possible with the Wada test.

Invasive Studies

When seizures come from the left temporal lobe, where speech may be involved, or when it is critical to know the extent of the epileptogenic region (where the seizures begin) and the location of motor function or speech, careful mapping of the cortex with grids can and should be done. Since this procedure requires an operation to lay the grid directly on the cortex (see Figure 14.1), it is called an invasive procedure.

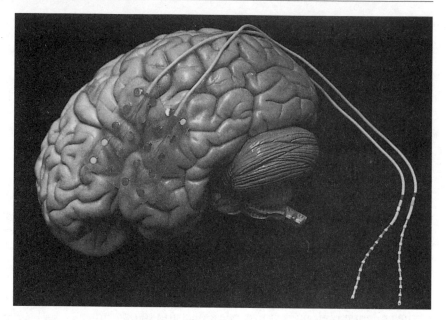

Figure 14.1 Invasive monitoring. The thin sheet of plastic with embedded electrodes, shown placed on a model of the brain, is called a grid. The grid is surgically implanted on the surface of the child's brain with wires running to the outside. The electricity is recorded by an EEG machine. The electrodes can also be used for stimulating the underlying brain, to localize specific functions.

Invasive procedures entail certain risks, which include anesthesia and infection.

A grid is a small plastic sheet with metallic electrodes embedded in it. The number of electrodes will depend on the area to be mapped, and several sheets may be used to cover the area of the cortex in question. The electrodes are connected by fine wires to the outside of the head and attached to the machine that records the electrical impulses, as in any EEG. The electrodes are 1 centimeter apart. Many, many electrodes (more than 100) may be used in assessing a patient's seizures. Depth electrodes, thin wires with spaced electrodes, are sometimes used to locate epileptic regions deep within the brain, where grids cannot reach.

The electrodes not only conduct the underlying brain's electrical impulses and permit recording, but they also can be used to stimulate the cortex with electrical input and thus to map speech and motor areas of the cortex. Electrical stimulation of the cortex, if in the motor strip, can induce the movement of a muscle in the finger, face, or foot, or, if the patient is moving that joint, can inhibit the movement. If the speech area is stimulated, speech can be inhibited; stimulation in the sensory area can induce sensation. By testing exactly which area controls which activities, a map of the cortex can be drawn.

With a map of the epileptogenic areas of the cortex (the areas where seizures start and spread), and a matching map of the eloquent areas of the cortex, we can indicate to the surgeon in precise detail the areas to be removed and the areas to be avoided. While expensive, time-consuming, and very labor-intensive, cortical mapping permits safer, more efficient surgery. It should be possible in the not too distant future to use this experimental technique to map brain function rapidly in the operating room at the time of surgery. Will this replace the week-long, tedious stimulation that is currently the standard of brain mapping? Probably. Will we be able to do this noninvasively at some time in the future? Maybe. Jeff's story illustrates the current process of invasive monitoring.

❏ Jeff was thirteen years old when he first came to us. He had had seizures since he was three and a half years old. His seizures were partial complex in type, typically beginning with a discomfort in his stomach, which he described as nausea, followed about fifteen seconds later by turning his head toward the left, then stiffening of his body, which progressed to a tonic-clonic seizure lasting thirty to forty-five seconds and was followed by a quick return to baseline. He had been tried on many medications and at one time he had had as many as one hundred spells per day. When he came to us his seizures were controlled on two medications. The family wanted to know if the epilepsy could be cured, or if he was going to require medication for the remainder of his life.

EEGs in the past and one video EEG had shown right frontal spikes, and an MRI had shown a suspicious pattern in the right frontal lobe. SPECT scan showed increased blood flow in that area during a seizure, and a PET scan also showed changes in that area. We thought that he might be a candidate for surgery. We had thought that these seizures were originating in the right frontal lobe, but where in the right frontal lobe? Could we take out the epileptic area without causing any damage?

Our medical team discussed with Jeff and his family the process of deciding the risks and benefits of the surgery. Jeff and his family were eager to get on with the surgical evaluation, and Jeff was scheduled for five days of video-EEG monitoring at Hopkins. Although we had reports from his original physician, we feel strongly that if we are to be responsible for the surgery and its outcome, we must also be responsible for making sure of the data at each step of the way.

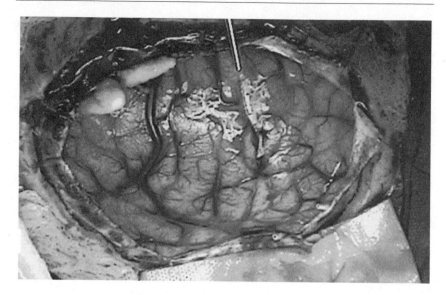

Figure 14.2 Photograph of Jeff's brain at surgery. The skull over the frontal portion has been removed and the brain and the blood vessels can be seen. This is the right side of the brain as seen from above. The back of the head is to the left.

In the monitoring unit, his medications were reduced to allow seizures, and video monitoring confirmed that the seizures were coming from the right frontal lobe; but they seemed to be deep, and not on the surface. How much would the surgery have to remove to take out all of the epileptic focus? Did the seizures involve any of the motor strip (see Figure 2.1) on that side? Was paralysis a risk?

Jeff was scheduled to have a grid applied so we could map the cortex to determine the "epileptic zone" and to identify exact locations in his motor strip. He was admitted to the hospital, and an operation was performed in which a large portion of the skull over the right frontal lobe was removed (Figure 14.2), and the grids (Figure 14.3) were inserted under the dura, the covering of the brain. The grids contained more than a hundred electrodes. Jeff, with the removed portion of skull replaced, the grids in place, and his head bandaged, is shown in Figure 14.4. A skull film showing the placement of the grids is seen in the inset of Figure 14.5.

Over the next seven days, Jeff's seizures were recorded and carefully analyzed to detect the area involved in the seizures, and a map of the cortex was drawn (Figure 14.5) documenting the epileptic area. During this week the cortex was also electrically stimulated through the grid and a map of the motor control

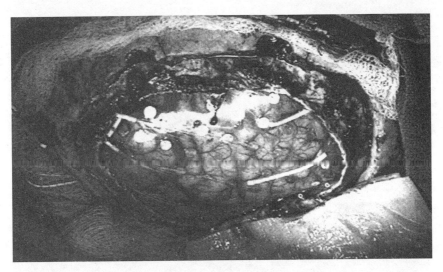

Figure 14.3 Photograph of Jeff's brain after the grid has been put in place. The grids are plastic sheets with multiple silver electrodes embedded in them. The electrodes come in contact with the surface of the brain and record the underlying electrical discharges. The electrodes can also be used to stimulate successive areas of the underlying cortex in order to map the location of specific brain functions. In the photograph the white connecting wires have been cut prior to removal of the grids. During the recording they were used to connect the grid to the EEG machine. The brain can be seen beneath the plastic of the grid.

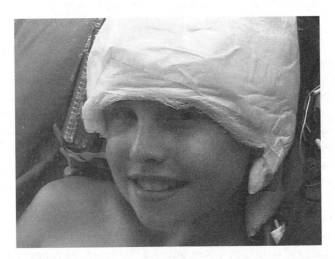

Figure 14.4 Jeff in the epilepsy monitoring unit several days after the grid was implanted. The section of skull has been replaced and the grid is in place beneath it and the bandage.

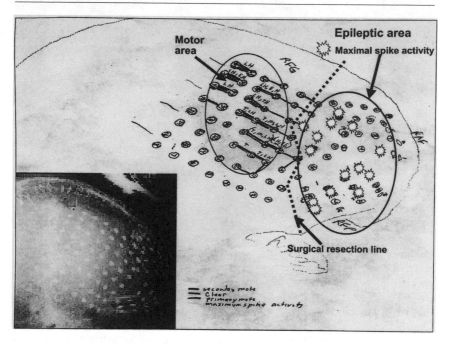

Figure 14.5 The inset is a skull x-ray showing the grid in place. The electrodes are visible. Our map of the cortex shows the areas of seizure discharges and the areas of motor activity located by stimulation. The dotted line is the guide for the surgeon to follow in removing the frontal cortex (the epileptic area) and avoiding the motor areas.

areas (face, tongue, hand) was made. On the basis of this information we decided where the surgeon would cut and what tissue he would remove. As expected, there was a gyrus, a convolution, between the "epileptic area" and the motor cortex, and the surgeon could remove the epileptic area. Since the surgery to remove the epileptic area, Jeff has had no further seizures. He was up walking two days after the surgery and out of the hospital in five days. We are gradually tapering him off his medications.

As we have seen, Jeff's epilepsy surgery was a two-step surgery. Step 1 was placement of the grid. Step 2, the surgery to remove the epileptic area, was planned in advance to be done one week later. At the second surgery the grid would be taken out and the carefully mapped epileptic area of the brain would also be removed, sparing the motor cortex. An important point here is that the basic decisions about doing epilepsy surgery in a case such as this must be made *before* the grid is placed. The grid is used only to determine which areas will be removed and which will be left. Only when unexpected findings make surgery difficult or impossible does excision of tissue not follow grid placement.

Special Techniques for Localization of the Seizure Focus

As we have pointed out, the first step in making decisions about epilepsy surgery is to find whether the seizures start from a single area, a focus.

- The first step in that process is a careful description of the seizure, especially its onset. Does it always start in the same fashion? From the same side? If so, it sounds focal.
- Is the EEG focal, that is, does it show either focal sharp waves or spikes or focal slowing? This would be further evidence of focality and that the child would be a possible surgery candidate.

CT Scanning and MRIs

A CT (computerized tomography) scan may show calcifications (mineral deposits) in a focal lesion, but it is far less sensitive than an MRI (magnetic resonance imaging) scan. As the MRI has become faster and better, it has begun to show lesions we would have missed before. A good MRI with thin cuts, and other sophisticated imaging techniques, can often pinpoint an area of abnormality; or it could show multiple areas of abnormality, which might rule out surgery. In young children, the brain is still developing, and abnormalities that are missed on initial MRIs may become apparent when the MRI is repeated at an older age.

A child with seizures that seem to be focal should have an MRI, even if one done several years earlier was normal. Today's machines are better, the imaging slices are thinner, and during the interval since the previous scan the brain lesion may have become more obvious.

Today's MRI scans can reveal mesial temporal sclerosis (scarring of the inner portion of the temporal lobe). This condition, commonly seen in adults with partial complex seizures and in adults often considered an indication for surgical evaluation, is very rare in children, even those with partial complex seizures.

New techniques with MRI functional imaging (fMRI), which looks at the blood flow in specific areas, are now being used. Functional MRI scans can be used to locate the increased blood flow associated with local brain activity such as moving a finger, visualizing an object, or thinking of words. It should be of increasing use in mapping the brain prior to surgery and perhaps in locating the seizure focus.

Modern computer technology allows three-dimensional reconstructions of both CT scans and MRIs, and these 3-D images may permit visualization of brain abnormalities that can be missed on the typical 2-D images.

Single Proton Emission Computerized Tomography (SPECT)

SPECT scans look at the blood flow in the brain. SPECT scans use a radioactive material that "lights up" in the area of the increased blood flow during the scan. Since blood flow increases immediately with a focal seizure, an injection of the material within the first minutes of the onset of the seizure may reveal the focal area. *The injection must occur almost immediately after the onset of the seizure, so someone must be at the bedside, with the radioactive material handy, when the seizure first registers on the EEG.* This is not as easy as it sounds. The ictal (during seizure) SPECT scan is then compared to the interictal scan to find the location of the increase in blood flow. Both scans must be done in the hospital or monitoring unit to ensure the appropriate EEG monitoring.

Magnetic resonance spectroscopy (MRS)

Magnetic resonance imaging (MRI), which we have previously discussed as a technique for visualizing brain structure, can be used with a slightly different computer program to study brain metabolism. Used in this fashion, it is called magnetic resonance spectroscopy (MRS). By using more powerful computer techniques, it is possible to "tune in" to the energy changes that occur as one chemical compound is converted to another within living cells. Thus, as energy is utilized to fire cells during seizures, the changes in energy can be detected and analyzed. As cell membranes change with this firing or with recovery after their electrical discharge, these changes can be studied. One use of MRS is to differentiate between tumors and scar tissue and between deteriorating tissue and healthy tissue. As the technology continues to evolve, it should be possible to understand better the chemistry and spread of seizures and to develop and visualize the effects of new drugs in blocking the initiation and spread of seizures.

Magnetoencephalography (MEG) and magnetic source imaging

If the U.S. Navy can use changes in magnetic fields to detect a submarine one thousand feet under the sea from a satellite many thousands of feet in the air, then we should be able to detect the changes in magnetic fields generated by a seizure focus two inches under the scalp. And we are beginning to do so.

Submarines, being made of metal, create a minute disturbance of the earth's magnetic field, a disturbance that can be accurately localized by the proper instrumentation in the satellite. Using similar technology, laboratory investigators are beginning to be able to localize the tiny changes in magnetic fields within the brain created by the firing of cells. It should be possible with this technology to localize accurately epileptic foci deep within the brain, but the usefulness of the technology for this purpose remains to be demonstrated.

Computerized mapping of brain function

When a person reads a word, she first sees that word. As the occipital lobe (see Chapter 2) identifies the letters, cells fire. By placing an electrode grid on the surface of the brain, we can now identify that firing of cells. For the word to be recognized, another area of the brain must fire (association cortex). The pattern recognized will be remembered in yet another area. *Saying* that word requires the activation of speech cortex and motor areas. With the availability of extremely powerful and fast computers, we are able to detect these changes occurring at individual electrodes on the grid that has been placed on the brain. In experimental fashion, we are currently able to visualize the electrical changes involved in such a function and its processing through the various regions of the brain.

Making the Final Decision

While each step in the process of evaluation of a child for surgery requires careful thought, it is at the conclusion of the invasive monitoring, when all the available information has been collected, that we decide exactly what would be done during surgery, and reconsideration of the potential risks and benefits is necessary. We accomplish this with a meeting of the whole team that has been involved in the evaluation. This team includes the epilepsy specialist who has been your child's primary physician, our group of monitoring specialists, those who have carefully assessed language and intellectual function, the counselor who has been working closely with the child and the family, and the surgeon who will be performing the operation. At this conference we carefully assess where the seizures appear to be coming from, what surgery can be done to eliminate them, what normal functions might be damaged by the surgery, and other potential risks and benefits of the surgery. At times we decide that surgery should not be performed. After the group reaches consensus, we then present our opinions to the patient and family, who must independently decide whether or not to proceed with surgery, whether their perception of the risks and benefits is similar to ours.

The family's considerations regarding surgery are different from those of the epilepsy team. It is the epilepsy team's responsibility to evaluate whether surgery is feasible and what the medical and physical risks of the surgery are likely to be. The team can also assess the likelihood of seizure control. The value of these benefits to you and your child and the acceptability of the risks must be determined by you and your child. Epilepsy surgery is never an emergency. There is always time to think carefully about the decision, to seek second opinions, and to talk with patients who have undergone the proposed surgery. We have often found it useful to have parents who are anticipating surgery meet with families and children who have previously undergone a similar procedure. It is impossible to conceptualize what a child who has undergone a hemispherectomy (removal of half the brain) will be like without seeing such a child.

There is often a disparity between how the two parents see the problem of their child's seizures and how they feel about the risks and potential benefits of surgery. At visits long before the surgery we discuss with both parents the need for agreement. We emphasize that a child's parents, even divorced parents, must be in agreement before we will proceed. If something goes wrong at surgery, or if the surgery is unsuccessful, we do not ever want one parent to be blaming the other. We often tell parents, "Every morning hereafter you will have to get up and look yourself in the mirror while you shave or put on your makeup. If the surgery goes well, as it usually does, you will smile and say, 'I only wish that we had done it sooner.' But, if things go badly—if your child has complications, if she is worse off than before the surgery, or if she dies (and that is a remote possibility)—you still have to face yourself in that mirror every day and be able to say, 'We made the best decision for our child that we knew how to make.'"

Including the Child in the Decision

Children are often left out of the decision-making process. Depending on their age and their level of function, however, they should be included. Older children should participate in the decision to do surgery. They must understand the probable outcomes of the surgery. Meeting another child who has had surgery may help them assess the situation. Unless the child agrees to the surgery, and unless both parents are in agreement, surgery should not be performed.

Jamie's story is an example of the importance of the child's participation.

❏ Jamie was twelve years old, part of a large loving family. Jamie had developed seizures two years before coming to see us, and the seizures had been progressive. They were occurring twenty times per day (if you only counted the big ones), with a thousand or more jerks of his left arm and leg each day. Jamie had been using a wheelchair, but his seizures had become so frequent and so violent that they threw him from his wheelchair. He now spent his time on the floor and crawled to get around. He had been out of school for almost a year. He had been home schooled and was obviously quite bright.

Jamie had Rasmussen's syndrome, an autoimmune process which eats away at one hemisphere like a Pac-Man and causes uncontrollable seizures and progressive loss of function on one side of the body. At that time the only treatment was removal of one-half of the brain, a hemispherectomy.

After long discussions with the family, and with Jamie, who agreed, the surgery was scheduled several months in the future. His folks had continued to talk with him, and Jamie was eager to get it over with. The day before the surgery was scheduled, we met with the family to go over last-minute questions. Much to our (and the family's) shock, Jamie said he didn't want surgery. Jamie was scared, although too proud to admit it. "I'm fine," he said. After considerable discussion, he remained adamant, so we said, "Okay. We'll cancel it." Then we added, "But you understand, Jamie, that you have a whole life ahead of you. You can't spend it at home, on the floor, with your family waiting on you. You *will* go back to school next week, in the wheelchair, tied in if necessary. You *will* do chores around the house."

Jamie went to lunch with his family and had a seizure, which threw him from the wheelchair. His older siblings pointed out that he *wasn't* fine. They reminded him of all the things he couldn't do and that they couldn't do together. After lunch he and the family came back and Jamie asked if he could still have the surgery.

The surgery went well and Jamie is back in school, walking, and without seizures.

Surgery for Other Types of Seizures

We have discussed the evaluation and decision making involved in surgery for focal lesions, but what if the lesion is not focal? What if it involves all or most of one hemisphere? What if it is multifocal and involves areas on both sides? What can be done then?

Hemispherectomy

For generations we *knew* that if there were problems during the development of the brain, then both sides of the brain would be affected. We *knew* that if a child was retarded, then both sides must be involved. We *knew* that if seizures looked like infantile spasm and the child had retardation, then the whole brain must be involved. All of these things that we *thought we knew* were not necessarily true.

- We now know that one side of the brain can have major developmental abnormalities but the other side can be normal or virtually normal. We know this because advances in MRI scanning have allowed us to see one-sided abnormalities. Removal of the abnormal side can relieve or eliminate seizures and allow a child to have relatively normal development. We must conclude therefore that the remaining hemisphere was normal.
- We now know that a congenital hemipareses (weakness on one side) due to newborn strokes can produce seizures *and* cause developmental delay. These seizures may be one sided, or may spread to both sides, or may be atonic or infantile spasm–like. Such seizures may be drug resistant but may cease with removal of the affected hemisphere, without increasing the weakness on one side and allowing normal intellectual development. The rate of development may actually improve after removal of the abnormal half of the brain.
- We know that unilateral vascular problems, such as Sturge-Weber abnormalities, can produce unilateral seizures and progressive intellectual delay which can be prevented by removal of the affected hemisphere.
- We now know that the progressive unilateral condition termed Rasmussen's syndrome can be cured by removal of the affected hemisphere.

Before we discuss each of these conditions, we know you are think-ing, "How can you even consider removing half of the brain?" "What will happen to the child's memory? To speech? To walking?" "I'd rather that my child be dead than allow you to take out half of her brain and leave her severely brain damaged."

Here are some facts that address these perfectly reasonable ques-tions.

- After removal of half of the brain all children are able to walk and run, and some even dance. Use of one leg is not normal, but the mild paralysis that results from the surgery is not handicap-ping.
- After removal of half of the brain, the arm on the opposite side is always impaired. Although there is some movement at the shoulder and elbow, there is no useful movement or sensation in the hand. It becomes just a helper hand.
- After removal of half of the brain there is a hemianopsia (no vi-sion to one side of the body.) Children largely compensate for this and do not bump into things, but the hemianopsia may be an impediment to driving a car.
- After removal of half of the brain, children do not forget any-thing they have previously learned. Old memories are retained. They remember McDonald's and Grandma's house and choco-late chip cookies. The remember everything they had learned in school. These memories remain regardless of which side is re-moved.
- After removal of the left side of the brain, where speech is usu-ally located, speech will return. Young children with congenital abnormalities of the left hemisphere may have better speech af-ter removal of the left side, since the electrical abnormalities of the left hemisphere will no longer interfere with the transfer and function of speech in the right side. Older children with a pro-gressive disorder, such as Rasmussen's syndrome, will lose speech facility if the left side is affected and will regain it only af-ter the diseased side is removed. The older the child, the longer it takes for speech skills to return and the more difficult they are to relearn. Even in the early teen years speech comes back and will be close to normal.
- After removal of half of the brain, children return to school. Some children who have had this surgery have made the honor roll, gone to college, and held a job.

• After a hemispherectomy many children are normal children with a paralyzed arm and without the incapacitating seizures.

Hemispherectomy is not a common type of surgery and should be done only in an epilepsy center that has experience with the procedure and its aftercare. The center should have a pediatric epileptologist with experience in the conditions treatable with hemispherectomy, a neurosurgeon who has done some of them, and a rehabilitation team that has worked with such children after the surgery. *The surgery and rehabilitation are not easy.*

Hemispherectomy is done for three types of problems: Rasmussen's syndrome, congenital vascular problems such as strokes or Sturge-Weber syndrome, and developmental problems on one side of the brain. Each has its own considerations and each its own outcomes.

For Developmental Problems

❑ Eva was a beautiful baby. Her mother had had a perfect pregnancy. But at two months of age Eva began to have seizures on the right side of her body. An initial EEG showed spikes on both sides of the brain, and an MRI showed the right side of her brain to be smaller than the left. Several anticonvulsant medications given over the next several months had no effect on the multiple seizures she was having each day. She was making no developmental progress.

Her parents brought her to an epilepsy center for a second opinion, and she was reevaluated there. Right-side seizures should mean a left-side brain abnormality. The second evaluation revealed that the problem was not that the right side of her brain was smaller but that the left side was larger and malformed. Eva had unilateral hemimegalencephaly (see Figure 14.6). Video-monitoring showed that most of the seizures were coming from the left side of Eva's brain, but the right side was thought perhaps to be involved as well. By now, at seven months, Eva was displaying obvious left-handedness, further indication that the left side of her brain was involved.

Removal of the abnormal left side was suggested, but the family was unwilling to accept the consequences of the surgery. They didn't want their child to have a paralyzed arm and only half a brain. "Eva's only problem is her seizures. There are many new medications. Perhaps they will help," they said.

Over the next nine months Eva's seizures continued and her development fell further behind. The weakness on her right side became more apparent. By eighteen months she smiled, laughed, and babbled, but she could not sit or stand and had no real words. Her loving family had become increasingly aware

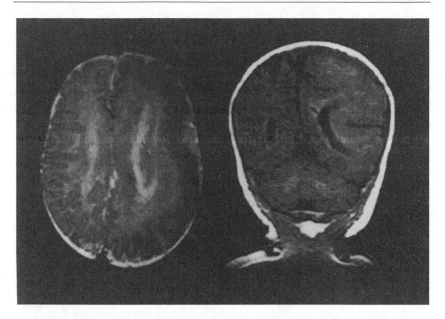

Figure 14.6 MRI showing unilateral hemimegalencephaly. In this case, unlike Eva's, the right side of the brain is larger, and it is very malformed. A hemispherectomy was performed to treat this condition.

of her deficits and increasingly apprehensive about the future. The newer medications were working no better than the standard ones, and they were affecting her personality. Another opinion confirmed the possible benefits of surgery.

A left hemispherectomy was done without problems when Eva was two years old. Since surgery she has had no seizures. Within six months, she was standing, beginning to walk, and talking in short phrases. After a year she was off all anticonvulsant medications.

Children such as Eva, who have developmental problems, often have difficult-to-control seizures within the first days or weeks of life. The abnormalities may not be readily apparent on an MRI scan at this age, because of the lack of brain development. They may become apparent only as the child becomes older. In young children, unilateral seizures that are frequent and persistent despite one or two medications strongly suggest a developmental abnormality. If the seizures persist, an opinion from an epilepsy center is indicated and video monitoring may be helpful. We advocate early surgery for such children and have done hemispherectomies in children as young as three months of age. Would Eva have developed better if she had had earlier surgery? We'll never know. Is her slight delay associated with mild but nonepileptic developmental abnormalities on the remaining hemisphere? We can't tell.

Evaluation of infants with developmental abnormalities has to be done very carefully. Although one side may be clearly abnormal, spikes may be seen on the other side on EEGs and may be only a reflection of the epilepsy on the bad side. We have often told parents: "One side is terrible. We are not sure about the other side, but it looks reasonably good. If both sides are bad, the future looks bleak. If this is mainly, or exclusively, coming from the bad side and we take it out, the remaining half will function better and may not have seizures." All of the children with congenital dysplasias on whom we have operated have done better, and most are seizure-free, although many still have developmental delay.

Hemispherectomy in very young children should be done only in one of the small number of epilepsy centers that has experience in the surgery and has a pediatric epilepsy team. The Johns Hopkins center has performed more than a hundred hemispherectomies. Among our early hemispherectomies on young infants we had three deaths and two near tragedies. Having gained more experience, our team has had no deaths in the past ten years.

The outcome for the child depends primarily on how normal the remaining half of the brain is. The health of that half cannot necessarily be accurately predicted prior to the removal of the "bad" half. It is our experience, however, that having *no* brain tissue on one side is preferable to having constant electrical interference coming from abnormal brain tissue. It appears that this constant electrical interference impairs the function of the better side.

For Vascular Problems

Strokes in very young children do not necessarily look like strokes in older children or adults. Strokes may occur prior to birth or in the perinatal period. They may be accompanied by some difficulty during delivery, or by a few seizures in the days after delivery. They may be silent and only detected if a scan or an ultrasound of the head is performed, as might be done if the child is slightly delayed in development and is found to be displaying handedness too early, during the first year of life. (Children do not usually show a definite hand preference until they are over one year of age.) Sometimes, looking back at baby pictures you can see that the child was splashing in the tub with only one hand or one foot.

Strokes in the newborn are usually of unknown cause, but they may be due to abnormalities of blood clotting, and your physician will want to check the child's bleeding and clotting factors.

Children who have had strokes may in most ways be normal, but they are sometimes slightly slow in sitting, do not prop themselves well on one side, and may be slow in walking or talking. Such children, even those who have had large one-sided strokes, are usually of normal intelligence. They may or may not have seizures. It is difficult to predict which of the children who have seizures (usually unilateral seizures or focal seizures which secondarily generalize) will go on to have difficult-to-control epilepsy.

If your child has a congenital hemiparesis (weakness on one side), *and* the child has seizures that are not controlled by the first or second drug (used appropriately), you may want to consider having the child evaluated for a hemispherectomy at an epilepsy center. Children with seizures due to structural abnormalities of the brain who do not respond to the first two anticonvulsant medications are unlikely to respond to others. Since that child already has weakness on one side of the body and probably has loss of vision on that side as well, removal of the bad tissue can eliminate the seizures without increasing the child's neurologic deficit. The surgery can eliminate the need for medication and can, if the left side of the brain is affected, actually improve speech by eliminating the electrical interference that may be influencing speech areas on the right side.

For Sturge-Weber Syndrome

Sturge-Weber syndrome (discussed in Chapter 8) is a unilateral congenital vascular problem that produces seizures, a progressive hemiparesis (weakness on one side), and often mental retardation. At one time the affected hemisphere was removed in early childhood to prevent the effects of the seizures on the child's development, since it was believed that the hemiparesis was inevitable. Few physicians now advise doing this procedure prophylactically, but if the seizures are difficult to control, a hemispherectomy may control the seizures and prevent much of the handicap. Some physicians advocate removing only the affected portion of the brain.

For Rasmussen's Syndrome

Rasmussen's syndrome (also discussed in Chapter 8) is a progressive condition that eats away one side of the brain. It is probably due to an autoimmune condition that destroys neurons. It produces weakness, mental deterioration, and, if in the left hemisphere, loss of speech, and it also produces very severe focal or unilateral epilepsy. These seizures may be constant in one portion of the brain (*epilepsia partialis continua*) or may be unilateral with hundreds of seizures per day.

Anticonvulsant medications are ineffective, and immunotherapy with steroids, plasmapheresis, or intravenous gamma globulin treatments provide only temporary relief from the progression. Brain biopsy may not prove the condition is present and may make the condition worse. If only the portion of the brain most severely affected is removed, the condition always recurs in the adjacent portions. The only successful treatment to date has been hemispherectomy. Beth's story is one case. (Jamie's story, on page 233, is another.)

❏ **Beth was a bright, vivacious almost five-year-old when she fell off of a see-saw and had a generalized seizure. A CT scan showed atrophy in the left hemisphere, but she had no neurological deficit. Shortly thereafter she began to have more seizures, these on the right side of her body. They did not respond to medication, and gradually she began to limp on the right leg and to have increasing difficulty with speech. Clearly something was continuing to happen to the left side of her brain. Another hospital diagnosed Rasmussen's syndrome and said there was nothing they could do, that this process would continue to destroy her brain.**

Six months later her seizures were occurring several times a day and her speech and right-sided paralysis had worsened. She was seen at Johns Hopkins, and we agreed that she had Rasmussen's syndrome. We told the family that this condition would become worse, that children with it become retarded and severely handicapped. The only treatment was to remove the left side of Beth's brain.

Since at this time Beth was walking, talking, and had only slight intellectual deterioration, the family, quite understandably, was reluctant to subject their daughter to a risky operation that would leave her paralyzed on one side and might cause a problem with her ability to speak. They decided to wait.

Six months later, when Beth was clearly having more difficulty with her seizures, with the right side of her body, and with school, they decided she should have the operation.

The operation was a success! After a stormy postoperative period, Beth has made a remarkable recovery. She is left-handed and uses her right hand only minimally. Her speech and reading are entirely normal. She has had no seizures since surgery and is on no medications. She has gone on to college, is doing well, and doing volunteer work with handicapped children. Apart from the lack of use of her right arm, she is a normal young woman.

We hope that before the next edition of this book appears we will have found a less drastic approach to the treatment of the autoimmune-like disease called Rasmussen's syndrome.

"What do you do when the epilepsy comes from both sides of the brain?"

Unfortunately, much of the difficult-to-control epilepsy is multifocal and involves both sides of the brain. We cannot take out both hemispheres or do brain transplants. We are making great progress in learning to treat these severe epilepsies with new medications, some of which will work when all prior ones have failed. However, there are, at present, only two surgical approaches in these cases, vagus nerve stimulation and corpus callosum sectioning.

Vagus Nerve Stimulation

The vagus nerve runs from the brain stem down the neck and controls heart rate and the diaphragm. Studies have shown that stimulation of it can have an effect on certain types of epilepsy. It appears that the impulses go up the vagus nerve to the brain and help the brain stop seizing.

The vagus nerve stimulator is a small device, roughly the size of a silver dollar but several times as thick, which is implanted under the skin of the chest. The stimulator contains a battery and can be programmed to send electrical impulses through small wires, also implanted, which run under the skin and wrap around the left vagus nerve, in the neck. The stimulation travels upward via the vagus nerve, ending up in the brain. The operation to implant the stimulator takes about an hour and the individual often returns home the same day.

The stimulator can be turned on by a magnet carried by the patient. If the patient has an aura preceding the seizures, activating the stimulator may prevent the full seizure. In addition, the stimulator is programmed to deliver small electrical discharges at set intervals. The settings of stimulator, such as the timing of the impulses, the interval between them, and the amount of the electrical discharge, can be modified to achieve optimal seizure control for each patient. The changes are made using a computer to send a signal through a wand placed over the battery. Every three to five years, the battery of the stimulator must be replaced, which requires a minor surgical procedure.

While the vagus nerve stimulator can decrease seizures in patients who have continued to have seizures despite most of the newer medications and who are not candidates for epilepsy surgery, less than 5 percent of patients are seizure-free on this treatment alone, and most remain on medications. Many of these severely impaired patients feel that their quality of life has been improved by the treatment. The size of the stimulator limits its use in very small children.

Corpus Callosum Sectioning

The corpus callosum is the major pathway connecting one hemisphere of the brain with the other. Some seizures that are focal or multifocal in origin will spread throughout the cortex by the pathway of the corpus callosum and become generalized tonic-clonic seizures. Others will spread by this pathway to deeper structures and lead to atonic and minor-motor drop spells. When an individual is severely handicapped by these generalized seizures, and when the seizures are unresponsive to anticonvulsant medication, sectioning (cutting) of the corpus callosum may prevent spread of the seizure and abolish the generalized component. Sectioning of the corpus callosum does not stop focal seizures, and indeed may sometimes increase them, but focal seizures are more easily tolerated than generalized ones.

After this operation, often done in two stages, there is usually a 50 to 70 percent decrease in the atonic and generalized tonic-clonic seizures. There is little experience with this procedure in young children, where its success rate and its effect on the child's developing nervous system are less understood.

This operation seems to be losing favor. Unlike hemispherectomy patients, who seem to make important gains in intellectual function after surgery and sometimes improve their motor function as well, after corpus callosum section, children and adults seem less likely to experience substantial intellectual or motor improvement. The life of these individuals may be dramatically improved with cessation of the akinetic seizures. Total seizure control, however, is uncommon.

Both the vagus nerve stimulator and sectioning of the corpus callosum may improve the quality of life for individuals severely impaired by bilateral or multifocal seizures who are not candidates for resection of brain tissue. The strong advantage of the vagus nerve stimulator is that it can be turned off or even removed. Sectioning of the corpus callosum is irreversible. Neither approach cures seizures. Virtually none of the individuals undergoing these procedures are seizure-free or medication-free. The quality of life for many is improved, however.

Summary

Surgery for epilepsy has made great strides, but it still has a long way to go. We are now able to localize epileptic cortex with EEGs, various scanning techniques, video monitoring, and grid mapping. We can remove small or large amounts of epileptic cortex while leaving the remaining cortex intact and functional. In general we advocate removing enough, but not too much. "Enough" in children, who have remarkable abilities to recover, is the largest area possible around the epileptic area without encroaching on "eloquent" functional cortex. The risks of the surgery must always be balanced against the benefits of freedom from seizures.

Perhaps our major advances have come from newer imaging techniques. Seizures once thought to be idiopathic are sometimes now found to be due to small areas of abnormal cortex. As newer and better techniques are developed for discovering and localizing these areas, more seizures may be treated successfully with surgery. When an individual has difficult-to-control seizures, brain surgery, once thought to be a last resort, should be thought of early. Perhaps surgery should become a consideration when any individual, child or adult, has seizures that do not respond to two medications used properly.

Tips for Parents of Children Undergoing Invasive Monitoring or Surgery

If your child is old enough to understand, be sure that you have prepared him or her well for the hospitalization and for the procedure. The unknown is always more frightening than something that has been explained.

Monitoring

Prior to the monitoring you should have a discussion with the staff on the monitoring unit. You should ask:

• What is the room like?
• Is the child allowed to move about the room?
• What clothes should we bring?
• What toys and videos may we bring? What will they have on the unit?
• How will the electrodes be placed?

Monitoring is a very boring time for the child.

• Bring a bag of inexpensive "surprises." Games, toys, books can be wrapped ahead of time. Each day allow the child to pick one as a reward for having done well that day. We call these incentives, not bribes.
• Bring a favorite stuffed animal or two and a favorite blanket.
• Bring clothes and pajamas that don't pull over the head.

Monitoring is a very anxious time for parents. Some common questions asked by parents are:

• Will my child have enough seizures for the monitoring to be useful?
• If they reduce the medications, will he have too many seizures? Will he have status epilepticus?
• How long will it take to get "enough" seizures? How many is enough?
• Will they get enough seizures and be able to operate?

Don't be afraid to ask these and other questions before and during the monitoring.

Surgery

If surgery is planned, preparing the child and the rest of the family (siblings included) is essential. No matter how calm your child may seem on the outside, on the inside the child, the siblings, and the parents are frightened. Appropriately so!

Sometimes presurgical counseling is useful for the child and for siblings. Ask your neurologist or neurosurgeon if they can help. Talking with other families and children who have been through the surgical procedure can be invaluable. Ask them how they felt. Ask how they dealt with specific problems. Ask what problems to anticipate. Ask for practical tips. Most parents are delighted and eager to share their experiences, both the good and the bad, and even their most personal feelings. We have found that our parent support network is one of our greatest assets and that every parent benefits from those who have gone before, and everyone is willing to help those who will come after. Older children are also willing to share their experiences with an individual of a similar age. Both children derive benefit.

For some children, particularly teenage girls, the most traumatic part of the surgery may be having to have their head shaved. Kids are often very concerned about how they will look with their head shaved. We often suggest that girls with long hair change their hair style in the weeks prior to the surgery, gradually adopting a shorter and shorter style. Some dads (and an occasional mom) have shaved their own heads as a mark of solidarity with their child. We suggest that you have the head completely shaved on the day prior to arriving at the hospital. (Our surgery staff are not very good at it.) Be sure to buy lots of hats prior to your arrival. We have not found that wigs are very useful for children, but their hair grows back amazingly rapidly.

❏ **Colleen was a charming twelve-year-old with a long black pony tail going down her back. She had difficult-to-control seizures due to a cyst in her right temporal lobe. When we recommended surgery and told her that her head would have to be shaved she responded, "No way, José! I'm not going to cut my hair. I'd rather have seizures!" We continued to try different medications without success, as Colleen remained adamant about not cutting her hair in order to have surgery.**

Finally, when Colleen was sixteen and her friends began to drive, she asked if we could still do the surgery and get rid of her seizures. Her parents bought her a wig and lots of hats, and she had her head shaved the day before the surgery. The surgery went spectacularly well, and Colleen was discharged five days after the surgery. The staples used to close the scalp incision were still in place, and they showed under her cap, but she felt so well when she went home that the next day she went to the mall with a friend. They encountered a teenager who had four earrings, a lip ring, and an eyebrow stud. "Cool," was the teen's comment on noticing the staples. "Where did you get those?" Colleen explained that she had just had brain surgery. There was a prolonged silence, and then a profuse apology.

We tell this story often, because it puts head shaving in perspective. The hair grows back rapidly. It does often grow back curly even if its was straight before surgery.

The Hospital Routine for Patients Undergoing Surgery

Every hospital has a different routine, and surgeons have different preferences. We are going to present the Hopkins routine for you as an example, but be sure to ask about the timelines and routines at the hospital where your child is having surgery.

- Our children usually have a preoperative evaluation on the day before surgery. They will be checked for infection, and blood will be drawn to check for bleeding and clotting abnormalities and for cross-matching. The child and the parents will see the neurologist and/or the neurosurgeon to answer any last minute questions that any of them may have.
- Instructions are given about eating and drinking on the morning of the surgery, where and when to report for surgery.
- The anticipated duration of the surgery, and why it takes so long, is also discussed. We explain that it takes time to put the child to sleep, to put in all the appropriate intravenous lines, and to shave the head and prepare the scalp. Often, two hours have elapsed *before* the operation even begins.
- Nurses or physicians come out of the operating room from time to time to update the parents on the progress of the surgery.
- When the surgery is completed it may take one to two hours to put everything back together.

Most of the time the child is in the operating room is spent getting the child ready for the operation and closing after the operation. *The time you spend waiting only* seems *to last forever.*

After surgery, all of our children go to our ICU (intensive care unit), where they have one-to-one nursing.

- We tell parents how much time will elapse before the child will be transferred from the ICU to the epilepsy monitoring unit or to the less intensive care floor, depending on the surgery performed.
- We warn parents to expect the child's eyes to be swollen and to expect him to have headaches, which we medicate.
- We try to prepare parents for the worst, since they are then relieved when it is not so bad.

• We warn families that when the doctors come around to check on the child they often do not linger, and that therefore they should write down their list of questions so they will remember to ask them. Under the stresses of the surgery and the postoperative period, questions can easily be forgotten.

We also tell parents to have discussions with the child's school administrators and teachers and with the other students so that they all will know about the surgery and about what to expect when the child returns to class with a shaved head and a scar. If the other children know, they can be very supportive.

We'll discuss postoperative rehabilitation in another chapter. Suffice it to say here that after some types of surgery rehabilitation is imperative, while after other types of surgery rehabilitation is unnecessary.

Part Four

Coping with Epilepsy

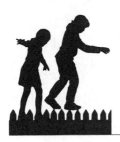

15. Coping with Seizures and Epilepsy

There are many different kinds of seizures, and each may affect you and your child in a different fashion. Some children will have only one seizure. Others may have many. You, the parent, will have to find a way of coping, and so will your child. The child's strategy will vary with his or her age, and the strategies of both of you will vary with your personalities as well as with the type and frequency of seizures. But common themes run through all these variations.

Since a single seizure usually has its greatest effect on the parent, it is parents of these children who need advice first. In the second part of this chapter, we discuss how parents and a child can cope with epilepsy itself.

The First "Big" Seizure

What You Should Know

"Richard had a seizure!" his mother shouted to her husband over the phone. "He's on his way to the emergency room in an ambulance! They said that he had a grand mal seizure! Meet me there right away!"

A generalized tonic-clonic, shaking seizure (once called grand mal) is the type most frightening to parents. This one seizure has changed your life. Can you ever look at your child the same way again? Can you really let him go out and play in the backyard without watching him? Suppose he has another seizure? Maybe he could hurt himself. What would the neighbors think if they knew? Will your best friend still let her son come over to play? Will she take the responsibility of watching him? How about the school? Do you want them to know? Do you want it on his records? Will the school allow him to be normal, to do all the things his classmates are doing?

The first thing you need is information. You need to talk to your doctor about what he thinks caused the seizure, about tests and treatment, and about your child's future. If your child's seizure was related to a virus or head trauma (a provoked seizure), it is unlikely to recur. When your child recovers and whatever caused the seizure is gone, the seizures will be gone. If the seizure was caused by a fever (a febrile seizure), your child will probably need a few tests but no treatment and will outgrow these seizures as he gets older.

"But what caused the seizure?"

After most first seizures, the doctor will respond, "I don't know." She may say, "It was idiopathic" (that's medicine's expensive word for "I don't know").

Physicians are very uncomfortable saying "I don't know." They are trained to search for reasons, for causes, so that they can treat or eliminate the cause. That is why, after a first seizure, many physicians will do unnecessary tests—CT scans, MRI scans, blood and urine tests—to look for chemical or metabolic imbalances. Only when most possibilities have been exhausted, maybe even when "an expert" neurologist also cannot find a cause, is the doctor willing to accept "I don't know."

Parents are also frustrated with "I don't know." Medicine has oversold its ability to find causes. Until all the tests are done and all the experts seen, many parents remain anxious, fearing the worst, and are unwilling to accept the concept of "idiopathic."

In almost three-quarters of the cases of children with seizures in childhood, no cause can be found. Under these circumstances, it is understandable for a parent to be very anxious. We emphasize to parents that the best thing is to *not* to find a cause. It is *best* if the seizures are "idiopathic." *Idiopathic* means there is no known cause. The *known* causes of seizures are: tumor, infections, structural problems, vascular problems, metabolic causes, and trauma. Would you rather that your child's seizures were due to a tumor? A structural problem like a cyst or a malformation? Of course not! You would prefer the child's seizures to be of unknown cause.

• Seizures of unknown cause are the least likely to recur.
• Seizures of unknown cause are the most likely to be controlled with medication.
• Seizures of unknown cause are the most likely to be outgrown, even if they do recur.
• Seventy percent of seizures in childhood are idiopathic.
• Seventy percent of first idiopathic seizures do not recur.

"Will my child be retarded?"

No! A single tonic-clonic seizure does not cause mental retardation or brain damage! Nor do recurrent seizures cause mental retardation or brain damage. It is true that tonic-clonic and other seizures occur more often among children who already have learning problems, brain dysfunction, brain damage, or mental retardation, but there is no evidence that seizures make these conditions worse. *Most* children with such problems do not have seizures, and *most* children who have seizures do not have these problems.

Of course you are afraid that seizures will recur, but don't let this anxiety control your life or your child's life. Don't allow it to make you so overprotective that your child can't play or go outside without your constant supervision. If no new seizure comes, think of the single seizure like a fall out of a tree, something frightening at the time but now over and not influencing your life or your child's life forever.

If seizures do recur, most likely they will recur within two to three months after the first seizure. It might be reasonable to be a bit more cautious during this brief period. Maybe your child shouldn't be climbing trees or be in other potentially dangerous situations during this time. But there's no reason why he can't swim, play most sports, go on field trips, and lead an otherwise normal life.

What Do You Tell Your Child after a Single Seizure?

Be truthful and be simple. What you should tell your child depends on your child's age, sophistication, and level of understanding. It is always best to be truthful. Otherwise, sooner or later you may get trapped in a web of lies and cover-ups that will only make things worse. If your child does not ask questions, it may be because he's too frightened and unable to articulate his fear. So don't take his silence as meaning he has no concerns. Remember that your child probably has no memory of the event that was so frightening to you. His first memory is likely to be of awakening in the ambulance or in the hospital emergency room. He is likely to be frightened because he doesn't know what happened—and is as fearful now of the unknown as you were.

To a young child, your explanation may be as simple as, "You had a seizure. You couldn't talk to me for a few minutes, and Mommy and Daddy got very excited and called the doctor, but he says that you're fine."

For an older child, you might talk about what a seizure is, about electricity in the brain, and tell him that a seizure is like a short circuit or a little static on the radio. The preteenager or teenager needs a more in-depth explanation. Your doctor or a nurse could do this, but you should discuss it with your child as well. He has heard about seizures and may have many misunderstandings. Give your child a chance to ask questions. Contact your local epilepsy foundation or the National Epilepsy Foundation (see Chapter 24). Get some of the Epilepsy Foundation's publications geared to his age.

Explain that while there is no guarantee that a similar episode will not occur, most children never have another one. He is still your normal boy (or girl) and everything is fine now. Be truthful and reassuring. Let him know that you were scared, too, but that when you understood what had happened you were no longer afraid.

What Do You Tell Other Children after a Single Seizure?

Using the same criteria we've discussed above about age appropriateness, reassure your other children. Brothers and sisters need to understand what happened, why you're upset, why you may be treating their brother or sister differently, and whether it will ever happen to them. Friends and playmates or schoolmates may or may not need to know, depending on whether they witnessed the seizure. If they did, you obviously need to explain. You need to reassure them that their friend is all right and that they can't catch a seizure as if it were a cold. If friends didn't see the seizure happen, you should consider the pros and cons of telling them about something that may never happen again. Remember that your child may tell them something on his own.

What Do You Tell Grandparents and Friends after a Single Seizure?

What you tell grandparents and friends depends on many factors. There is no right answer. After a single seizure in a child who is otherwise well, you might decide to tell them nothing. Or you might decide to give them the same frank, simple explanation that you give to older children. The most frightening thing about seizures is the uncertainty. At this stage no one knows if or when they will recur. This frightening anticipation of the unknown is often far worse than the reality of a second seizure itself.

There is something to be gained and something to be lost by discussing the seizure with family and friends. Saying nothing may prevent some overprotection and the constant observation and anxiety. But informing them about the seizure may allow them to cope better should another seizure occur. Reassurance to grandparents and friends that seizures are common, benign, not life threatening, and do not necessarily indicate a brain tumor or any other bad disease of the brain may be an important ingredient in helping your child lead a normal life.

What you tell others depends on who the others are, their relationships to you and your child, and the frequency of their contact—and their personalities. You will have to use your own judgment, but, in general, we prefer openness.

What Do You Tell the School after a Single Seizure?

In the best of all possible worlds, clearly you would tell the school about the seizure. Unfortunately, this is not the best of worlds. Prejudice, misconceptions, overconcern, and fear of seizures still exist. Therefore, there is no simple correct answer to the question. In general, there is no need to tell the school about a single seizure. There is nothing school officials can do, or should do, about your child. They need not watch him more carefully unless he is participating in gymnastics that would place him at heights or is swimming. They should not restrict him from playing on sports teams or at recess. He should be allowed to go on field trips and to do everything the other children do. Since there is nothing special school personnel need to do after a single seizure, it's probably not necessary to let them know about it. What or whether you tell the school about the seizure may depend on your assessment of the teacher, the principal, and the school nurse and how you think they will react to the information. If your son or daughter does have another seizure, and if it occurs in school, you will wish that you had told them if you did not. After a second or third tonic-clonic seizure, or with epilepsy, it's a different matter, which we will discuss later.

This same philosophy applies to day care and to babysitters. Individuals acting as surrogate parents should have the same information and philosophy about overprotection you have.

Schoolteachers and school administrators are apprehensive about what they don't know or understand. In today's suit-prone society they are even more nervous. This is why we don't necessarily recommend telling them about a single seizure. The same is true for day care workers, babysitters, sports coaches, and others who come in transient contact with your child. Although there could be another seizure, and you might wish that you had told them in advance, remember there is a 70 percent chance that another seizure will never occur.

"My step-father (mother, aunt, etc.) thinks that I should get another opinion. What do you think?"

Your physician should never be hesitant about referring you to another physician for a second opinion. If he or she is hesitant, then we would recommend that you get another physician. However, after a single seizure is probably not a time to get a second opinion. There is general consensus among physicians that no treatment is needed at this point. If your child doesn't need medication or further testing, and you don't need to place any restrictions on your child, then a second opinion isn't going to tell you anything you don't already know. But sometimes hearing it again can be reassuring. If your child has another seizure, or if there are other things about your child that are of concern, then talk further with your physician. Perhaps he or she can be of help, or perhaps he can recommend a specialist in your area of concern.

Recurrent Tonic-Clonic Seizures: Epilepsy

If seizures do recur, your response will be different from your reaction after the first seizure. You have already been through the initial shock of seeing tonic-clonic shaking. You have probably come to terms with your initial anxiety. Perhaps you know what to do this second time and are less frightened than at first. But you may be discouraged. Your hopes that a seizure would not recur have been dashed. What is worse, your physician has now used the word *epilepsy*. Although *epilepsy* simply means recurrent seizures, the term still carries a lot of baggage—myths, mystiques, and prejudices—as we discuss earlier in this book.

When many people think of epilepsy, they think of the child who is severely handicapped by continuing seizures. Yet those children are a small subgroup of children with epilepsy. The largest group are those with "benign epilepsy of childhood," who have seizures that can be controlled with medicines and that are usually outgrown. In most children with epilepsy (eight out of ten), seizures can be controlled—

yes, completely controlled. When a child's epilepsy is under control, it shouldn't significantly alter his life or yours. The myths are wrong!

For one in five children with epilepsy, however, seizures may be difficult to control. Control will require trying out different medications, coping with their side effects, and perhaps even surgery. If your child has difficult-to-control epilepsy, your life and your child's life are obviously going to change in significant ways.

Which group will your child fit into? After only a second or even after a third tonic-clonic seizure, it may be difficult to tell. We are beginning to be able to predict this, as we indicate in Chapter 11.

Benign Epilepsy of Childhood

Once upon a time epilepsy was considered a chronic disease. People who had two or more seizures were declared to have epilepsy, and it was believed that they were doomed to seizures forever. The real situation now is quite different:

- Seventy percent of children whose seizures are controlled for two years can go off medication and remain seizure-free. These children have either outgrown their epilepsy or have been "cured."
- Only one in five children who have one tonic-clonic seizure and a normal EEG will have a second seizure, whether or not they are treated.
- Children who are otherwise normal, who have no evidence of prior damage or dysfunction of the brain, are likely to outgrow their epilepsy.

"Benign epilepsy of childhood" is a new concept, one not universally accepted, but one we are convinced by observation really exists. Our conviction is reinforced by the fact that the threshold for seizures increases as the young child's brain matures and is more resistant to seizures, and also by the fact that genetic tendencies toward seizures are influenced by age—most children "outgrow" their epilepsy, whether treated or not.

How do you know if your child has benign epilepsy of childhood? After a second seizure neither you nor your doctor can be sure, but, if your child is neurologically and intellectually normal and if the EEG does not show a lot of abnormalities, then there is good reason to hope. Only time will tell.

Controlled Epilepsy of Childhood

Even if your child has a number of seizures, and even if it is difficult to find the best medicine to control them, there is still a substantial chance that they will be controlled. There is also a very good chance that after they are controlled for two years medicine can be discontinued. Your child will have outgrown his seizures. The seizures of 80 percent of children will be controlled, and most of those children will cease taking medication. Thus, most children will not have epilepsy forever.

Even with these encouraging thoughts, when your child has had recurrent seizures, many emotions come into play. It is not uncommon for a parent to vacillate between fear, grief, and anger. The first emotion most people experience is fear.

Coming to Terms with Epilepsy: Fear, Grief, Anger, Acceptance

Fear is parents' *normal* response to hearing that their child has epilepsy. You are fearful because of your concerns about what epilepsy might do. You fear that the seizures may present difficulties: you will now have to take time to go to the doctor; it will interfere with your job, your activities, your interests. You fear that your child's life—and your life—have changed forever. This is really fear of the unknown. Information helps make the unknown known. Reality is always less frightening than what you imagine.

Grief is another emotion that parents must go through when faced with epilepsy. You are sad and you grieve for the child who you think no longer exists as before. You grieve for yourself because you're embarrassed and fearful. All of these feelings are common and normal. Indeed, we worry about the parent who shows no signs of grieving. You have to go through grief before you can achieve acceptance.

How do you cope with this grief? It's all right to cry, to feel sorry for yourself and your child. You need to realize that you may not be able to cope all alone. Grieving is much easier when it is shared with someone else. Another person can help you put your grief in perspective. You need to reach out and find support. You may find this within your own home, by talking about your fears and concerns with a member of the family. You may find it from another parent or group of parents. The Epilepsy Foundation or your local affiliate may be able to put you in touch with resources that will help you deal with these feelings. While grieving is a normal stage, it has to come to an end and ultimately be replaced by a more productive approach to living with epilepsy.

Anger is often the next stage. You're angry at your child for having done that terrible thing, even though you know the seizure was not his fault and that your anger is irrational. You're angry because the ambulance took so long to come, angry that the emergency room was so crowded and inefficient, angry that the nurse was not more considerate, and angry that the doctor didn't take more time examining your child and explaining things to you. You are angry at the system and the world, at your husband (or wife) because he or she is not more concerned or involved or is too concerned and involved, angry at yourself for being angry.

Again, all these reactions are perfectly normal. Different people handle them differently and at different speeds. Your spouse may be at a different stage than you are. He or she may be more fearful and not yet have progressed to the stage of grieving or anger. Occasionally a person moves through these stages rapidly, but more often it takes weeks and sometimes months; eventually you will get through them. You can deal with anger in many of the same ways you managed to deal with grief. Talking to others may help you to put your anger in perspective. Communication between parents can be difficult; your spouse may not understand your feelings. You may resent a seeming insensitivity. Openness and communication are the only way to deal with these feelings of anger. You may need someone to help you find a way to talk with your spouse about your feelings.

Anger is often long lasting, but it can be made productive. If you're angry at the school because of their attitude toward your child, perhaps the best way to handle it is to educate the school system, so that they may treat the next child better. If you're angry at your doctor, it may be important to discuss with him why you are angry. Discuss what he said, or what he didn't say, that made you upset. Sometimes your doctor may have said things that were inappropriate, but often parents misunderstand what physicians say or mean to say. Communication is always difficult, particularly in times of stress. Talking should improve matters.

Anger, of itself, is not productive. A person who continues to be angry ultimately alienates those who could be supportive.

Acceptance also takes time. It, too, has many different stages. We suggest the power of positive thinking and will discuss it more extensively in Chapter 16. Some parents would like to deny that a seizure ever occurred. These parents might say, "It won't happen again, and I won't let the seizure affect my life or my child's life." But it did occur, and it may recur, and it did affect your life. Whatever approach you take—and different individuals take different approaches—all of these phases should eventually lead to acceptance.

Acceptance means that you can consider your child a normal child who happens to have seizures. It means realizing that your child is not "an epileptic." Lack of acceptance, by comparison, can lead to over-protection, overpermissiveness, lack of discipline, and an inability to set appropriate limits for your child.

❑ **Butch was sixteen when he came to us. Butch had had three generalized tonic-clonic seizures in the previous several years. He had been taking phenobarbital and had recently had a fourth seizure. Butch had given up football and was barely passing in school. The family told us that they just couldn't control him. He was staying out late with his friends, drinking beer, and they suspected that he was experimenting with drugs. They asked us if there wasn't some medication that would control his seizures so they could get their old Butch back.**

As we talked with his parents, it was apparent that the seizures and medication were only minor issues. His behavior problems were partly related to his feelings about himself and his seizures. But epilepsy had paralyzed this family. They felt so sorry for Butch because of the seizures that they could not bring themselves to put normal restrictions on him. They were unable to set limits on his behavior. They overcompensated for what they saw as a major disability. Butch was far more handicapped by the lack of discipline, an important element of good parenting, than he was by his seizures.

We were able to help Butch's parents realize how their attitudes, although well intentioned, were handicapping Butch. Butch had taken control of the family and was neither ready for that control nor comfortable with it. He had gone so far that he was also manipulating the medical situation. He refused to let us draw blood for routine work that would have been necessary in changing to a more appropriate medication—one that might have had less impact on his behavior. Counseling took weeks, but eventually we were able to develop a contract with Butch. We helped his parents to set limits. We helped him to focus on the possibility of driving, a much desired goal. We enabled him to be a participant in the control of his epilepsy and his life, so that neither he nor epilepsy was the dominant force in his family.

It was the overcompensation by his loving family that had led to this intolerable situation and had handicapped Butch.

When your child has had only one seizure and has recovered, it is hard to accept the truth that he is unchanged, that he's no different from the child he was before the seizure. It will take time to accept the fact that the seizure is in the past, that the world has not collapsed, that your child is not retarded or brain-damaged. Indeed, he probably has forgotten that anything ever happened. It will take time for you to accept the fact that your child *can* go out and play, *can* go to the neighbor's house, *can* go on camping trips.

When your child has had recurrent seizures, epilepsy, it is even more difficult to realize that often very little has changed. Since most seizures can be controlled, children can return to their normal lives and, in an important sense, nothing need change. Children, of whatever age, still require the same love, attention, limits, and goals.

But in a different sense everything has changed. Your child has to take medicine, at least for a time, and is reminded, at least for a time, that a seizure could happen again. He feels different and may be treated differently by teachers and classmates. He may have some side effects from the medications that he is taking, or he may think that an ordinary upset stomach or school problem is caused by his epilepsy or medication. Both you and your child must find a way to accept the situation. Acceptance may come quickly if seizures are brought under control. *Acceptance comes when you realize that you can't change the past and that the future holds many opportunities.*

Helping Your Child Cope with Epilepsy

Your child will go through the same emotional stages you do. The manifestations of these stages will vary with the child's age and maturity and with the kind of seizures involved.

Fear is real for many of these children. Children may fear dying even if they have no concept of death. This fear of dying should be dealt with forthrightly. All people fear losing control, and people who have seizures are made anxious by the fact that a seizure could happen at any time. Educating your child about what actually happens during his seizures, what they look like to others, and that he will always return to his previous normal state may help him to adjust to this fear. For the older child, the fear of embarrassment may be even worse than the fear of death. "What will my friends think of me? Suppose I wet myself? Suppose this happens at a dance or in school?" Acceptance by one's peers is critical in adolescence. The worst thing that can happen to most teens is that somebody will notice that they are different.

Helping your child to understand epilepsy and accept it to the point where he can explain it to his friends and classmates is the most important element in overcoming these fears.

❑ **Judy told us that seizures had ruined her life. She felt she no longer had friends. She had given up field hockey because she was afraid that a seizure might happen on the field. She now hated school. Even though her seizures had come under control, she was an unhappy young lady. We finally got her to begin to accept her epilepsy by encouraging her to tell the field hockey coach that she had seizures and that they were controlled. Getting her to go back out for the team was the first step in rebuilding her life. Since she could play with the team, she began to realize that she wasn't different from her teammates. As she felt better about herself, her school work improved and her attitude shifted. When she was able to tell classmates about the seizures and what it was like to feel different, Judy began to realize that the rest of the kids never really felt she was different. She realized that her isolation was self-imposed, constructed because she was worried that they *might* feel that she was different. Once she became aware that the problem was within her and not them, she could work to regain her self-esteem.**

Grieving also occurs in children. Initially the older child or adolescent will think that life has ended, that he can no longer do the same things others are doing. If you impose unwarranted restrictions, the child will not be able to continue his usual activities and there will be loss of a previous lifestyle; then there may truly be reason for grieving. This is one of the reasons why it is so important that your child be allowed to participate in his chosen activities to the fullest extent possible. Even when restrictions are needed because of the frequency or severity of the seizures, it is important that you find activities in which your child can participate and achieve safely. Achievement and participation are very important ingredients in helping people develop self-esteem.

Here are a couple of examples of how children can be helped through these stages of adjustment to having epilepsy:

❑ **Melissa was still grieving. This bright, articulate, theatrically talented teenager had had staring spells for almost nine months. Although she had been to many doctors, she was trying to deny that there was anything wrong, and she refused to take medicine. We were the ones who finally told her that she had** epilepsy. Even though she had begun to take her medicine reliably and had had no seizures in two months, she felt sad. Seizures no longer interfered with any of her many activities, and there were no side effects from medication; but she still felt different, and she was still angry. We helped her move toward acceptance by offering her an opportunity to meet with other young people who had seizures, youngsters who had already been through some of these stages. We began to see a difference—a willingness to channel these feelings in a productive way. We saw a young lady who was beginning to believe that she was not handicapped by her seizures. Now, three years later, she has been abroad and is in college majoring in drama.

❑ Sean felt sad. Although only nine, he had coped with his seizures by talking about them incessantly to all his classmates and friends. Unfortunately this was not productive; it resulted in negative reactions. Most of his young peers didn't care, and so they ignored him or were angry at him for bothering them. We let Sean know that there are lots of people who have seizures. It had a profound impact on him when we told him that the Orioles' baseball stadium could be filled with people from Maryland who have epilepsy. Also, meeting another child with epilepsy who understood his feelings made it possible for him to begin to put his seizures into perspective. He no longer feels alone.

Both of these children were grieving and had not accepted their epilepsy. Melissa had internalized the problem and withdrawn, while Sean had externalized his difficulties and was making himself a nuisance. Neither response was productive.

Children, like the adults around them, ultimately need to accept their epilepsy if they are to be happy and productive citizens. They need to realize that epilepsy is only one part of their life and, for most children, not the dominant part. *People should be defined by the kind of person they are, not a condition they have.*

Perhaps most important to a child's acceptance of epilepsy is a feeling of self-esteem. For anyone to achieve his full potential, he must feel good about himself and be able to achieve.

One aspect of self-esteem is a child's feeling of control over his epilepsy and his life. This is why the child should participate in his treatment. Certainly the older child must know why she is taking medicine. A parent who tells his child that she's taking medication because, "It's good for you" or "It's a vitamin and will make you stronger" has not accepted his child's epilepsy and is not allowing the child to accept it either. Also, we encourage parents to let the child, from almost any age, be responsible for taking his own medication. The younger child will require supervision. The older child and adolescent can supervise himself, or learn to, and, in doing so, gain a feeling of control over his epilepsy. We realize that it is scary for parents not to make sure the child has taken her medicine, not to ask, not to hand it to her. But it is crucial that children learn responsibility. They need to learn that it is their epilepsy, not yours, and that the consequences of not taking medicine are theirs, not yours—as much as you wish otherwise. This is the beginning of their ability to control the frightening uncertainties of their condition, and of life.

An individual is known by what he can do, not by what he can't do. If you focus on your child's limitations and wish for things that are not realistic, your child is likely to become a failure in your eyes and in his own and may fail to achieve his potential. Recognizing your child's potential for achievement is a first step in helping him to recognize his own capabilities. Rewarding achievement is far more productive than focusing on failure.

What Do You Tell Grandparents and Friends When Seizures Recur?

When your child has had a second or third seizure, family and friends need to be informed. Your child has probably been started on medication and could experience side effects or even temporary changes in personality from the medication. The likelihood of your child's having a further seizure is now high enough that those close to him should be aware of the situation. They should know what these "frightening episodes" look like and what they should do if another occurs. They should have the various myths about epilepsy dispelled. Most of the time your child will be normal. Make sure his epilepsy is not blown out of proportion. Don't let your friends and relatives dwell on it. If they understand, perhaps they can avoid the overprotection and inappropriate restrictions that deprive your child of normal experiences.

What Do You Tell the School and Classmates after Additional Seizures?

Teachers are an important part of your child's environment and can be enormously helpful to a child with epilepsy. If they are informed and properly educated, teachers will know what to do and what to say to classmates should a seizure occur in school. They need to be prepared should a tonic-clonic seizure occur. They can be very helpful in alerting the parent and physician to changes in performance or personality that might be related to drug toxicity.

One of the prevailing myths is that children with epilepsy are stupid or have learning problems. According to many studies, children with epilepsy do tend to have more difficulties in school, but this may be a consequence of fear or anxiety, their own and others'. This does not mean that all children with epilepsy have learning problems. Most children with epilepsy do not. Some teachers may see learning problems that aren't there. They may be responding to the myths. But often, the teacher is sensitive to your child's needs. If she points out problems, your physician can evaluate whether they are related to medication. The school may be able to devise an individual educational program to meet your child's needs, if one is required.

Learning problems may not be the result of epilepsy at all. Many children who never had epilepsy don't learn easily. Or, as noted, problems may be a side effect of medication. A change in your child's personality or in his abilities when medication is started may signal such a cause. Early identification of this possibility may allow the physician either to reduce the dose of the drug or to change the medication (see Chapter 20).

To be sure that teachers, school nurses, and principals have accurate information about epilepsy, you may provide some of the excellent pamphlets available either directly from the Epilepsy Foundation or from a local affiliate. Many pamphlets are written so that a young child can understand them and are available either free or for only a nominal charge. Pamphlets that explain epilepsy in simple terms can be given to a young child's siblings and friends and, when appropriate, can be used in the child's classroom. Your local epilepsy association can probably provide speakers or perhaps the wonderful puppet show "Kids on the Block" and will try to help educate the school. A brief classroom session may help your child's classmates be more understanding, helpful, and friendly should they see your child have a seizure. There is a lot of help out there, but you have to ask for it.

Absence Seizures

If your child has staring spells, or absence seizures—instances where he or she briefly stops and stares, perhaps with some smacking of his lips, picking at his clothes, or confusion—the chances are that he or she has not had just a single episode. These brief spells are usually diagnosed only after many have occurred. Since it is likely that you are recognizing the problem after the fifth, the tenth, or the hundredth spell, it is obvious that the spells are likely to continue, to recur, unless treated with medication.

While less frightening than the tonic-clonic seizure, staring spells cause a particular type of anxiety. Parents are worried that they won't even know when their child is having a seizure. "Is Jane just daydreaming, as all children do, or is she having an absence seizure?" "Should I have yelled at Billy for not taking out the garbage? Did he not hear me? Did he disobey, or was he having an absence seizure?" Since these seizures are brief and subtle and therefore difficult to recognize, it is probably even more important to tell neighbors, friends, grandparents, and the school about them. This awareness will permit other people to notice when they occur, to be more tolerant of "daydreaming," and to be a bit more careful when the child is crossing the street or in a situation where loss of awareness could cause harm. Also, because this type of seizure is likely to occur far more frequently than tonic-clonic seizures (sometimes many times each day or several times per week), staring spells are *more* likely than the single tonic-clonic seizure to interfere with the child's functioning.

Again, it is important to be truthful, but since the child will be unaware of these spells unless someone tells him, the explanation needs to be handled with sensitivity. "You have little blackouts, episodes when you don't know what is going on. They're like static on the radio, a brief second or two when you can't hear the music." It is important to use terms appropriate for the age and understanding of the child and to make sure that the words you use are not frightening. Better for you to tell him than for him to be asked awkward questions or be told disturbing stories by other children.

You need to give your child the opportunity to let you know he's missing things in school—for example, instructions or the end of a story. We know of one child who assumed that life was just a series of blank spaces. His class was making a movie about a train going by, and he wanted to cut out frames of the film. When asked why, he told his teacher that's how he saw it—with short blank spots between the pictures. It was then that his teacher became aware that there were frequent, very brief, gaps in his attention. The diagnosis of absence seizures was eventually made.

These simple absence seizures can usually be brought completely under control with medication, although it may take several weeks to gain control. Until then, the child's activities should be more carefully supervised, with caution and concern but without overprotectiveness or panic.

Teachers are a very important, perhaps even crucial, part of the evaluation and treatment of a child who has absence seizures. School classes are one of the few times when a child is consistently under observation and when brief lapses in attention can be readily recognized. It is not uncommon for the teacher to be the first to recognize these lapses of attention. Some parents feel guilty that they did not notice these lapses themselves, but in the structured atmosphere of the classroom, they are often easier to see and recognize than in the more informal atmosphere of a family. And once they are recognized, the teacher can be your child's best ally, by noting spells and possible side effects of medication.

On the other hand, because of the myths about epilepsy, an uninformed or biased teacher may begin to treat your child as if he had a learning problem or were stupid. Normal daydreaming may be misperceived as staring spells. A child who is daydreaming may or may not respond if called, but will certainly respond if the teacher goes over and touches him. When a child does not respond when touched, he is more likely to be experiencing absence seizures.

Complex Partial Seizures

In complex partial seizures, as with absence seizures, the child stops, stares, and is unaware of his environment. But in this case there is often a period of confusion after the child stops staring. Also, during the spell, he may get up and wander around the room, pick at his clothes, and fail to respond appropriately. These "peculiar" episodes are likely to be misunderstood by the other children in a classroom and by his teacher. As with absence spells, it is important that the teacher understand what is happening. The teacher needs to realize that if your child is wandering around and someone tries to restrain him, the child may lash out or even become highly agitated. Providing gentle guidance and supervision at such times is far better than trying to force him to sit down. The teacher needs to be able to be comforting and reassuring both to the student having the seizure, who is not aware of what is happening, and to the other children, who may be confused by the behavior. It is important that the teacher alert you to changes in your child's performance. You can then alert your doctor.

As with other recurrent seizures, your child needs to understand what is happening during these episodes when he is not aware. He may remember the beginning of the seizure; he may feel an aura (for example, fear, a rising feeling in the stomach), and he may be vaguely aware of people responding to his behavior during and after the seizure. Or he may only be aware that something happened and that now things are different from what they were a few seconds or minutes ago. Since these spells usually follow a pattern, let him know what has been going on, so that he will be less upset and confused. If he does have an aura, point out that it can be a useful warning. Encourage him to pay attention to it, so that he can avoid harmful situations when a seizure may be coming on.

Is Your Child Disabled or Handicapped?

There is life with and after epilepsy. Let's talk about the important things in your child's life—about all the times when he is *not* having seizures.

Society glibly says that everybody should be able to do what they want if they try hard enough. Clearly this is foolishness! Some people are too short to be basketball players. Others are too tall to be jockeys. Some people are not beautiful enough to be fashion models. Some wear glasses and can't, therefore, be astronauts. In this global sense, all of us are handicapped. However, we should all have the opportunity to achieve our full potential, whatever that may be. Neither society, nor parents, nor our own attitudes should be allowed to interfere with this.

Is epilepsy a "handicap"? For some it clearly is. For most, it need not be. The child whose seizures are well controlled with medicine need not be handicapped. He can achieve his full potential, even if there will be some limitations on his choices. Crucial for your child's future is that you not impose unreasonable limitations on his activities or aspirations, nor allow others to do so.

"Can I let my child go out and play?"

Of course! You not only can but you must let him go out and play, go on trips, sleep at a friend's house. "But suppose he has another seizure?" That's a risk you have to take. A careful analysis of risks is an important part of raising any child. It is a particularly important part of raising a child with the uncertainties of epilepsy. It is the crucial ingredient in avoiding overprotection. His ability to run around and his intelligence are the same as before the seizures. Most children with epilepsy are neither retarded nor learning-disabled. For most such children, the only impairment is that, from time to time, they may experience a seizure. For 99.99 percent of the time your child is the same as always.

"But isn't he disabled?"

The answer is *no!* He can still run and play, go to school, sleep over at a friend's house. There is virtually *nothing* that a child who has had a few seizures cannot do. "Can he ride a bike?" Sure. The chances of having a seizure while riding his bike are very small, and if he is wearing a helmet, he is at only minimally greater risk than before his seizures. "Can she swim?" Absolutely, but her swimming must be supervised, just as *every* child's swimming must be supervised. "Isn't there a higher risk that she could drown or have a seizure in the water?" Yes, but only a *slightly* higher risk, since she has had only occasional seizures and may never have another one. Technically, your child may have a disability. He or she may fit the government definition that enables a person to obtain special services if the seizures interfere with education or work. But having a disability is very different from being disabled.

A handicap is often superimposed by society, parents, friends, or schools. A person can also impose it on himself.

"What do I write on all those school or camp forms now that she's had several seizures? Is she 'an epileptic'?"

No! Your child is not "an epileptic." She is a child who has had seizures. She's a child with epilepsy. First of all she's a child, a person, an individual; she is not defined by her disorder. Most of the time she does not have seizures. Most of the time she is her normal self. Seizures, or epilepsy, are a brief interlude in her life. But labeling is a big problem. The terms *epilepsy* and *epileptic* carry many myths and misconceptions. Unfortunately, the labels are often used in the pejorative sense. Labels are to be avoided unless they have some clear benefit for your child. One expert has stated that a good reason not to treat after a first seizure (other than that it isn't of any benefit) is that having to take medication once or twice a day is a constant reminder that you are different. It is a reminder to the parents, and a reminder to the child. It is a label, and cannot help but affect the child's self-esteem.

"I've heard that the local epilepsy association runs a camp just for children with epilepsy. Is that a good idea for Johnny? Wouldn't he be better off with normal kids?"

See? You've slipped already. Kids with epilepsy *are* normal kids. They just have seizures in addition. Many of our children with epilepsy think that they are the only one in the world who is different, even if their classmates can't see the differences. They do not know anyone else with seizures. They have never even seen a seizure. Camps for children with epilepsy can often help develop a child's self-esteem. Johnny will find that there are children with seizures who are far more handicapped than he. He may also find that there are children who are brighter or more athletic than he is. He will find that he is just like all of the other children in many ways, one of them being that they all have seizures. Good self-esteem is the greatest gift you can give to your child, perhaps especially if he has seizures.

We find that the best approach to a child who has had several seizures, who has now been labeled "epileptic," is for you to gain a realistic acceptance of your child's limitations (if any) and to focus on his potential. This requires a conscious effort to put aside your anxiety and concern about all of the things that could happen. This is not an easy thing to do. It requires acceptance of the fact that there are risks inherent in rearing any child and that most children with epilepsy, especially those whose epilepsy is controlled, face only slightly greater risks than other children.

Children who have severe or difficult-to-control epilepsy and those who have additional impairments, such as mental retardation, cerebral palsy, or learning disabilities, also require realistic acceptance. It is important that these children, too, be encouraged to reach their full potential and that additional handicaps not be superimposed (see Chapter 17).

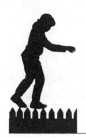

16. Coping with the Uncertainties of Seizures and Epilepsy:
The Power of Positive Thinking

A Tale of Two Parents

❏ Melanie White's mother was thirty-two and had struggled hard to achieve this, her first, pregnancy. She was, naturally, quite anxious when she went into premature labor and delivered a three-pound baby girl. Problems with breathing led to Melanie's immediate transfer to University Hospital. Dr. Richards, Melanie's intern, seemed very competent and conscientious. After a thorough examination and after Melanie was settled in the isolette with all the tubes and the respirator, the doctor spent a lot of time with Melanie's father explaining the problems and the potential problems of a premature infant. She told him that it was really too early to predict the outcome and that most children with such respiratory problems could be saved without permanent lung disease. Other problems could occur: intestinal problems, seizures, bleeding into the head. "Small babies like this can have a greater chance of mental retardation, cerebral palsy, and epilepsy," she said. "However," she reassured him, "at the moment Melanie looks very good. We have reason to be hopeful."

Mr. White relayed this information to his wife, who was still in the community hospital. The nurses there tried to be as reassuring as possible. They all had seen premature infants who had done well. On the fourth day, Mrs. White was discharged and was able to see her daughter for the first time. Melanie was unbelievably tiny, but Dr. Richards reassured her mother that everything was going well, so far. Actually, the next five weeks in the hospital nursery went very well. Melanie did not develop any major complications. She grew and thrived and went home weighing four-and-one-half pounds.

This was the end of one story, but it was the beginning of another tale—or rather two different tales: one is the mother's, the other the father's.

Mrs. White was an accountant for a prominent firm in town and had worked very hard to achieve her senior position. Indeed, this was one of the reasons she had deferred having children. She was also a worrier. The doctor had mentioned the possibility of mental retardation and cerebral palsy. "Is Melanie all right?" she would repeatedly ask her pediatrician. "Shouldn't she be smiling by now?" "When should she be rolling over?" Reassurance that premature babies were a bit slower to do these things only made Mrs. White more anxious, particularly when she saw other infants beginning to sit at six months and walk around furniture before they were a year old.

Melanie was able to sit when she was ten months old, began cruising around furniture when she was fourteen months, and said her first words at about a year. "All of these are normal, particularly for a baby who was born five weeks prematurely," the pediatrician said. But Mrs. White knew that they were at the lower end of normal and she worried. "Isn't she supposed to be using her thumb and index finger to be feeding herself by now?" she would ask. "I think that her right foot turns out when she walks. Is that normal? I'd like to take Melanie to the pediatric orthopedist to see if she has CP."

Mr. White was a college professor who did much of his writing and research at home. By nature, he was more laid back and less of a worrier than was his wife. He spent a lot of time with Melanie while his wife was at work, and he thought that Melanie was just fine. "Einstein did not talk until he was three," he was fond of reminding his wife.

The orthopedist found no deformities. "She's just a little slow in gaining control of her muscles," he said. "She'll be walking soon." And she was.

When, at two, Melanie had a cold and a sore throat, she experienced a convulsion. It was over before the ambulance got there, and the pediatrician met them at the hospital's emergency room. After an examination, he reassured them that this was a febrile seizure and that she would be fine. He said she did not need medication because there was only one chance in about three of her having another febrile seizure. Mr. White was delighted that Melanie did not need medication. By contrast, his wife thought that one in three was a high likelihood, and she was less happy, particularly when her daughter had a second convulsion with fever four months later. An EEG, done to assuage Mrs. White's concern, was normal, but Melanie was placed on phenobarbital "to prevent still another one." Unfortunately, phenobarbital made Melanie a terror. She was irritable, overactive, fussy, and had problems going to sleep. After two weeks, everyone agreed that she was far better without the medicine, and it was stopped.

When she entered nursery school at three, Melanie seemed less mature than her peers. She was less ready to play in the groups, less interested in hearing stories, not as good at coloring within the lines. In the spring the teachers expressed their concerns at the parents' conference. Mr. White's reaction was: "Let's keep her in the play group another year. There's no need for her to be the youngest in the next group. In another year she'll be older, wiser, and more mature. After all, she did start this world early." Mrs. White insisted on psychological testing; it showed that Melanie was "low normal," more like a two-and-one-half-year-old than her chronological age of three years and four months. The report also stated that "Melanie's strengths are in the personal-social area. In fine motor coordination and the perceptual areas she lags slightly behind." A visit to the pediatric neurologist confirmed that she was not mentally retarded and that she did not have cerebral palsy. "She is just slightly slow in development, as are many premature babies. They usually catch up as they enter school," he said.

Melanie's mother found a speech therapist who would see the child at about five in the afternoon, so that she herself wouldn't have to leave work early. She and her husband would alternate taking Melanie for therapy and practicing speech sounds. An occupational therapist also saw her once a week, and Mrs. White took Melanie to a Saturday morning gym class for "exceptional children." She considered that "together time."

When Melanie was five, she had her first generalized, nonfebrile seizure. That brought the family to our office. Most of the questions came from the mother. "Why did she have a seizure? Will she have another? Shouldn't she be on medication? Can she still go to the gym class? They do all these exercises swinging on bars. What about riding her bike?" They were the questions you may have asked your own physician. Mr. White had few questions; he mainly listened as we tried to explain seizures and the uncertainties of the future.

"Why can't you doctors ever give a straight answer to a simple question?" Mrs. White finally cried out in anguish. "I thought you were supposed to be scientific." We tried again. We explained the potential side effects of treatment, and they agreed not to start treatment at that time. Every week or so, Mrs. White would call our coordinator to describe one thing or another. "Melanie was sucking her thumb, and I had to call her three times before she responded. Is that the absence seizures the doctor mentioned might occur?" "Melanie has fallen twice this week and skinned her knee. How do you tell if she just tripped or if this was an akinetic seizure?" "The teacher tells me that Melanie is not paying attention in school this week. Could she be having seizures, or do you think it is just her cold?" "I was watching while she was sleeping last night and she was really very restless. Could these be seizures during her sleep?"

"This is driving my wife crazy," Mr. White told us on one visit. "I think that Melanie is doing fine. She's a delicate flower who is just taking her own time to bloom. She is sweet, lovable, affectionate, but my wife is so concerned about seizures and about Melanie's future that she's unable to enjoy her any more. She's stopped worrying about the mental retardation and cerebral palsy, or at least she's not focusing on those things any more, but the uncertainty about future seizures and about what is or is not a seizure is affecting my wife's work. It's ruining our marriage, and it's hurting Melanie. We've got a wonderful little girl here, and my wife is spending so much time being concerned that she's missing all the fun."

When Melanie had a second generalized seizure one year later, things got even worse. She was started on medication, and concerns about the side effects were added to the confusion about what were and what were not seizures and the fears about the possibility of injury when she was out playing. The already troubled marriage was now more so. Melanie herself became more manipulative. When she did not get her way, she would sulk and stare. Was she having an absence seizure? With her mother's fear of the effects of punishment—of getting Melanie upset and causing another seizure—Melanie's behavior grew worse. Problems she experienced in learning to read in the first grade led to concerns about the possible effect of the medication on her learning ability, and then to changes in medication. During the change-over, Melanie had a complex partial seizure, and this, in turn, led to additional concerns.

The frequent visits to our clinic became increasingly difficult for everyone. We couldn't satisfy Mrs. White, because we could not give categorical answers to her questions. "Was this the best medicine?" We could only answer that this medicine worked on many children with this type of seizure and did not often have serious side effects. "But how do you know that Melanie wouldn't do better on ____?" "We don't, but this is what we would choose first." We would try to point out the potential risks and benefits of switching. "Will she have another tonic-clonic seizure?" We would reexplain the uncertainties of epilepsy. "If we take her to visit my parents in Alabama, what do we do if she has a seizure during the long drive?" "Could she die during a seizure if she had one during the night?" "How do we know that she isn't having seizures during the night that we are not aware of?" The questions were endless, as were the doubts, and both were unanswerable.

Two or three years of counseling these parents and of patiently answering and reanswering the same questions, and also of marriage counseling, finally led to Mrs. White's acceptance of the facts. Melanie was by then a lovely young lady—beautiful, well dressed, very sociable. She was an adequate student who required special resource teaching, a little slow, the lower end of normal, but not retarded. She was not graceful, but she participated in a children's ballet class. We would have called her a child with learning disabilities and sort of clumsy, with what neurologists call "soft neurological signs." We would not have dignified her minimal deficits by calling them either cerebral palsy or mental retardation. Melanie's seizures remained under control with medication.

Mrs. White finally came to accept the state of affairs and to accept Melanie for what she was, not for what Mrs. White had once hoped she would be. And what she was, on her own terms, was terrific. How much easier Melanie's earliest years were for Mr. White, who had accepted her on those terms all along.

In all chronic conditions there is a need to be realistic. There is also a problem in defining "reality" and in accepting it. One of the most difficult realities of epilepsy is that no one can predict when and where (or even if) a next seizure will occur. This is "the uncertainty factor." It is this uncertainty factor that differentiates epilepsy from most other chronic conditions. It is this uncertainty factor that is most disturbing to older children with epilepsy and to parents. "Could I have a seizure while crossing the street?" "Is it all right for me to go to school today, or will I be embarrassed by another one of those things?" "Suppose he goes to the prom and has a seizure?" Uncertainty leads to anxiety and worry. Coping with anxiety is the principal task for a parent of a child with epilepsy. Worry must be contained. It cannot be allowed to permeate every waking moment of your life. It cannot be allowed to be the master, dictating overprotection of your child.

But how can worry and anxiety be contained? It's useless to be told not to worry. You need to be helped to see the reality of your child's epilepsy. For some, that reality may be a few seizures, likely to be controlled, and epilepsy that eventually disappears. For other parents, the reality may be continuing seizures or retardation or other disabilities. No one can predict with absolute certainty what the future holds for a child with epilepsy, any more than we can predict with certainty what the future holds for a child without epilepsy.

It is the lack of ability to influence the future that can be the most disturbing to people with epilepsy and to their loved ones.

The Power of Positive Thinking

When your child has had one seizure, and even when a child has been diagnosed as having epilepsy, it is important for you and your child that you both develop a positive approach. One way to achieve a positive approach to dealing with this uncertainty is to focus on the low probability of another seizure. A second way is to recognize that another seizure may occur and accept that possibility. It's important to find what approach works for you and your child, what approach leads to acceptance.

You might say to yourself: "She's going to be one of the lucky ones with benign epilepsy who will, or has, outgrown it." Or you might say, "Chances are that she will *never* have another seizure." Never is a long time and it might be more useful to say, "She's not going to have another seizure today." If you said that to yourself, the chances are overwhelming that you would be correct. If you said, "I don't think she will have another seizure this week or this month," you still have an enormous chance of being right. Many people with epilepsy have only two, or three, or four seizures in their lifetimes.

If you live your life *as if* your child isn't going to have another seizure, then you can avoid the extra handicap superimposed by worrying about another seizure and its possible effects. If you allow your child to live as if another seizure will never occur, you can avoid the overprotection that may accompany the fear that it will. Thinking that another seizure will not occur can be called "denial." But it is not a denial that your child has epilepsy: for many people, at most times, denial that another seizure will occur is realistic. Most of the time you will have been correct.

What happens if your confidence is wrong and your child has another seizure? You and your physician will explore why that seizure occurred. Did your child forget her medicine? Not get enough sleep? Does she have an infection? Does the medication need adjusting? You may find a good reason. If you don't, you will have to begin your positive thinking all over again.

However, you'll be right about her not having a seizure far more often than you'll be wrong. And, since the consequences of being wrong are not within your control, this framework may help you and your child achieve a positive approach to living.

Another approach involves the realization that the medical risks of a recurrent seizure are minimal and that, as in the past, your child will quickly recover from the seizure and resume her normal activities. You may even be able to accept the social consequences and not be overly concerned that you or your child will experience embarrassment. It may be easier for your child to do this if she has a good understanding of seizures and if you have been able to educate her school and her friends that, although having a seizure is unpleasant and interrupts activities for a short while, these activities usually can be resumed without any real harm.

Communicating

When we initially wrote this chapter, two of us almost came to blows. We discovered, to our surprise, that we used, and advocated, different strategies for coping with anxiety. We also found that, although we had worked together closely for many years, in this nonmedical sphere we were having difficulty communicating. It was only after prolonged discussion—argument, really—that we discovered that we were exhibiting the variation that exists between men and women in the way they use language and in their strategies for coping. We had accidentally stumbled across this verity, but several authors have written about the differences in communication and use of language by men and women. Deborah Tannen, for one, has written extensively on these issues. Coping and communication styles also differ among various groups and cultures. As you communicate with your spouse, your family, your physicians, and others, be sensitive to the potential problems in communication created by these variations in style. You and your child will also have to find your own way to communicate effectively, and to cope with anxiety.

Anxiety, the Greatest Enemy

Coping with anxiety is a crucial step in acceptance of your child and his condition. You may have sensed the teacher's anxiety when you first told her about your child's seizures, or perhaps you simply worried how she might react. Maybe her anxiety is a consequence of lack of information. Perhaps she has been exposed to the myths. Perhaps she once had a child in her classroom who fell and hit his head during a seizure.

You may be able to reassure the teacher by saying, "I know that you're worried that Steve will fall and be injured and that I'll be furious and accuse you of not looking out for him. But I won't. We'll both be upset that it happened, but we both have to realize that Steve needs to be in school with his classmates. His seizures are really infrequent, and he usually has a little warning. We need to convince him to let you know that warning has come, so that he can be in a safe place. We have to let him take some chances if he's to have the opportunity to be a normal child."

This kind of dialogue is critical to an understanding and working relationship among parent, child, and teacher. Teachers often need help in coming to terms with their anxiety, just as you do. Accepting the realities and receiving accurate information can do a lot to relieve anxiety for everyone. It is important, in this litigious society, to remember that teachers, schools, day care workers, and others are not only anxious about the seizures but anxious that, should a seizure occur, they will be sued for what they did or did not do. This fear of lawsuits often paralyzes the system and works to your child's disadvantage. Assuaging these fears, sometimes in writing, can often help your child.

There is a familiar prayer that asks for the serenity to accept the things that we cannot change, the courage to change the things we can, and the wisdom to know the difference. If your child's seizures have been controlled, acceptance of the reality that your child is back to his normal state is easier. If your child continues to have seizures, you may not be able to change that reality. If so, you and your child must have the courage to change your own perception of that reality and to help change the perceptions of others.

One kind of acceptance, however, is totally unacceptable. It is virtually never appropriate to accept that your child must be significantly limited by his seizures. You have to believe that your child can fulfill his own potential. If learning problems or physical problems exist, they must be recognized and solutions sought to optimize your child's ability to function.

Realistic acceptance of the multiply handicapped child is crucial. This does not mean that this acceptance should not incorporate a positive attitude, or that hope should be abandoned. Seizures that were intractable only a few years ago may today or tomorrow respond to new medications or to new combinations of medications, to the ketogenic diet, or to surgery. Focusing on what your child can do now rather than on what he cannot do, looking at the glass as half-full, rather than half-empty, will help you and your child through the rough times. Encouraging the child to be able to say, "I'm all right now, I can go back to class" or "I know that I had a seizure, but now I want to go out to play" is part of the same positive outlook. A positive attitude discourages the invalidism that can accompany a chronic disability. It encourages your child to have as much control as possible over his life. It maximizes his self-esteem.

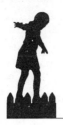

17. Coping with Substantial Handicap:
Mental Retardation, Cerebral Palsy, and Difficult-to-Control Seizures

Seizures can be controlled in 80 percent of children with epilepsy. For those children and their families, epilepsy should not be a substantial handicap. In the remaining 20 percent of children—those who have difficult-to-control epilepsy—there are often underlying brain abnormalities. This brain damage or dysfunction is frequently the cause of the mental retardation or the cerebral palsy as well as the epilepsy.

Here are some important definitions:

• *Symptomatic* epilepsy is epilepsy that is due to an underlying cause. The epilepsy is a symptom, not the cause, of any brain damage that may be present.
• *Cryptogenic* epilepsy is epilepsy in which we suspect underlying brain damage but cannot prove it. Symptomatic and cryptogenic epilepsies may be more difficult to control and may require surgery or the ketogenic diet.
• *Idiopathic* epilepsy is epilepsy whose cause is unknown. It is more likely to occur in otherwise normal children, to respond to medications, and to be outgrown.
• *Cerebral palsy* is defined as damage to motor areas of the brain. Cerebral palsy may or may not be accompanied by mental retardation and seizures.
• *Mental retardation* alone is most often of unknown cause. Mental retardation with cerebral palsy is usually due to damage on both sides of the brain and may be associated with difficult-to-control seizures.

• *Epilepsy* rarely causes damage to the brain and rarely causes mental retardation. When epilepsy is associated with mental retardation and cerebral palsy, it is usually the underlying brain damage which has caused the cerebral palsy, the mental retardation, and the epilepsy. Epilepsy never causes cerebral palsy.

Coping with Labels

Labels should be applied when they are useful. If being called "green" gets you or your child an advantage, then your child looks green to us. If your child is labeled "artistic" and this enables her to receive special art classes, then the label will have been useful. If calling him "retarded" or "autistic" enables your child to receive the special help he needs in school, then the label may be useful. Correspondingly, if a child is labeled "normal" but has a learning style that requires special help, then the label "normal" may be a disadvantage. However, labeling him "retarded" may be a disadvantage if what he has is a specific learning disability and he just needs focused help for that trait. If the label "handicapped" places your child in a large class of children with severe handicaps, then the label may not be useful.

Children with mental retardation (of whatever degree), with cerebral palsy, and with epilepsy are all children with special needs. Labeling your child is only useful if it helps him or her to receive the appropriate services so that he or she can fulfill his or her own potential.

It is also important that your expectations for your child be realistic. Putting a handicapped child in a regular class may or may not be to that child's advantage, depending on the child, the class, the nature of the handicap, and the alternatives. Mainstreaming (inclusion of children with special needs in regular classes rather than special classes) has many advantages, but it may be a disadvantage for an individual child. The stresses of inappropriate placements may be overwhelming for some children.

Remember, you can be the best advocate for your child, but be realistic about your child's needs and about what special labels you wish him to have.

Mental Retardation

Mental retardation is a handicapping condition defined as having less than average intelligence. Children with mental retardation may

Table 17.1   Terminology, IQ, and Academic and Vocational Potential of Children with Mental Retardation

Degree of mental retardation	IQ (approximate)	Academic potential*	Vocational potential
None	>80	Normal	Normal
Borderline	70–79	6th grade level	Employable
Mild	55–70	4th grade level	Employable
Moderate	40–55	May read and write simple words	Noncompetitive employment
Severe	25–40		Sheltered/supported "employment"
Profound	<25		

Source: Modified from H. J. Cohen, "Mental Retardation." In H. M. Wallace, R. F. Biehl et al., eds., *Handicapped Children and Youth* (New York: Human Sciences Press, 1987), p. 354.
*Academic potential levels cited are approximations; function will vary within each group and with each individual child.

also have less than average personal independence and less than average social responsibility. Ninety-seven out of every 100 children have an intelligence score between 70 and 130; children with IQs (intelligence quotients) below 70 are said to have mental retardation. There are varying levels of retardation, each of which may have different levels of academic and vocational expectation (see Table 17.1).

In a child handicapped by mental retardation, seizures may further impair function and therefore require treatment. Even in the most profoundly retarded child, seizure control may be possible and if attained will result in an improved quality of life for the child and the caretakers.

Commonly Asked Questions

"If my child is mentally retarded, what are her chances of developing epilepsy?"

About one in ten children with mental retardation also has epilepsy. The figure itself is, however, virtually meaningless, since the risk of epilepsy varies markedly with the cause of retardation, its severity, and the age of the child. The severely or profoundly retarded child is far more likely to have seizures than the mildly retarded child. With children who are severely retarded, seizures are likely to begin, if they begin at all, in infancy or early childhood.

The child whose brain damage is caused by brain trauma or lack of oxygen, whether sustained during birth or later, is more likely to have seizures than a child whose retardation has an unknown cause. Severe retardation of genetic origin has a significantly different risk of epilepsy, depending on the specific cause. In one condition, Rett's syndrome, epilepsy occurs almost universally; in Down's syndrome, however, the risk of seizures is only slightly higher than average.

"If my child has epilepsy, what is the chance of mental retardation?"

The risk of retardation in a child with epilepsy depends primarily on the cause of the epilepsy and to a far less extent on the type of seizure itself. A previously normal child who begins to have seizures of unknown cause will virtually never become retarded. However, if these seizures are caused by a progressive or degenerative disease, the risk of retardation is high. Children with developmental delay or neurological handicap seldom become more retarded because of seizures, the two exceptions being infants with infantile spasms and children with the Lennox-Gastaut syndrome. Both of these types of epilepsy are often associated with retardation.

"I don't believe my child is retarded; I think his problems are due to all those medicines he's taking. How can I tell for sure?"

Parents may prefer to believe that a child's slowness is a result of the medication, but the effects of medication overdose seldom resemble mental retardation. Children with retardation who are on medication tend to progress at their own prior rate, while drug toxicity usually causes a new decline in function. Overmedicated children often are sleepy during the day or unsteady; mentally retarded children are neither.

The only way to rule out medication as a cause is to decrease or eliminate one or all of the drugs in use. *Do not do this on your own.* With your physician's advice, you may want to consider tapering medication slowly, decreasing a single type of medication at a time. *If,* on tapering medicine, your child's function obviously improves, *then* the slowing *may* have been drug related. You and your physician will have to decide whether the risk of decreasing or changing the medication, as well as the chance of recurring or worsening seizures, is outweighed by the possible benefit of improved intellectual function.

Barbiturates like phenobarbital and benzodiazepines like diazepam (Valium), clonazepam (Klonopin), clorazepate (Tranxene), or lorazepam (Ativan) may cause slowness, dullness, sleepiness, and depression, symptoms that may resemble the characteristics of retardation. Any anticonvulsant, even when in the therapeutic range, may, on occasion, interfere with mental function.

"How should I treat my child who has both retardation and epilepsy?"

The answer depends on the child's level of retardation, particularly for the child with mild or moderate retardation. The natural tendency of most parents and grandparents is to overprotect a child with epilepsy. However, overprotection, particularly of a mildly mentally retarded child, leads to infantilization, ultimately a greater handicap to the child than seizures. It is crucial for such a child to be as independent as possible. The retarded child needs every opportunity to achieve his optimal potential.

When your child has multiple problems, such as mental retardation and epilepsy, the family has a lot of compensating to do. With epilepsy alone, you can usually maintain your expectations for his future—assuming, of course, they were realistic to begin with—since most epilepsy can be controlled or outgrown. Even when epilepsy occurs in children with retardation, your expectations for your child should rarely be changed.

Helping your child to cope with mental retardation depends greatly on the degree of retardation. The severely retarded child may not be clearly aware of his disability. Today many moderately retarded individuals function in noncompetitive employment, are able to live in the community with assistance, and engage in a variety of social activities. The process of developing these capabilities begins in childhood with mainstreaming in schools and socialization through churches, scouting, and athletics. Developing these capabilities begins within the family as well—seeing a child's potential, encouraging him to learn to participate, helping him to achieve his full potential.

Cerebral Palsy

Cerebral palsy (CP) is a condition in which the brain's control of motor movements or posture is abnormal. It is caused by damage within the motor areas of the brain or spinal cord which has occurred before or during birth or during childhood. It is not caused by a tumor or by degeneration of the nervous system. Cerebral palsy is not progressive—it does not continue to become worse—although it may become more obvious or its symptoms may vary slightly as the child matures.

"Will my child who has cerebral palsy be retarded? Will he have epilepsy?"

Not quite half of children with cerebral palsy are retarded to some degree; a number of others may have behavior and learning problems. Some have no such problems and are of normal intelligence; indeed, some children with cerebral palsy have superior intelligence.

Approximately one in three children with cerebral palsy will also have epilepsy, but few children with epilepsy will have cerebral palsy. *Epilepsy does not cause cerebral palsy; it does not cause mental retardation. Nor does cerebral palsy* cause *epilepsy. When cerebral palsy and epilepsy do occur together, underlying damage to the brain has caused both.*

There are various forms of cerebral palsy, and the present classification is far from satisfactory. One scheme for classification, shown in Table 17.2, indicates, broadly, that both the frequency and type of seizures vary with the kind of cerebral palsy, as discussed below.

Spastic Hemiparesis

A spastic hemiparesis is a form of cerebral palsy that is characterized by stiffness on only one side of the body. It is caused by damage to the

Table 17.2   Types of Cerebral Palsy and Risk of Seizures

Type of CP	Frequency (approximate percentage of all cases)	Risk of seizures
Stiff (spastic)		
Both legs (diplegia)	30	low
One-sided (hemiparesis)	25	moderate
Both sides (quadriparesis)	25	high
Abnormal movements	10	low
Athetoid		
Dystonic		
Mixed (spastic and dyskinetic)	10	variable

opposite side of the brain by a stroke, bleeding into the brain, trauma, or a problem in the brain's development. The arm is usually more affected than the leg; there may be major problems with the use of the hand. Most such children will be able to learn to walk, although they will usually have a limp. Since the damage is focal (one-sided), these individuals are less likely to have mental retardation. Although we do not understand all of the factors that cause one person's damaged brain to provoke seizures while another's does not, and we cannot predict which child will have seizures and which will not, in general we do know that a child with a hemiparesis whose CT or MRI scan shows brain damage is more likely to have seizures than one whose scan does not. We treat the seizures as we do other focal seizures. Unlike the child with a spastic quadraparesis (see below), the child with a hemiparesis may be a candidate for focal epilepsy surgery to remove the damaged tissue causing the seizures, if they are uncontrollable otherwise.

A child with a hemiparesis and difficult-to-control seizures on the paralyzed side should be evaluated for possible epilepsy surgery by an epilepsy center. Seizures due to congenital strokes or to developmental abnormalities of the brain may be very difficult to control with any combination of anticonvulsant medication. Surgery to remove the affected portion of the brain may give that child the best chance for seizure control and for more normal function without medication. When such a child has not responded to the first two medications, that may be the time to consider a surgical evaluation.

❑ **Sarah was five years old, a bright young lady with a congenital left hemiparesis. She was five months old when it was first noted that she was not using her left arm. She was diagnosed as having delayed development and cerebral palsy. A CT scan and later an MRI scan showed evidence of a stroke in her right cortex caused by a thrombosis (blood clot) in the right middle cerebral artery. At four years of age she had her first seizure; it was status epilepticus. Over the next few months she had more generalized seizures despite several different medications, and she developed myoclonic jerks and drop spells so that she could barely stand or walk. She was tried on the ketogenic diet and did well for several months, but the seizures broke through.**

The family finally agreed to allow us to do a right hemispherectomy to remove the whole damaged area. Sarah is now ten and in the third grade in a regular class. She walks, runs, and plays with her classmates, wearing a short leg brace. She uses her left hand only as a helper hand. Physically she is no differ-

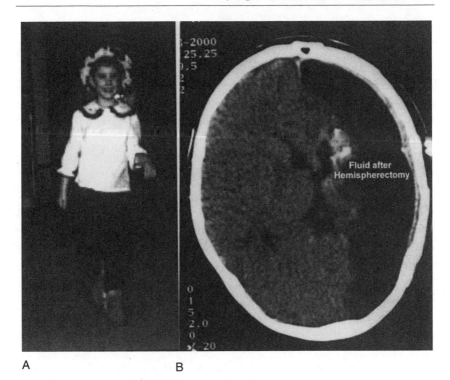

A   B

Figure 17.1 (A) Sarah after hemispherectomy. Note the posturing of her left arm as she walks. (B) An MRI scan of Sarah's head shows the intact left hemisphere. Fluid has filled in where the other hemisphere was removed.

ent than she was prior to surgery, but she has had no seizures in three years and is on no anticonvulsant medication. Perhaps we should have done the surgery far earlier. (See Figure 17.1.)

Spastic Quadriparesis

Children with stiffness in all four limbs (spastic quadriparesis) usually have sustained severe damage to the entire brain. They are likely to have severe or even profound retardation. They often have experienced seizures in the newborn period (neonatal seizures) and may have had infantile spasms during the first year of life. They will have a high incidence of generalized tonic-clonic seizures as well as of atonic attacks and the Lennox-Gastaut syndrome. Seizures in children with spastic quadriparesis may be very difficult to control with medication.

Diplegia

Diplegia is the type of cerebral palsy in which both legs are stiff. It is far more common in children who were born prematurely than in children carried to full term. These children are usually of normal intelligence and are less likely to develop seizures. Their principal handicap is a difficulty with walking. Physical therapy, bracing, and orthopedic surgery can often be of help.

Abnormal Movements

When brain damage affects areas of the brain that control the coordination of movements, the child may be athetoid; movements are performed slowly and in a writhing fashion. Damage to other areas of the brain may cause more rigid movements, that is, dystonia. Since these control areas lie deep within the brain in regions less likely to cause seizures, epilepsy is uncommon among such children. They are also less likely to be retarded.

Children with damage to multiple areas of the brain may have both spasticity and either athetosis or dystonia. Such children are said to have mixed cerebral palsy.

"How can I help my child who has cerebral palsy?"

How you help your child to cope with cerebral palsy depends on whether or not there is mental retardation. Many children with cerebral palsy are of normal intelligence, and for these children the motor dysfunction can be enormously frustrating. To be unable to dress or go to the bathroom alone or to feed oneself can create such a sense of helplessness and dependence that depression is not uncommon among such children. And yet children with cerebral palsy are increasingly able to find areas in which they can become competent and ultimately develop self-esteem. Appropriate use of computers assists learning and communication. Motorized wheelchairs and special adaptations may permit mobility and independence. It is amazing what can be done to help unlock the real person who is within these handicapped bodies.

For the child with cerebral palsy, as for the child with mental retardation, the most important ingredients in successfully coping are motivation and self-esteem. Motivation can be stimulated by hard work and activities, such as those involved in preparing for the Special Olympics. The joy of successfully participating in sports promotes self-esteem.

The Special Olympics are a model of what can be achieved in other areas of life, with patience and persistence. Such children need role models of successful handicapped adults. Their ability to become achieving adults begins with small successes in the family and in the school.

Helping your handicapped child to cope with the accompanying psychological problems is still an art, not a science. There is no how-to manual, although there are many sources of help. Your child and you will need help in articulating your frustrations and concerns, your anger and your hopes.

There has been amazing progress in recent years in enabling both retarded persons and those with cerebral palsy to participate more fully in the community. The old stereotypes of institutionalization and handicap persist, but these children, while *dis*-abled, are not *un*-able.

Difficult-to-Control Seizures

For most children, seizures are not *un*controllable, they are only difficult to control. There is good reason to hope for control. The next medicine may be successful or a combination of medications may bring control. The ketogenic diet or surgery may offer a solution. You may need to get a second opinion, and you may decide to consult with an epilepsy specialist or an epilepsy center. Many times, parents of children with difficult-to-control seizures who persisted in looking for the right therapy turned "uncontrollable" seizures into controlled seizures.

❑ **Margo was a bright ten-year-old with intractable seizures. Her hemiparesis was not disabling, but several seizures each week and the effects of all of her medications were interfering with her progress. She came to us looking for surgery to remove the epileptic focus. Unfortunately, we found that there were abnormal areas on both sides of the brain and that surgery was not an option. She had had good trials of virtually all of the anticonvulsants. After a lot of discussion with her parents and with her, and despite her age, we decided to try the ketogenic diet. Margo said she would do almost anything to get rid of those darn seizures.**

Margo faithfully stuck to the diet. She had no seizures. After two years on the diet, it was gradually stopped. It's been more than ten years now; Margo is seizure- and medication-free and doing superbly well. She says the diet was really tough, but worth it. She has gone on to college and is an active volunteer with her local epilepsy association.

Families need to persist in looking for a solution, and physicians also need to be willing to keep trying. Both need to be willing to take risks in order to achieve benefits. Unfortunately, not every family finds such a happy ending.

❑ **Greg is a fifteen-year-old boy whose seizures began in very early childhood. Although his development was delayed, seizures came under control with medication and the family came to accept their mildly retarded son. At age five, the seizures recurred and Greg appeared to become more severely delayed developmentally. The family again went through grieving, anger, and frustration while the physicians tried new medications. Eventually the seizures were again controlled and the family readjusted to their new circumstances. At age nine, atonic seizures began, and Greg made frequent trips to the emergency room for stitches. During the brief periods of time when these seizures were brought under control, Greg could function in the moderately retarded range, but the frequency of seizures or the side effects of medication continued to handicap him. An abnormality on the MRI scan led us to hope that surgery might control his seizures. Surgery was successful even though his minimal hemiparesis increased. Greg had only rare seizures, in his sleep—at least he wasn't falling—and his language and function improved. Both his family and Greg were delighted. This honeymoon lasted for six months, then the seizures recurred. Had the vagus nerve stimulator been available, it might have been useful.**

In Greg's case, we and the family have a dilemma. We know of no other combination of medicines likely to control his seizures. We are considering further surgery to section the corpus callosum. Will further surgery be of benefit? Are the risks of new surgery worth taking? What are the chances of success? The answers are unclear.

There are many lessons in Greg's story. One lesson is that even if parents do develop a realistic acceptance of their child's limitations, that acceptance may be challenged when the situation changes. For those families whose children have multiple handicaps, adjustment may be a roller coaster. A second lesson is that often trying a new approach might succeed in controlling intractable seizures. Deciding whether or not to take the risks of these new approaches when you don't know their benefits in advance can be difficult for both the family and the concerned physician. There may be a time when you and your physician must accept the status quo, but the question will be, when has that time come? Not all of our stories have a happy ending.

Coping with Severe Handicap with Epilepsy

Parents may come to accept the limitations, even the severe limitations, of their child's cerebral palsy or mental retardation, realizing that there is no medicine or surgery that can reverse the condition. "But if you could only get rid of the seizures," they may say to us, "life would not be so difficult. I thought you could control seizures with medicine for most children. Why is my child still having seizures?"

Seizures in a child who has other evidence of brain damage may be much more difficult to control. Still, your physician should try new medications, the ketogenic diet, or vagus nerve stimulation (VNS); and even if your child is retarded, surgery may not be impossible. You may need to find a physician who is willing to consider new options.

If your child's damage is primarily in one portion of the brain, removal of that portion could be of benefit. However, most children who are retarded have damage on both sides of the brain; removal of one portion will not be of benefit. Still, even in the child who has bilateral brain damage, VNS or, rarely, section of the corpus callosum can sometimes be of benefit in controlling the atonic seizures that lead to injury.

We treat seizures because they interfere with a child's function. For the otherwise normal child, occasional seizures that interfere with function require treatment. For the severely handicapped child, however, an occasional seizure may be less handicapping than the toxicity of medications. The risks of treatment and its potential benefits must, therefore, be evaluated carefully in light of your child's other handicaps. When seizures interfere with your child's behavior or interfere with placement in otherwise optimal programs in school, every reasonable effort should be made to control them. Schools may be reluctant to accept the responsibility of a child who has seizures. Parents should first try to convince the school that the seizures are not a major problem. It will require persistence, information, and lobbying. It may take legal action. The solution will require both strong advocacy and compromise.

❑ **Katie was two-and-a-half and severely handicapped. She functioned like a one-year-old. She was not able to walk or talk. Fortunately, her local school system had a superb program for handicapped children. This program had occupational therapists, physical therapists, and speech therapists. Katie was an ideal candidate—except for her seizures. The school claimed that they had no** one who could cope with her frequent generalized tonic-clonic seizures. What would happen if a seizure was prolonged? What were they to do? Katie would require far more time than the other children, and if a seizure occurred, they had no one with the special training needed. Katie's mother had no problem coping with her child's seizures, although she had had no special training. To put it frankly, the school was afraid of accepting the responsibility. Katie was deprived of her right to an optimal program. The school's solution was a home teaching program with visits several times a week. Clearly this was not optimal. Finally we helped Katie's mother to achieve a compromise. She agreed to go to school to handle the seizures while the teachers taught. Over several weeks the school came to realize that Katie's seizures did not pose a major problem, and no longer required that her mother be present.

The end of this chapter in Katie's story is that she was found to be a candidate for surgery, her damaged hemisphere was removed, and she no longer has seizures.

A Parent's Special Needs

As parent of a child with severe disability *you* have special needs as well. We have talked about success stories, about children who have been cured of their seizures. Magazines are full of such success stories. The epilepsy movement has concentrated on a message of hope in its campaign to eliminate the stigma associated with epilepsy. But for parents of multiply handicapped children or children with intractable seizures the message of hope is frustrating. These parents feel left out of the mainstream. They are angry, worried that their children will not get the help they need, and fearful that they themselves will be unable to cope.

"My God! How do I cope with all this?"

You need help! Every parent in a situation like this needs help. Each faces a terrible feeling of loneliness when confronted with the overwhelming dual problems, for example, of mental retardation and epilepsy. The initial stages of grieving, denial, and anger that any parent with a disabled child experiences are compounded by a feeling of shame, of wanting to tell no one, of feeling that you are the only person in the world who has faced such overwhelming problems. Nor do you want to bother your physician with your sense of hopelessness. "He is always so busy." Or maybe the way he has explained things to you has simply confused you. "Did he really say . . . ?"

There are several places to turn. *First,* give your doctor another chance. Ask him to explain again. *Write down your questions* before the appointment; in the stress and intimidation of an office visit, anyone can forget what questions they wanted to ask. A second place to turn is the local affiliate of the Epilepsy Foundation. There are many such affiliates around the country. If you have difficulty finding one, contact the national office of the Epilepsy Foundation in Landover, Maryland. Their toll-free number is 1-800-EFA-1000. Either your local chapter or the national office can provide information that will answer your questions.

A third and important step is to contact a local support group. Since your child has mental retardation or cerebral palsy as well as epilepsy, a local organization for retarded citizens or for individuals with cerebral palsy can be immensely helpful.

"I don't want to be part of a group. I don't need them, and I don't need to hear about someone else's problems. I have enough of my own."

We often hear this statement from parents. Or else one parent will say, "I'd like to go, but my husband (wife) won't have anything to do with it." Groups are generally helpful, but some people are just not ready to join a group at a particular time in their lives. Some people are embarrassed to talk about their feelings or problems in public. But you are not the only one who has had to deal with such problems. Hearing how other parents have coped is often far more helpful than hearing similar advice from your physician. Parents choose different words, have a different tone to what they say. And they have "lived" it, not just learned about it. Talking about your problems can help put them in perspective.

If you feel you do not need a group, or feel that you can't cope with counseling just now, reconsider it later. Remember: If you have adjusted so well that you don't need any help, perhaps you are the person who can help someone else.

Children who have cerebral palsy and/or mental retardation as well as epilepsy need considerable support. And so do their families. The combination of these disabilities may seem overwhelming, but remember, you are not alone. There are many organizations to help you and many available services. Every child, regardless of disability, is entitled to an appropriate education, for example. Handicapped children are eligible to receive services as soon as their handicaps have been identified, at whatever age. Ask your doctor, your school system, or your local health department about these services. You don't have to wait until your child is old enough for school.

For the child who has cerebral palsy, and for the parent of that child, United Cerebral Palsy (UCP) provides excellent support services with appropriate guidance and advice. The Association for Retarded Citizens (ARC) can provide similar services for the retarded child and his family. Parents' groups sponsored by these organizations talk about managing mental retardation or coping with cerebral palsy. They don't talk about seizures, and for parents of children who have intractable seizures, even when mental retardation and cerebral palsy coexist, the focus is often on the seizures. "If only the seizures were controlled, it would be easier to deal with the other problems," such parents often say. It's important for you to decide what is really most important for your child. Maybe it is the seizures. But maybe it isn't. For some children the problems of mental retardation are far more important than the seizures. For some children with cerebral palsy, mobility may be the principal problem. For parents of these children, UCP or the local ARC may provide the most important resources. If seizures are the central problem, you may need to educate these organizations about epilepsy and about the special needs of children who have recurring seizures.

For children whose seizures are the dominant disability and mental retardation, for example, is of lower priority, at least for now, parents have often had difficulty finding help. There has been a gap in support services for the multiply handicapped child who also has seizures. Fortunately, many local Epilepsy Foundation affiliates have recognized this need and, as part of their commitment to serving *all* families, are developing new programs.

The medical community also has failed to serve this population well. Developmental pediatricians trained to help manage the multiple problems of the disabled child and to help families find needed services frequently have less expertise in epilepsy than in other conditions. Further, neurologists and epileptologists who do specialize in treating children's seizures often have inadequate expertise in managing family problems and in finding services. We need to develop better one-stop shopping for this comprehensive care. But until we do, parents of a multiply handicapped child must continue to advocate and seek services with persistence and determination.

Coping with Shattered Expectations

Parents of a newborn child have great expectations. These expectations are dashed when a child is diagnosed as having multiple severe handicaps. But such a diagnosis should not mean that expectations for your child must be abandoned. It means that your expectations must be modified, although your hopes may persist. Your expectations for your child need to be individualized. You should discuss them with your physician, but your doctor does not have a crystal ball. He may not be able to foresee with any great precision how well your child will be able to do.

Parents often tell us that their physician had said that their child would never walk. Their child is now walking, and they are angry that the doctor underestimated their child's abilities. Others are angry because their physician did not tell them that their child would have troubles in school or be retarded. When a child is only one year old, it may be difficult to predict how well he will talk, walk, or learn. When your child is three, your doctor may be able to be more precise in making predictions. By age eight, you and he will have a much better idea about learning problems. The more severely handicapped the child, the earlier accurate predictions can be made. Betting on children is like betting on race horses; the more they've run, the better you will be able to predict their future success.

But in addition to the imprecision of foretelling the future, parental frustration and anger at the medical professions are frequently the results of miscommunication. We have all played the game "telephone" as children and know how distorted verbal communication can become. Often there are misconnections in the communication process: between what a physician *intends* to say, the words he or she uses to say it, how the words sound to you, how you interpret those words, and then how you remember them.

This is not to excuse the medical professions. Some health care providers are very good counselor-communicators. Sometimes staff members other than the doctor serve as counselors, since good counseling is very time-consuming and often requires repetition. Sometimes a physician does not like to be a bearer of bad news, however, and may assign this task to someone else. Some are optimistic that the young, developmentally delayed child will outgrow her disabilities—and many children do. Sometimes for this reason the physician keeps the discussion nonspecific and imprecise, leaving the listener with an unintended (or intended) confusion. On the other hand, some physicians see the dark side of the future and, while trying to be "honest," succeed in dashing parental hopes.

When you recognize that your child is delayed, make certain that the physician explains what is known—and what is uncertain—in terms that you can understand. Don't be afraid to ask questions. When you have recovered from the initial shock, write down any new questions that come to mind and then make another appointment to continue the discussion.

Do not hesitate to ask for a referral to another physician for a second opinion. Any physician who refuses or discourages such a second opinion is probably providing a good reason to obtain one.

You should remember that a misunderstanding may not be because of what the physician said or didn't say, but rather because of what you heard or didn't hear. No one likes to hear bad news, and we often forget or deny it. In contrast, some people focus on the bad news, ignoring the hopeful signs.

We see so many parents who are trying to obtain the "best" services for their child, but in doing so are only wearing themselves out and exhausting their resources. Occupational therapy to improve feeding on Tuesday and Thursday afternoons, speech therapy Wednesday and Friday, sensory integration therapy Monday and Wednesday mornings. All this for a child who is only seven months old.

- "If there were only more hours in the day we could get more therapy and he would start to walk."
- "I know he's only one year old, but he's not talking. He needs more speech therapy."
- "The therapist said that she lacks sensory integration and needs therapy."
- "What about the Institute for the Development of Human Potential?"

The learning process is like a bottle with a narrow neck. You can only pour in so much so fast. Despite your desire to do more, you can do only so much and things can progress only so fast. Development goes at its own pace, and therapy can only help a person around roadblocks. Therapists may help you and the child find a way to solve a problem that was preventing some function: an adapted spoon may make it possible for the child to feed himself. Therapy cannot make development go faster, but specific therapies introduced at the developmentally appropriate stage can be very useful. You wouldn't obtain speech therapy for your normal ten-month-old to help him talk sooner. If your child is developmentally at a ten-month-old level, speech therapy is not going to help him to talk until he is ready. Gait training is not useful until the child has achieved the ability to sit and stand. Often it is better when therapists see the child only once a week, or once every two weeks, and teach you how to interact with your child. Then you can provide the therapy several times each day, as you play with your child. Therapists are used most effectively when there is a specific, realistic goal to be achieved.

There may come a time when neither you nor your physician can do enough, or any more. There may come a time to stop your search for the physician who will tell you what you want to hear, for the school that will provide the perfect services and the ideal program for your child. The time may come when you have to accept that you are a good parent, you have been a good advocate for your child, and you have done your best.

No child stays the same forever. All children make progress. In a brain-damaged child, the rate of that progress is a measure of the severity of the neurologic damage. For the parents of a profoundly handicapped child, progress may be measured in terms of smiling, feeding, head control, or reaching—or even just an awareness that you are there. These milestones that parents of more normal children take for granted can be major achievements for profoundly handicapped children and their families. When your child is severely handicapped it may be difficult to hold great expectations for the future. Take pleasure in small accomplishments; deal with the bad things, and then set them aside. If you cope in small ways, day by day and week by week, coping in general will become easier.

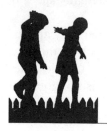

18. Epilepsy as a Psychosocial Disease

Epilepsy is usually considered a medical disorder. But for centuries it has been a psychosocial disease as well. This is not because of anything intrinsic to the disorder. Epilepsy is not confined to any social group, nor is it contagious. Epilepsy is a psychosocial disease because of the reactions, or perceived reactions, of society to persons with epilepsy and because of the psychological and social problems often associated with the disorder.

Epilepsy is a chronic condition, but unlike most other chronic health conditions, which cause constant problems, the recurrent seizures of epilepsy wax and wane over time. Dr. William Lennox, considered one of the fathers of the American epilepsy movement, characterized the disorder as "a recurrent tidal wave" compared with the constant rough seas of many other chronic health disorders. This is an apt metaphor.

Most of the time, *most* people with epilepsy are normal, subject to the same stresses and strains as everyone else. *Most* of the time, seizures do not complicate their lives. Most individuals with epilepsy take their medication and go on. But then, usually without warning, some of these individuals with controlled epilepsy are suddenly swamped by the tidal wave of another seizure. After the seizure they usually right themselves and pick up where they left off, not knowing when, or if, another tidal wave will strike. Thus, epilepsy is complicated by an uncertainty factor.

Where will your child fit on the broad spectrum of the epilepsies? Will he or she have "benign" epilepsy of childhood or one of the other chronic epilepsies in which recurrent seizures vary in frequency and severity? Will she outgrow her seizures or develop the disabling drops of the Lennox-Gastaut syndrome? Will he have the staring spells of petit mal (simple absence) seizures, which will usually be outgrown, or the staring of partial complex seizures, which may be more difficult to treat? Will he have one of the additional disabilities sometimes associated with epilepsy?

The underpinnings of possible future difficulties for people with epilepsy are set in childhood and are, to a large extent, the result of the psychosocial impact of epilepsy on the child and on the family. If the physician and the parent are sensitive to the possible development of these problems, many can be avoided.

The Child's Self-Perception

Self-image and self-esteem, as we have often said, are important ingredients of success in later life. How does your child's self-image change after a seizure? The answer to this may depend on his self-image before the seizure. The change, if any, will depend on the type of seizure and its immediate effects on him, on his developmental age, and on what, if anything, follows the seizure. Most important, self-image and self-esteem will depend on how your child and the seizure are treated by you, by your friends and family, and by your doctor.

The response of family and friends is perhaps the principal determinant of the eventual outcome for the young child, and for children of all ages, your response is the principal factor under your control.

Accurate and honest information appears to be an important ingredient of any child's self-perception. This has been best documented in adolescents. In many studies, the adolescents who were the least well-informed were the ones with the poorest psychosocial adjustment. The quality of their adjustment did not correlate either with their seizure control or with their neurological normalcy. The adolescents who were most physically normal—who had no neurological abnormality and whose seizures were under control—often were most negative about their social adjustment, because they were fearful about "being discovered." Those individuals who had had a seizure in public were better able to adapt than those who still feared being discovered. Compared to children with other health-related conditions, children with epilepsy had lower self-esteem, higher levels of anxiety, and felt less in control.

Most of these psychosocial problems can be prevented if your child is included in discussions of his epilepsy and its treatment. Having age-appropriate discussions with your child about epilepsy, his particular type of seizures, and the reason for taking medication is an important first step in his understanding and accepting his condition. In one study, it was revealed that many children still believed they could swallow their tongues during a seizure. They feared that they might die. Unfounded apprehensions seem to be more damaging than the reality. Shielding your child from the facts to prevent him "from being scared" is more likely to lead to worse, but unspoken, fears than is honesty and openness.

Your attitude toward your child and his seizures will affect his own attitude. If you are frightened, he may be too, even if he doesn't understand why. If you are overprotective, he may respond by becoming either dependent or rebellious. Your understanding that he is normal most of the time and your honest calmness will allow him to get on with the process of developing independence and competence.

It should be the job of your physician and the rest of the therapeutic team to be sure that issues of honesty, overprotection, and dependency are discussed with you and your spouse and that you come to terms with them. The epilepsy team should also discuss the seizures, medication, and reasonable restrictions with your child and make sure that you also have discussed them with him in age-appropriate terms.

Remember, ultimately epilepsy is your child's problem. If the seizures continue or if he must continue to take medication, then he will have to assume responsibility for his condition and its treatment. If your child is given a sense of control from the beginning, he will feel more responsible for his future life. We try to have these discussions with children when they are as young as five or six years of age. Responsibility clearly increases with age, but participation can rarely begin too early.

Overprotection and Overindulgence

Overprotection often causes more handicap for a disabled child than the underlying health condition itself. Protection of their young is the natural reaction of parents. Even in the absence of disability, parents raising children must tread the fine line between protection and overprotection. This line changes with the age of the child and is challenged by the independent adult trying to emerge from the child during adolescence. Your natural reaction to protect your child is greatly magnified when he is injured. You naturally want to protect him from the cruelties of the public and his peers. You want to shield him from further physical and emotional injury. Your overprotection is magnified by your anxieties, fears, and often by an unwarranted sense of guilt. These are normal reactions, but they may deprive your child of the rewards of having coped with the challenges himself and been successful.

❏ **Roberta wanted to try out for cheerleading. It was very clear to her mother that her poorly controlled seizures and her general clumsiness would not allow her to make the squad. Rather than preventing her from competing, her mother helped Roberta to realize that many people try out but are unsuccessful and that while trying out was terrific, she needed to be able to cope with the possibility of not being selected. Her mother went to the try-outs and took lots of pictures. Indeed, Roberta did not make the squad, but she was thrilled to have been part of the process. She was not terribly disappointed, and she had some wonderful memories for her scrapbook.**

Growing up requires risks to achieve benefits. Your child with epilepsy, like any child, needs opportunities to achieve independence. Opportunities necessarily entail risks. Think carefully about how much the epilepsy has really increased your child's risk.

The other side of overprotection is overindulgence. It can be equally destructive. "But if I yell at him, he might have a seizure." "He throws a tantrum when he doesn't get his own way, and I don't want to upset him." "She's been through so much, I don't want to keep her from . . . ." We hear these types of statements from many parents. When the seizures are subsequently brought under control with medication, these parents are left with a miserable, spoiled, undisciplined child or adolescent who is not handicapped by epilepsy but is socially handicapped.

Attitudes of Brothers and Sisters

Sibling love, as well as sibling rivalry, is normal. The reaction of a child's brother or sister to a sibling with epilepsy will depend on age and developmental stage but most of all on your reaction to epilepsy and to each of your children.

All children fantasize, and it is not uncommon for a child to believe that he caused his sibling's seizures by playing with him roughly or pushing him and causing a fall. Children often wish for things to happen to their brother or sister. If something does happen, then guilt is a common response. These feelings may be compounded by jealousy because you are giving so much attention to the child who has seizures. Brothers and sisters may show these feelings by "acting out," by withdrawing, or by displaying signs of depression, any of which may affect the sibling's school performance and sleep patterns.

Children often believe that epilepsy, like measles, is contagious and that they might catch it, too. This fear should be discussed openly within the family.

Your other children may be drawn into a pattern of overprotection or overindulgence. Either you or they may say, "Don't play so roughly, you might bring on a seizure." "Don't let him get so excited." "Give him the toy, or he'll get upset and have a seizure." Such statements give enormous leverage to the child with epilepsy to manipulate the people around him.

Most of these problems can be avoided by your sensitivity to the effects of your child's epilepsy on his brothers and sisters and openness and honesty about your own feelings about the epilepsy and expression of your continued love for all of your children. It is important that you initiate discussions with your other children and that no matter how time-consuming and preoccupying your child's seizure problems may be, you find some time to spend individually with the others, talking and doing something special with them and for them.

While there is always an impact on siblings whose brother or sister has a disability, studies have shown that, if handled appropriately, the impact is positive. Brothers and sisters can become stronger, more sympathetic, more empathetic, and more caring.

We have found two other ways to be helpful to siblings of a child with epilepsy.

Sibling Workshops

Sibshops, as they are called, meet periodically under the leadership of the local Epilepsy Foundation affiliate. The Sibshops are led by a person who is well versed in epilepsy and its effects and adept at working with children and adolescents. Sibshops allow the siblings to talk about the problems of having a brother or sister who seems to get more than his or her share of attention, who requires special handling, who doesn't do an equal share of the chores, who may receive less discipline and more praise. Many of these complaints are common to all siblings, even when there are no medical problems in the brother or sister, but these feelings are stronger in siblings of children who do indeed require different care.

Allowing siblings to talk about their problems and their perceptions, to hear that others are facing difficulties also, and to find out how others have coped with them can only be of benefit. Brainstorming about solutions is also helpful. Every child thinks that he or she is the only one to have suffered such a fate. Particularly when such discussions are led by a good counselor, they can be invaluable.

At times, older siblings are given undue responsibility for the child with epilepsy or other handicaps. This is often true when the affected sibling has multiple handicaps. It is important to recognize when this extra responsibility is becoming burdensome for the sibling, and to be sensitive to the responsibilities placed on a youth or adolescent. Keep the lines of communication open, and be ready to help siblings avoid or solve problems.

Camps

Many Epilepsy Foundation affiliates run summer camps for children with epilepsy. The camps are of varying length and expense. Some are only for the children with epilepsy. Others include siblings. Some are for children with lots of seizures, others also welcome those whose seizures are controlled or outgrown. Camps for children with epilepsy are often held at the same time as a camp for children without epilepsy. The inclusion of children with little or no handicap allows everyone to develop a realistic perspective on epilepsy and allows them to teach and become role models for one another.

While requiring more staffing and volunteers, these camps can be a very rewarding experience for adolescents and adult volunteers. Siblings and parents might participate as counselors. The camps offer an opportunity to talk with other people who have epilepsy and often provide an opportunity for a child who has epilepsy to see for the first time what a seizure looks like to someone else.

If your Epilepsy Foundation affiliate does not have a camp, a group of parents might like to get one started.

Attitudes of Friends

It is up to you and your child to tell friends about her epilepsy. The information conveyed, and the persons to whom it is conveyed, should depend on the type and frequency of the seizures. For the child with absence or partial complex seizures that occur with some frequency, it is far better for the friend to understand the seizures than to assume that the child is "weird," "on drugs," or "going crazy." One of our teenagers with unrecognized absence seizures had been nicknamed "Spacey" by her friends. It is more useful for a friend to understand what to do should a seizure occur and not to panic.

Unless the seizures are frequent, it is unnecessary to inform everyone with whom your child comes in contact. However, her good friends and those families with whom she spends time should be aware of her seizures and how they are controlled. In general, the fears and apprehensions that are consequences of ignorance are far worse than any reality.

"Should I tell my date?" is a question we are often asked by teenagers. Again, this depends on the frequency and type of the seizures. Certainly if a relationship begins to become serious, your teenager should be self-confident enough to talk openly about his or her condition.

How Common Are Psychosocial Problems?

It is hard to tell how common psychosocial problems are, since there are biases in all studies: children with psychosocial problems are far more likely to be identified and included in studies than those without problems, and children with continuing seizures are more likely to be identified than the 80 percent whose seizures are completely controlled or outgrown.

Whatever the true incidence, such problems are sufficiently common that they should be monitored. Problems with learning and even with retardation are usually caused by brain dysfunction rather than the seizures themselves. Learning problems, as well as hyperactivity and behavioral problems, may be caused by medication. Close monitoring of your child's school performance is the parents' responsibility, and if you have concerns, you should discuss them with your physician.

Depression is not uncommon in children. It may be hard to identify.

Symptoms of depression include sleep disturbances, school problems, fatigue or listlessness, lack of enthusiasm, easy crying, and irritability, among others. Depression can be due to the anticonvulsant medications. But depression also may be a consequence of a child's or family's reaction to the seizures and their treatment. If you are concerned about these problems, you should discuss them with your doctor. Early identification of depression can lead to earlier help.

Psychosocial problems are sufficiently common in children with epilepsy that families and physicians should be alert to them. Preventive discussions with members of the family and the school may avoid problems or permit early identification of them. Psychosocial problems should not be allowed to become a handicap.

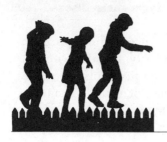

19. Counseling:
A Dialogue

Guidance and counseling, commonly used as synonymous terms, have somewhat different connotations to us. Guidance is something one person provides to another. It implies, to us at least, something actively given and passively received. Counseling, on the other hand, implies something done together and requires active participation by both parties. We believe this distinction is important.

Physicians often speak of patients as compliant or noncompliant, meaning they have or haven't followed the instructions of their medical practitioners. Implied in the word *compliant* is a sense of submissiveness. We often assume that a person with seizures should do exactly what we tell them to. We forget that it is the patient who experiences the seizures, who is encumbered by the stigma of epilepsy, and who may experience side effects from medication we prescribe. We forget that the disorder is the patient's and, therefore, that the patient must ultimately exercise his own control. However, in a more positive sense, compliance should not constitute submissiveness but rather should reflect a partnership in which the patient agrees with a recommended therapy and therefore follows it willingly.

If the patient or, in the case of young children, the family is to exercise the control, then they must be educated, so they can become active partners in the decision-making processes. They must be informed about their condition or their child's condition and about the likely future. The patient—or the parents of a young child—must assume the responsibility for that future. They must determine their own goals and aspirations. Some people use phrases like "owning your own disease" or "empowering the consumer." We prefer to talk in terms of a partnership and counseling. Then the physician and his team are in the more appropriate position of teachers, counselors, and supporters on this road to seizure control and to medical as well as psychosocial well-being.

Below, Diana Pillas shares some information and insights about counseling patients and families dealing with epilepsy.

Who Needs Counseling?

I believe that everyone touched by epilepsy needs education and information. Each person should understand the medical information about epilepsy and the social ramifications of the disorder. Many people have a difficult time coming to terms with the diagnosis of epilepsy, whether for themselves or for their child. For most, the diagnosis is overwhelming. The enormous amount of information initially given is hard for parents and children to comprehend and absorb. Often they find it difficult to stand back from the immediate situation and achieve a perspective. A counselor may be able to help them sift through the information the physician has provided, to explain it again, perhaps in different terms, and then to help them begin working on a process of coping. Parents, often numbed by the initial diagnosis and the overwhelming amount of information, worry that in their numbness they may appear unable to comprehend, unable even to think of appropriate questions. Parents voice concern that the doctor may think they are stupid. A counselor can step in when this numbness subsides and help them voice the questions they were too stunned to ask before.

In working with people who have epilepsy, the counselor has to develop trust. In developing that trust, the most important ingredient is total honesty. I emphasize to parents and children that I am speaking to them as a counselor, not as a person who knows what it is like to have a seizure, since I've never had one. I tell them that I don't walk in their shoes but that what I offer are some tools, developed by working with lots of people, the tools which they need to deal with epilepsy so that it does not take over their lives.

What most people want is some control over their lives. What I want for every person with epilepsy is for them to have ownership and control over their seizure disorder. Counselors can't give them complete control over the medical aspects of their disorder, but we can help them to gain the best control possible over the social ramifications of epilepsy and of their own self-image.

A referral for counseling can come from the family itself, if they recognize their own need for help; it may come from the physician or anyone in contact with the child or family who recognizes that they need additional help in understanding or coping.

Many people have their own way of coping and do very nicely. But often when the family is under stress things can just come apart. Sometimes the stresses are due to misperceived guilt or an effort to fix blame; sometimes fears or jealousy among siblings are the cause; occasionally, people who seem to be coping well just get tired of pretending that everything is okay, that nothing has changed. They need to unload and say, "I'm sick of pretending that I'm coping well. My child is sick of pretending that everything is still fine in school." This pretending that everything is okay may work for awhile, but it is useful only until acceptance of the epilepsy and of its problems ultimately occurs. These are some of the things that bring a person or family in for counseling.

Counseling should be part of the initial educational process, not just directed at working out later problems. Preventive counseling should begin at the time of the diagnosis. If the patient and the family don't understand that treatment will require trial-and-error medication adjustment, they may lose trust in their doctor when other seizures occur. They will often feel that the doctor hasn't "fixed" the epilepsy. If the patient has side effects of the medication and has not been made aware of that possibility, they may feel the medicine is no good, rather than considering that it needs to be adjusted. Children or adolescents who have never seen a seizure will have trouble understanding their friends' reactions when a seizure occurs or the fear that others may have of a seizure's occurring. If the family hasn't been warned about the dangers and consequences of overprotection, then they naturally overprotect their child and have to suffer the consequences later.

Counseling is not for everyone. Some don't need it, and some don't want it. If a person or a family doesn't want it, then it will be of no use to them. All you can do is leave the door open for them to come back later. Another possibility is to try to connect a family with another family or a support group. Talking to other parents and other children may be less threatening than talking to a member of the treatment team.

Sometimes counseling is crisis intervention; something catastrophic has happened and the individual needs to talk about it. Sometimes families just need help understanding the information the physician has given them. But sometimes, while intervening in a crisis or reinterpreting information, a can of worms is uncovered. Suddenly the counselor finds underlying stresses in the family that need to be addressed. Families who are dealing with epilepsy are just like other families, with all their stresses and tensions. Epilepsy is an additional stress, one that can exacerbate and expose the others.

All families need to be able to communicate, and a counselor gives both the person with epilepsy and the family an opportunity to do just that. They need to talk about the epilepsy but also to talk about all of the other things that affect families, things like expectations, fears, responsibilities, restrictions, and feelings about themselves and others.

Counseling and education should involve the child, even a child as young as five or six. It is a disservice to leave him out. Involving children early begins the process of ownership of their condition which, over the long run, will be so important in helping them to cope.

The counselor doesn't cope for others. The child, the teenager, the adult, the family will have to cope for themselves. All I'm there to do is to be the catalyst, to give them the tools to achieve the benefits of confidence and independence.

Where Counseling Helped: An Example

❏ Karen is one of the best examples of the importance of counseling. Karen had her first seizure when she was about ten. It was a tonic-clonic seizure, and then she had a few complex partial seizures later. Medication controlled these for about two years, but when she was about twelve she again began having seizures and first came to Hopkins. The doctor wanted to change Karen's medicine, but he was also very concerned that things were going poorly for her in school. He thought the problem might be with the school's lack of acceptance of her seizures. The doctor asked me to see Karen and find out what was going on.

Karen was a very shy young lady, and during our first visit all she did was cry. I couldn't get her to talk at all. So I asked her to keep a journal, to go home and write down her thoughts about everything she felt, so that when she came back we could talk about them. What we discovered was that the problems weren't in school, they were at home. The major problem was her father, who blamed Karen for the strife, arguing, and financial problems that the family was experiencing.

Eventually we asked her parents and siblings to come in to talk. Her father refused to participate. He was a very domineering type, her mother a rather meek lady. The counseling, which went on weekly for over a year, helped Karen gain control and do better in school. This may have had less to do with understanding epilepsy than with the fact that the family situation changed. Her mother, who ostensibly came to counseling to understand more about epilepsy, gained insight into her own problems. She ultimately decided to divorce Karen's father. This led to an additional need for family counseling, as they adjusted to being a single-parent family.

It took a long time for Karen to realize that the problems were really due not to her but to the dynamics of her family. She finally realized that she was not responsible for having epilepsy. She learned that her medical bills were not the cause of the family's financial problems. She eventually saw that her father was just using the epilepsy as an excuse, and that she was suffering from both his need to blame and her own feelings of guilt.

Karen's seizures were not a major problem, but she had had no education about epilepsy. She was surrounded by all of these family arguments and strife, and she said to herself, "Hey, I'm the only one who is sick. I'm the only one who is different. Therefore, all of this must be my fault." This also led to her doing poorly in school, which made her think that she was not as smart as her friends, which she attributed to her epilepsy. All of these things contributed to a terrible self-image. So we had to work on these issues. We also had to work with her brother and sister, who were jealous that she was getting a disproportionate share of attention. They needed to see that Karen was the victim, not the cause, of the parental discord.

Helping Karen took a year. We would reexamine the thoughts she recorded in her journal. I challenged her to do things. At the start, she was tired all the time, had no energy, wanted only to sleep. We wondered if this was medication, but it probably was depression. Karen enjoyed athletics but had given them up because of her epilepsy and her school problems. We got her involved in just one sport and watched her energy level increase. When she found she could participate despite her epilepsy, things began to go better.

Initially Karen was having seizures every few months. With medication adjustment (and as she got older) she would go for almost a year without a seizure. Karen really wanted to be able to get a driver's license when she was old enough. Our state then required a person to have been seizure-free for one year to get a driver's license. It would seem as if she'd almost made it, then she'd have a seizure, and the rug would be pulled out from under her each time. But, through counseling, she had become a stronger person and was able to deal with the recurrence of seizures and her frustration about not getting her license. With each recurrence she was, of course, disappointed and angry, but most of all she was determined. She figured out that most of the recurrences happened when she had tested the limits of how little sleep she could exist on, or how much she could drink, or of how long she could miss her medication. Gradually she learned to pay attention to those limits and that the seizures and the driving were under her control.

When Karen would come back to see the doctor and me after a recurrence, she would be angry and extremely upset, but I could support her. I never made light of her problems, and that is very important. What may seem to be small problems to the counselor and possibly to the parents can be big problems to the teenager.

How Do You Help Teenagers Cope?

I ask teenagers, "What are your choices?" They could go in their rooms, close the door, and never come out again. That would be a choice. If you help people discover alternatives and allow them to make their own choices, eventually they can find the best way to deal with their problems. There really isn't anything to do but to pick yourself up and go on, is there?

But sometimes things don't go so well. People with epilepsy have to walk a fine line between hope and reality. Life is not always fair, but what are you going to do about it? You just have to deal with it. Counseling often can be very helpful in enabling people to see that.

I saw Karen every week at the beginning, but later, as things got better, our meetings would be less frequent. She would call just to let me know how things were going or if there was a problem. We got through her first date (she learned that girls with epilepsy could date and be attractive, like everyone else). We discussed whom you tell about your epilepsy and when. She didn't tell every date, but when she began to be serious about one person she made certain that he knew about her seizures. She told her close friends and also the coach of her team.

Karen first went to junior college to prove to her father, who was still visiting with her and sharing in her financial support, that she could do it, and then he agreed to let her transfer out of state. She did very well. She now has a good self-image. Her seizures are under control, although there is still an occasional seizure when she tests the limits. Then I just say, "Hey, you've got to pay the piper. You know the rules and what you can do. It's your choice."

Teenagers want to be in control, and all children and adolescents need to test limits, to explore. That is a time-tested way of growing. It's no different for kids with epilepsy, but they have additional boundaries to test. They don't like parents or anyone else telling them what to do. They don't like having to take medication, because it doesn't seem to be under their control. Now that Karen is more mature, she really understands. She knows it *is* her choice whether she takes medicine and how she treats her body. That gives her ownership of her seizures, and she should exert as much control as possible.

Another thing which has been a big help for Karen's self-image is that she has become a counselor to other teenagers. We have asked her to participate in conferences for parents and others. On occasion, we have asked her to talk with teens, either individually or in groups. She has been a role model, and that works out well for everyone.

Karen has recently married. The confidence to go away from home for the last years of her education, to find and keep employment, and to marry, all despite occasional seizures, was established during the years when she was seeking help, learning to cope, and reaching out to others with epilepsy.

Her progress came partially from her mother's willingness—albeit reluctant at first—to allow her to participate in counseling, and her mother's eventual participation. Parents should not underestimate their role in helping their child develop self-esteem. Much of this is rooted in respect for the child and allowing the child to be a full partner in the seizure management team.

"Is there much difference between counseling teenagers and counseling adults with epilepsy?"

I work mostly with children and teens, so I'm more likely to talk about them, but I counsel adults as well. Every person is an individual. Some are more mature than others. Sure, teens have their own hang-ups and you need to help them achieve independence and get over the hump from child to adult. While there are many similarities in counseling adults, it is sometimes more difficult, especially if they've had seizures since childhood. Too frequently, adequate counseling and education were not available to them; they've spent so many years with a poor self-image. Reconstructing self-confidence is more difficult than building it right in the first place. These persons need to learn how to take control of their epilepsy and also of their lives. That's one of the reasons why I feel so strongly that children need to take ownership of their seizures at the earliest possible point.

Adults need to be careful not to patronize young adults and teens. Young people are very sensitive to how you say things as well to what you say. I say, "I don't have epilepsy. I've never had a seizure, so I don't know how you feel, but I've got some tools to help you and they have come from talking with hundreds of other kids. The information comes from them. I think you may find some of the ideas useful. I can arrange for you to talk with another kid around your age, if you would like to do that, or I could refer you to our peer network." When approached in this manner, kids seem to respect you more, don't feel that you are patronizing them, and are more likely to open up.

"Does counseling always work out well?"

Not for everyone, but it does for many. Sometimes you have to take different approaches. We treated one teenage boy whose seizures were under complete control for long periods of time, and then he would have another tonic-clonic seizure. He swore that he took his medicine, but at the time of each seizure the blood levels would be low. He was never interested in counseling. He thought he was too macho and that he could handle his epilepsy. He was really a good kid. Off at college, he wanted to get his own car. In Maryland you now can drive when you have been seizure-free for three months. Finally, after he wrecked the family car in what was presumed to be a seizure, the doctor said to him, "Look, you are wasting my time and your parents' money. I don't care if you have seizures or if you never drive. I don't want to see you again until you can look me in the eye and tell me that you have been taking the medicine regularly and not drinking. If you have a seizure under those circumstances and the blood level is good, then I'll work hard with you to get the seizures under control. Then perhaps we'll try another medication, but not until that time. What's more, I'm going to suggest to your parents that they not let you drive until you've shown that you can take responsibility."

The doctor told this to the boy and then told this to the parents in the boy's presence. He has not had any seizures since. Sometimes tough love is necessary, and putting the responsibility in the patient's court gives a person the control they need to feel. It's their epilepsy, not their parents', not the physician's, not the counselor's.

This concept of control can apply to other issues as well. We recently saw a teenage girl who had not had seizures for two years. We suggested that she begin to taper the medication, in advance of starting to drive. She wanted to be off medication but was afraid she would have another seizure and, worst of all, that she might have one at school. We talked about her fears, but we left the decision about stopping the medicine to her. Several months later she decided to try it, and she has done well. She wouldn't discuss her fears with the doctor but would discuss them with me. I seemed to her to be less threatening.

Counseling the Younger Child

Whether counseling a younger child is different from counseling a teenager depends on the age of the child, the child's level of understanding, and the child's problems. Let me tell you about Jenny, who was nine years old when I first met her. She was a bright youngster, one of four children. Her mother was a former nurse and had a fair amount of medical knowledge about epilepsy. The father was attending law school at night. The family was under real financial stress. In addition to caring for the family, Jenny's mom was working two jobs. Let me tell you, tensions in that family were really high.

Jenny had several seizures, but that wasn't the reason she was referred to us. She was initially referred because her doctor thought she might have a degenerative brain disease. Over the previous year, she had deteriorated dramatically, both at school and at home. She was always sick with headaches or stomach aches and was missing a lot of school. Visits to the doctor's office weren't helping the family's financial problems, either. Neither her mother nor her physician could tell which of her symptoms were related to the seizures, which to the medication, and which were psychological. She had become a very belligerent and disruptive child, causing havoc in the family. Her actual seizures were not that bad, but the family was disintegrating, even though they wanted to stay together.

Jenny's behavior was the main issue at our first meeting. She didn't like taking medicine. She didn't like being sick and going to the doctors.

All kids seek attention, but some do not distinguish between attention for the positive things they do and attention for negative behavior. Jenny was not always aware of what she was doing. Her temper outbursts and not feeling well took up much of the limited time this family had for each other. Her brother and sister resented all the attention and concern Jen was getting, and they let her know it; they also began to manifest the same symptoms in attempts to draw attention to themselves. The family was a mess. This is a good example of how epilepsy can become a family problem, not just a problem for the affected individual.

Jenny, although only nine, had many long-range questions: "Do big girls have these seizures? Can they have babies?" Things like that. I arranged for Karen to have lunch with Jenny and me. The two of them just talked. They talked about seizures, about medication, about boys. What Karen provided for Jenny was something I couldn't provide; she was the role model Jenny needed. Actually, it was as good for Karen as for Jen; it provided Karen with a sense of self-esteem, a sense of helping.

Out of counseling come many good things, but sometimes it takes a while to see all of them. Greta was another young lady who had a rough time as a teenager. She had very frequent, mixed seizures, and she had a very overprotective father. It took many sessions for Greta, and even more for her father, to learn to cope with her epilepsy and her teen behavior. She is now married and has a baby. Her parents recently called me after a scare, when they thought that Greta had cancer. The family really panicked, but Greta remained cool. She handled it far better than her folks did. The diagnosis proved to be wrong, and when we talked about it recently she said, "You know, I went through so much while learning to deal with my epilepsy that it made me a much stronger individual. I was able to deal with that potential bad news much better than my dad."

One of the best things about this job is the relationships you establish with the kids. They'll call you up years later, as Greta did, just to say hi or to touch base and tell you what's going on in their lives. It makes you feel as if you've genuinely made a difference. Real friendships have been formed, and that is gratifying.

There's another child I want to tell you about. Jeb was only six. He had the mildest of seizures, just a few absence seizures, and he was adorable. But what an anxious family. Mom, a former nurse, read everything available and learned of allergic reactions to medication the doctors had never seen. Jeb was having some stomach problems and had become a monster at home. His mother thought he was not doing well in school. He had taken to fighting at school and misbehaving at home. Mom felt that most of these problems were due to the medication. Jeb was very verbal, bright, and had lots of questions. Both the doctors and I took him aside and explained his epilepsy to him. We asked him to write down his questions and we asked his sister, who was a year younger, to have her mother list hers. We promised to discuss them at the next visit. Jeb knew the family was very upset, but he didn't know why. He felt that he was different and asked, "What's wrong with me?" His mom was extremely knowledgeable, but she couldn't step back and be objective in her son's case, and so she became very nervous. She called me every day for several weeks. (Another way we do counseling is just to provide reassurance by phone.)

Jeb was given permission to call me also. He didn't always need to have his mom interpreting things for him. He could tell me, "I don't like this. I'm sick of that. Do you want to know how I did in school today?"

What he did was to take responsibility for his condition, his medication, and his young life. That's pretty remarkable for a six-year-old, and it is also remarkable for a parent to permit it and still provide appropriate supervision.

Jeb's sister, who also played an important role, had her own questions. Her first question was, "Will I catch this?" That is a typical question I hear from brothers and sisters. Her second question was, "Why did this happen to Jeb?" Only after she knew that she was safe could her concern for her brother come out. There were other questions, "Do more boys than girls get epilepsy?" The questions themselves were less important than the fact that both children had the right to ask them. Each child was important, and both were an important part of Jeb's getting well.

Too often, doctors and even counselors get caught up with the parents' concerns about their child's epilepsy and with the child's own concerns. We forget the brothers and sisters. Epilepsy is a family problem. It touches everybody. It's important to let brothers and sisters express their concerns. It's important to help them to ask questions that they can't articulate easily. In our experience virtually every sibling has fears, misunderstandings, and resentments. It's imperative that they talk about them and be part of the family's acceptance of epilepsy.

When it was time to discontinue medication, Jeb was the one who was allowed to make the final decision. It was discussed with him and his mom. He went home to think about it and discuss it with the family. Even at seven, he understood that there was a risk of having more seizures and that he might have to restart medicine. I strongly believe that it is important to be honest with people, especially with children.

When he was scheduled to come back and tell us his decision, I was out of town, so Jeb changed his appointment because he wanted me to be there, too. He said that I was a part of all of this, and he wanted me to hear his decision.

The important thing to understand about counseling is that it is not a routine thing. It has to be individualized for each child, for each adult, for each family, and for each problem. Education about epilepsy underlies much of it, but understanding kids and family dynamics is probably the largest part. There is also a large element of common sense.

Particularly Difficult Circumstances

One of the distressing facts one must face as a counselor is that you can't save the world. There are some people out there who don't seem to want to be helped. There are some who enjoy being unhappy. As hard as it is to believe, there are some who derive their pleasures from saying "poor me." There are those who just don't have any motivation, and some who don't have enough motivation to change at the time you see them. You have to try to keep communications open, so if their motivation develops later, they can come back and get help.

There are also parents who are reluctant to see their child get well, although this is generally a subconscious need. One parent or both parents may totally invest themselves in their child's illness. Their role in life becomes taking care of their "sick" child and protecting that "poor, unfortunate child" from embarrassment, pain, failure, and all of the other "traumas" that are part of growing up. If you help the child to be successful, the parent loses the role of protector and may feel lost without that mission. This makes it very difficult for the counselor to be successful.

This "sick child syndrome," as it is often called in medicine, is not necessarily related to the severity of the seizures or to the child's degree of impairment. Rather, it is related to the parent's personality and to family dynamics.

One approach to this problem is to begin to get the parents involved with activities outside the home. When prompted, parents recognize that they and their child each need some space. We try to get them to begin to focus on themselves, on their spouse, on the other children in the family. We may even give them "assignments": Spend one hour this week alone, apart from your child, doing something—or nothing. Call us next week to tell us what you did. Get a sitter and go get your hair done. Go to dinner with your spouse. Go to the movies. It is amazing the number of couples who have done none of these things since the child was born or since the seizures began.

In a support group, which you can locate through your local epilepsy association, not only do parents give and get support through talking, but often they set up exchanges, in which another parent knowledgeable about seizures will care for your child for half a day or one evening and you can do the same for that family. It's called networking.

We ask a mother and father to arrange a "date" with each other one night a month without children—to get reacquainted and refresh and replenish themselves. It may seem impossible to you at first, but your children will survive your brief absence. Remember, if you don't take care of yourself, you can't take care of anyone else.

One of our mothers created a "mothers' night out." One weekday night the fathers committed in advance to being home with the children, and a group of mothers of handicapped children, most with epilepsy, went out for dinner and drinks. Each month they would go to a different restaurant. The only rules were that there was to be no talk about children or medical problems. It started with only two women, but the group quickly grew and became a major source of respite and support. It's an idea you might consider starting in your community.

We live in a difficult time, and the divorce rate is high. When a child with a chronic disability is added to the normal family strains and stresses, families often become even more fragile. Communication with spouse and children becomes even more important. Suffering in silence or blaming or laying guilt can be a prelude to disaster. Communication takes hard work and practice. Group support can help establish lines of communication and bring families closer together.

Children are very sensitive to their parents' emotional states. They can sense when you are worried, unhappy, angry. They need to communicate their fears and concerns to you, and they need to understand your anxieties.

Parents who struggle with guilt and overprotectiveness often have difficulty imposing restrictions on their child and fail to discipline the child, who quickly learns to manipulate the parents. This role reversal further increases family tensions. Discipline is the core of competence and self-esteem. Modification of behavior takes consistency and patience. The earlier it is begun, the easier it is to achieve. We encourage the use of calendars, stickers, prizes, and rewards. Rewards need not be expensive, but at the start they must be awarded frequently. For an older child, you may want to let him pick the restaurant when the family goes out or get a favorite CD or pick the video to rent. This should be used not as bribery but rather as a reward for a job well done.

We were recently successful in changing a parent's approach to her child's epilepsy by having the *child* give the *parent* a star on the calendar for every day she did not ask of the child, "Do you feel all right?" or "Did you take your medicine?" An additional reward was given at the end of the week, determined jointly by parent and child, if the mother earned sufficient stars during the week. They loved it, and it gave a goal and a bonding not centered around epilepsy. Many of the techniques for coping with epilepsy are developed not by medical research but by applying common sense to solving problems—to achieving success.

The successes I've been talking about are primarily among the 80 percent of children whose seizures can be brought under control and who don't have other handicaps. In this group it is easier to give hope. You can easily and honestly say to them, "Look, most people like you will have their seizures completely controlled. You will probably outgrow your epilepsy." I can give them some positives to look forward to.

Families who have a child with retardation and epilepsy, or with cerebral palsy and epilepsy, or a child with some other combination of handicaps, may have to define success and failure differently. We often are faced with families with a severely impaired child who also has seizures. They come to us before they really recognize how damaged the child is and how limited that child will be. The parents will focus on the seizures and the medication and overlook the other underlying problems. Parents like this will need a lot of support over a long period of time. Everyone needs to maintain some hope, but parents of a multiply handicapped child need to become realistic, gradually to come to terms with the child's problems and to accept them. Realistic acceptance, coupled with hope, is the goal I set for these parents.

These parents need to be helped to see and appreciate the small successes every child achieves. These little successes—smiling, responding, turning over, making a sound—may seem minimal achievements to you, but they are major achievements to the parent who has waited for them a long time. Parents' reactions to severely handicapped children often will depend on ethnic background and on the social context in which they were raised. There is also a lot of individual variation. But it is amazing the reserves of strength that reside deep in many people.

I don't know how I would respond if I were thrust into the situation that faces many of these parents. And I don't think anyone knows how he will respond until he actually has to face it. But, somehow, virtually all of them do respond in a positive fashion. Somehow, virtually all of them learn to cope.

What they require most of all is support. They need to realize that they aren't the only ones who have faced a tragedy. They need support from husband or wife, from grandparents, and from friends. The counselor can be a major source of that support but must also help in finding other community and family sources. I try to make sure that the grandparents are educated about the epilepsy and about the child's other problems; if grandparents do not understand, they can be very destructive instead of supportive of the family.

In many cases fathers are more fortunate than the mothers, because they don't have to live with the problem twenty-four hours a day. They go to work and have other distractions and other responsibilities. Too frequently the burden (and it can be a burden) falls on the mother, who may have given up her job to stay home with the child, and that's not fair. One of my jobs is to try to make sure that the father stays involved, that he comes in for the counseling sessions, and that he shares some of the burden. I don't mean just the physical care of the child. He must shoulder some of the emotional burden, as well. Men often handle grief in a different fashion from women. They can bury themselves in their work and avoid having to face their grief and their emotions. This is less common with women, who seem to take on the responsibility, even when it grinds them down. They have to face the problems hourly, without a refuge.

Working women can have an even worse problem. Rather than using work as a refuge, work becomes an additional responsibility. They still have the child and the problem back home. We find that many parents don't share these problems very well. They need help in communicating with each other and in learning to share the burdens. It is important to try to keep the lines of communication open between the husband and wife. It is surprising how often they just don't talk. It is essential that the wife get some relief from her role, even if it is just an hour or two to go out to the market without the child, to go shopping on a Saturday when the husband is off work, to go away for a weekend or to a movie and dinner. A brief respite can make things more tolerable.

When there are other children, it is critical that each get a share of the parents' insufficient time. Each child should be made to feel special for a period of time, however brief. They should be taken out, played with, anything that is special for them, so they feel they still count. Parents need to be reminded that the handicapped child, who could consume thirty-six hours of every day, is not the only one who is important in the family.

Parents also need to understand that it is all right to be angry—angry at the doctors, at the system, at society at large. It's all right to be angry at the child, even though you know that the disease is not his fault. These are normal feelings, and you're not a bad mother or father for feeling them. But you can't let the anger be the controlling force in your life. You have to learn to keep it in its place. It's just as I tell some of the teenagers: "Hey, life is unfair, but what are you going to do? What are your choices?" When you explore your choices you realize that they are very limited. You can't give the child back, although there are times when you might wish you could. There may even be times when you wish your child was dead, but he isn't. These thoughts are not incompatible with your basic love for your child. It's hard to put your child in an institution, even if you want to. Usually you feel trapped.

"What do you find is the biggest problem for parents of multiply handicapped children?"

There's little question in my mind that the biggest hurdle is acceptance of the child. I don't mean that the parents don't love him or her right from the start. They do! They love the child, but they also love the image of the child that they carry in their minds. As I said before, none of us knows how we will cope with a child who doesn't meet our expectations. Even those who have had contact with handicapped children, who say they could cope, don't really know. Everyone has to go through the stages of grieving for the child who isn't as you planned, forgetting the child who is the image in your mind, before you can reach the stage of acceptance. For some parents, this can take a long time. But gradually people come to the realization of what their child can and can't do. Counselors and physicians must wait for the parents to come to those realizations themselves. They don't listen if you just tell them. You can help them to see, but, ultimately, they have to see for themselves before they can accept.

In the meantime, the treatment team has to be supportive. It's important to praise parents for what they are doing and to reassure them that they are doing everything possible. It is important to nurture their hope but to try to temper that hope slowly with realism.

It's my job to help parents find and use whatever resources are available. Solutions to some problems are obvious, but it's hard for families to think of everything on their own. I've usually heard the problem before. It's much easier for me to make suggestions about what they can do and where they can go for help. The work and follow-up is up to the family.

Some of the state-run preschool early-intervention programs, like Child Find, are helpful in getting the parents of handicapped children, and the infant or young child himself, involved with appropriate stimulation and physical therapy. Schools now integrate handicapped children at a young age, at least for part of the day. These programs give the parents some hope, some respite, and more realistic expectations about their child's progress and future.

"What about the handicapped young adult?"

One of the saddest experiences for a counselor is to encounter a young adult with limitations whose seizures are under control but who has been so overprotected by loving and caring parents that as a child he never learned to care for himself, never learned survival skills. The parents are now getting older and finally realize they won't be around forever to care for him. They begin to worry about what will happen.

Local epilepsy affiliates often teach these individuals independent living and survival skills. Learning these skills may offer young adults alternatives to living in their parents' home. Group homes may offer varying levels of supervision and more companionship and independence. Having these skills may enable a handicapped individual to make the transition to work. The skills are much harder to teach and to learn at an older age. It is difficult to break patterns of dependency that have built up over the years. Much of the overprotection and the resultant handicap could have been prevented if the family and the child had had good early counseling. It is rarely too early to begin work on these skills of independent living. The life of the whole family is much better when teaching independence is begun early.

While counseling is fun and rewarding when you're dealing with a teenager like Karen (who you know will be a winner if only she'll get her act together), at times counseling can be even more challenging and more rewarding when you have a family with a severely impaired child. Just think what you have accomplished when you help them to cope, to grow with the situation, to make the best of it, whatever that is, for themselves and for their child. If you look at bleak alternatives such as the family breaking up, leaving a single parent facing that future alone, or the child going into a foster home and the family disintegrating, then anything you can do to help the family to cope and to make a reasonable life for themselves and for their child is a success. If you define success in these terms, yes, we are usually, although not always, successful.

Acceptance and Responsibility

There are a couple of things that I would like to emphasize. First, people, particularly parents, have to remember that kids with epilepsy are kids first. You can't ascribe all of their problems to epilepsy. Kids fight, they sulk, they rebel, they don't do their chores. Epilepsy is not responsible for such behaviors. Epilepsy can influence and increase the magnitude of problems. But how the child handles the epilepsy and how the parents handle both epilepsy and the child will influence that child's future. Much of the counseling I do is the same counseling I would do for any parent of any child who had some problems. I have to help the child and the family deal with the problems in the context of the epilepsy and how everyone has reacted to it.

❏ **Jasmine was almost 13 and in the eighth-grade class for gifted and talented students. She had had a first generalized tonic-clonic seizure nine months earlier, followed by some staring spells. We had seen her in the spring and changed her medication to Depakote, and while her seizures had improved, she still had some eye fluttering and staring. One month later we increased the dose by phone, then saw her again in the fall. She had had no more spells and had had** a good summer. She had taken poetry-writing classes at the local university over the summer and received awards. Neither her mom nor Jasmine had any complaints, and we told them to return in another six months.

As she was leaving, Jasmine's mother said, "I do have one concern. This fall Jasmine seems more depressed at times. There are times when she doesn't have the energy she had last year. She is moodier, and on weekends she wants to sleep later. I wonder if she's depressed. Do you think that she's on too much Depakote?"

If she hadn't been on medication for her seizures, if she hadn't been such an exceptional young woman, if she hadn't had such perceptive parents, this information would have inspired the observation that she was entering middle school, puberty, and adolescence. We would have ascribed her symptoms to those changes rather than suspecting the dosage of the medication. We suggested that they wait a few months and see how things worked out in the new school rather than changing medication at that time. While medication could have been part, or all, of the problem, the likelihood was that the changes were due to one, or a combination of the other factors. We wanted to see.

A concept I find useful in counseling is the contract. My part of the contract is to be open, honest, and available. The other person's part depends on the person's goals and age. A reward system is always useful, regardless of age. Setting small goals which can be achieved is very important. For children, goals may be little things like brushing teeth, making their beds, doing one chore. These goals give children an area in which to succeed; they get their reward, and slowly they learn to take responsibility. When the child demonstrates responsibility in one area, then we can begin to work on another. Perhaps they are then ready to begin to assume responsibility for remembering to take their own medication, without the parent reminding them or giving the medication. This is then the child's first step in assuming control over seizures and over his or her own life.

For adolescents, the goal may be something in school or small things at home: washing the dishes, cleaning their room. For adults it would be a different goal, but something they clearly could achieve and for which they would receive a reward, even if the reward was just winning praise. Gradually they learn to take control and to assume responsibility, and ultimately that responsibility is extended to their epilepsy.

I want to emphasize again the words *control, self-image,* and *ownership*. Everyone wants control. You have to help children and adolescents with epilepsy to take control. You can't do it for them. It's not the counselor's epilepsy. It's not *my* problem. They have to do the work. It's their choice. They have to develop their self-image, and giving them small things at which they can succeed is a first step. They have to develop the self-image before they can achieve the control.

I've certainly seen good counseling done by nurses, psychologists, social workers, psychiatrists, and doubtless many others. But I've also seen well-trained counselors, who may be excellent with other types of problems, who feel uncomfortable working with kids or with adults who have epilepsy. To be a good epilepsy counselor, a deep knowledge about epilepsy and how it affects people is important. Many counselors are just not sufficiently familiar with seizures and their effects and so are unable to help families become comfortable and cope. Sometimes the personalities of the counselor and the parent or child do not mesh. If working with one counselor is unsuccessful, try another. Counselors must remember that, unlike other handicapping conditions, epilepsy is not present all the time. It is not a visible handicap. It's not like cerebral palsy or mental retardation. You have to help the kids and the families to cope in a different fashion, with an episodic condition.

I don't think there is any more rewarding job than helping these children and their families achieve their full potential. What keeps me doing this is that the rewards are so great. Can you imagine how it feels to have people like Jenny's family tell me that they would not be a whole family if I hadn't been there? That's pretty big stuff. And the kids—I've become a part of their lives. While I may not need to continue to see them or counsel them, they'll just call up to touch base and let me know how things are going. It's hard to beat that feeling.

Part Five

Living with Epilepsy

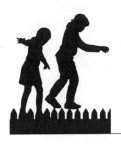

20. School:
Learning and Behavior

"Will my child have problems in school?"

"Are my child's school problems due to his epilepsy?"

There are no easy answers to these questions, since no one has a crystal ball to see how your child will do in the future. Even if your child is having school problems, your physician can't make a blanket statement that the child's school problems are or are not due to epilepsy. Answers to questions such as these require plenty of accurate information.

Why does one child do well in school and another have school problems? A child's "doing well in school" or "school problems" depend, in part, on his intelligence, on whether he has a learning disability, on his attitude toward school and about himself. They depend on the teacher's and the school's attitudes toward him and toward epilepsy. Let us reassure you first that

- there is *no* reason to worry about the possibility of school problems, if your child is not encountering and demonstrating problems.
- *most* children with epilepsy do well in school.
- *most* children with epilepsy *do not* have learning problems or social problems in school.
- there *is* reason to be aware that school problems could occur, since they do occur more frequently in children who have epilepsy.

You should also remember that lots of children without epilepsy have problems of various kinds in school. Thus, even if your child does have problems in school, they may not be related to epilepsy itself.

Intelligence

Most children have "normal" intelligence; the "average" IQ is given the number 100, and 95 percent of children have IQs between 70 and 130. While there are many questions and much debate about the meaning of an IQ score and about the tests by which it is determined, in a rough way it is shorthand for how a child will function in school. Most children with epilepsy have IQ scores within this normal range. However, if psychologists look at the range and distribution of the IQ scores for a large number of children with epilepsy, they find a larger than expected number with scores in the low-normal range. This is not because of the epilepsy itself, but usually because of what has caused the epilepsy. If the child had meningitis or brain damage or problems with the brain's development, then those problems could both have affected the child's intelligence and caused the epilepsy.

Intelligence is the result of many factors. The intelligence of parents and the environment in which the child is raised are the most important. Thus, one factor to consider, if your child is having difficulties in school, is his IQ. If his IQ is toward the lower end of the normal range, learning to read or doing math may be more difficult for him than for the rest of the class. The frustration associated with these difficulties could cause behavior problems and "acting out." Since these problems might be easily solved by a different class placement or by special help, it is important to recognize their cause early. Knowledge of the child's intelligence might also change your expectations and those of his teachers, removing undue pressure.

A very bright child, in a class that is beneath her abilities, may also be bored and not do the work or might act out. So, occasionally, a child's school problems are because the child is too smart for the class and requires more challenge.

One wonderful first grader was referred to us by his teacher because he was having difficulties reading and was not participating in class. The teacher wanted him tested for neurologic dysfunction. His parents couldn't understand, since he had no reading problems at home, only at school. A few questions to his family revealed that his favorite activity at home was reading *Popular Mechanics* and trying to build some of the things he found there. His response to the school problem was, "I'm not going to read about Dick and Jane and Spot. They're for babies." This young man clearly did not have a reading problem or a learning problem, he had a classroom problem.

Medications may also affect a child's performance in school and on IQ tests.

Learning Problems

Intelligence is only one of the critical factors in a child's ability to learn. For example, reading is a complex task. The child must first see the letters and the seeing must then be translated into electrical signals in the eye. These signals are then sent to the occipital lobe of the brain. From there the message goes to the association areas of the brain in the parietal lobe where the symbols are interpreted. Meaning comes from association with something that the child remembers, memories which must be retrieved from the frontal and temporal lobes.

Problems with reading could occur at many levels. A child with vision problems, who needs glasses, may not be able to see the letters. A child with damage in the occipital lobes might have normal eyes but might not "see" the letters. One with damage in the association areas of the brain might be able to see the letters but might not be able to recognize them. Problems in other areas might keep him from being able to retrieve the memories that give the words meaning. These varied difficulties with reading often go under the heading of "dyslexia." *Dys* means not working properly, and *lexia* means having to do with words. In most children the basic cause of the dyslexia is not understood. There clearly is a higher incidence of this type of learning problem in children with epilepsy.

Learning by listening is also a multistage process. It involves hearing and paying attention to what is said. It involves transmission of the electrical signals to the association cortex, where they must be recognized and associated with memories and actions. Thus, another type of learning problem might be associated with problems in hearing, attending, word recognition, and the association of words with memories.

Learning by seeing and learning by hearing are but two of the many multistep processes that may pose difficulties with learning. It is rare for anyone to have a complete block in one of these learning channels.

More commonly, a child will function poorly in one or more processes, and a learning problem will result. Some children learn better by listening to information, others by reading information. Most children will find their own best learning style. Some children with greater weaknesses in one area will require special help to get around their areas of difficulty and to maximize their strengths.

A child who is having learning problems in school, whether he has epilepsy or not, should receive a careful psychological and educational evaluation to identify his strengths and weaknesses. Only then will the teachers be able to find the best way to help him learn. For some children this will mean extra help. For others it may require resource teachers with special training. For still others it may mean repeating a grade, being placed in a slower class, or being placed in a special education class. Each child and his problems are unique. The child and his problems must be individually assessed and a plan developed to meet that child's specific needs. All of these statements are true for the child with learning problems, *whether or not that child has epilepsy.* They are not different for the child with epilepsy, the problems are only more common.

We have spoken about the learning problems caused by various medications. One should be aware that these problems can vary with the individual and with the medication. If your child has a learning problem, and if it has become worse after starting medication for epilepsy, the medication may be causing the learning problem, or making the problem worse. It is difficult to tell and, as we have said, learning problems may have many different causes. The only way to be certain that the learning problem is due to the medication is to take the child off the medication. This can cause the seizures to recur, so the decision should not be made lightly. Switching to another medication may resolve the issue, or you may find that the alternative also causes learning problems.

Sorting out the causes of learning problems in a child with epilepsy is, at best, difficult, and should be done with great care, often with the assistance of an educational psychologist who can carefully evaluate your child's learning problems—and *always* with the help of your doctor.

Attention Problems and Hyperactivity

In order to learn, one must pay attention to what is being taught. Teachers know that the attention span of young children is short. Therefore they teach in short blocks of time interspersed with activities such as marching around the room or recess. As the child gets older (as the nervous system and attention span mature), the child is able to sit and to concentrate or attend for increasingly long periods of time. A potential cause of a learning problem in the early years of school is that the child's nervous system is not yet sufficiently mature to allow the child to attend for long periods of time.

Another cause of attention problems could be that the child is not sufficiently bright to keep up with what is going on in the class and, therefore, is easily distracted. The other side of that coin is the very bright child who is bored by the slow pace of the class, her mind wandering to fill the time. A child who hasn't eaten and is hungry may also be less likely to pay attention. A child who hasn't had enough sleep may have similar problems. There are many different reasons for a child's not paying attention in school.

A cause that has received much attention is a condition called organic hyperactivity or, more recently, ADD, attention deficit disorder. Although this condition is common, we know surprisingly little about its source. It may or may not be associated with physical hyperactivity. ADD is more common (or more easily recognized) in boys, where overactivity is a more common accompanying symptom and more likely to draw attention to the child. Attention deficit disorders are not uncommon in children during the early school years; they are perhaps more common in children with epilepsy. They are also frequently associated with "immaturity" of the nervous system and with the learning disorders described above.

While its cause is unknown, we like to think of ADD as a problem with "filtering." Everyone is constantly bombarded by multiple different stimuli. As you are reading this chapter there may be children playing in the room, the TV may be playing, the clock ticking, and someone else talking. And yet you are able to filter all of these other stimuli out and concentrate, pay attention to what you are reading. We do not know exactly how this filtering takes place, but it seems to be to be partly a learned skill and partly a result of maturity of the nervous system. (By the way, did you notice the repetition of the words *to be* in the previous sentence, or weren't you paying attention?) Infants and young children are easily distracted by the many stimuli around them; they have difficulty paying attention (except to TV). As they get older, they can attend better. Some children mature faster in this respect than others. Some have far more difficulty paying attention than others and are diagnosed as having attention deficit disorders when the problem interferes with their work in school.

Some medications decrease a child's ability to pay attention, others appear to increase the child's ability to attend. Perhaps the actions of these drugs are on the "filter," either allowing more stimuli to reach consciousness and thus to be distracting, or increasing the filtering so the child is less aware of the distractions and can concentrate better.

Phenobarbital is known to increase the inattentiveness of some children and to cause hyperactivity as well. One of its actions may be to depress the "filter," allowing more distractions to reach conscious levels. Other drugs, such as methylphenidate (Ritalin) and dextroamphetamine (Dexedrine) may act by improving the "filter" of inattentive (or hyperactive) children, allowing them to concentrate better. These drugs are often called stimulants, because in older children and adults they seem to boost energy.

There are many new medications for ADD and for the hyperactivity that may or may not accompany it. A discussion of these medications is beyond the scope of this book. We can tell you this much, though. In every study of drugs for hyperactivity there has been a very large placebo effect. For instance, if you tell the teacher or the researcher or the parent that the medication being given is used to increase attention or to decrease hyperactivity, the adult will often perceive improvement in the child's problem, even if the medication is only a sugar pill.

Children (and adults) often rise to meet expectations. Therefore, when we begin medicating a child for attention and hyperactivity, we often do a small experiment. We tell the parent to try a small dose of the medication on a Saturday and again on Sunday morning. If there are no adverse effects (like making the child wild), they can give the child the medication on Monday, Tuesday, and Wednesday before school; then, on Thursday, call and ask the teacher how the child is doing. If the teacher responds, "He's been just wonderful this week," tell her that you started medication for ADD and you need her help. Gradually increase the morning dose to see what is the best dose. Then, since many of the medications do not work all day, find the best dose for the afternoon.

When you have worked with the teacher to optimize the response, leave the child on that dose (or doses) for a month or so. Then "forget" to give it to him on Monday, Tuesday, and Wednesday, and check with the teacher on Thursday. If she says, "It's been a terrible week," admit that you forgot to give it to him and promise never to forget again. If she responds, "He's been fine," say, "Thank you." You now know that the effects were those of a placebo. This is called a "blinded" experiment, since the teacher has evaluated the child without knowing whether or not he is receiving the medication.

Not all children with learning problems have attention deficit disorder. Not all learning problems are due to medication. Some children with and without medication, and with and without epilepsy, have problems in school. Not all children are the same height and the same weight, or have the same learning styles or the same learning capacities. Children should not be treated identically in school; every child has special needs and every child needs to be treated as an individual to bring out that child's special needs and special assets.

Sometimes all that is required is a bit of creativity. One of our patients was in a very expensive private school. His seizures had been controlled, but he was about to be expelled because he couldn't pass his tests. It turned out that he was smart enough, but he couldn't complete the tests in the allotted time. Arranging for him to take untimed tests showed that he knew the material and had learned what was taught. If a test in school is to see if the child has learned the material, why does he have to reproduce it in a fixed time? Ask about untimed tests. Ask about using a computer if writing is a problem. What about oral tests? What about a tape recorder for the visually impaired? What about using a tape recorder for those with reading problems? Creativity can be an answer to many children with learning problems.

When a child with epilepsy is having difficulty focusing his attention, we need to ask if his anticonvulsant medication may be the cause. All anticonvulsants are capable of causing both attention and learning problems. Phenobarbital seems to be the most frequent offender. Every parent of a child with epilepsy should be aware of his child's school performance and note if there is a change (for better or worse) when the child is started on medication, when the medication is changed to a new drug, or when the dosage is changed.

Psychological and Social Problems

A child's performance at school is, to a large extent, determined by the child's feelings about himself. The child who thinks that he is stupid will frequently act and perform poorly. He is unlikely to perform at his best level. The child who is depressed because of her seizures, because of her family's reaction to the seizures, or for other reasons is likely to do less well in school. Indeed, a drop in school performance may be one of the early signs of childhood depression.

But a child's school performance is also affected by what others think of him. Children, and even laboratory rats, tend to perform up to the levels of expectation placed on them. In a classic psychological experiment, researchers who were given rats to test, and who were told that they were studying "dumb rats," found that the rats did less well on testing than when they were studying "smart rats." This was true even when the "smart rats" and the "dumb rats" were from the same litters and had identical intelligence.

The effect of expectation can present a problem for the child with epilepsy and for that child's parents. If the child's teacher expects the child with epilepsy to have learning problems, then such problems are more likely to be perceived, whether they are present or not. On the other hand, a teacher who is aware that your child could have a learning problem is also more likely to identify the problem early and to be more sensitive to it. Therefore, telling the teacher about your child's epilepsy and about any concerns you may have about your child's learning could be an advantage to your child.

Make sure that the teacher understands about your child's type of seizures and that she makes you aware of any concerns she may have about your child and of any differences from your child's past performance. These could be due to changes in medication or in the frequency or type of seizures. Mutual trust and exchange of information and concerns between you and your child's teacher can benefit your child.

Here are some school problems typical of what we have seen.

Mrs. Christiansen brought us a letter from Billy's teacher. It said, "We have enjoyed having Billy in our kindergarten this year. He is a charming, adorable little boy. However, he did so poorly on his reading readiness test that we all feel he should spend another year in kindergarten. We would like you to come in for a meeting with us at your convenience." Mrs. Christiansen asked, "Should we tell her about Billy's epilepsy? He hasn't had a seizure since he started taking phenobarbital more than a year ago."

The first thing we would recommend is that she and her husband meet with the teacher, find out more about Billy's problems in school. Have there been other problems, or did he just do poorly on the reading readiness test? Is he immature in other ways in school? How does his ability to learn games and other things compare to that of his peers? Does the teacher think that this is just a problem of immaturity, which would be solved by repeating kindergarten, or are there other problems as well?

Teachers usually have a great deal of experience in identifying school problems, and the teacher's impressions can be of great help to you and to your physician in sorting out the problems and in finding the proper directions in which to proceed.

The second step would be to meet with the physician, to get his advice about the teacher's impressions and suggestions. Do we all agree with the school? Is Billy one of the younger children in the class; might he benefit from another year there? Is he immature in other social ways? Does he act more like a five-year-old than the usual six-year-old who is starting first grade? Is he intellectually slower than normal? Is he a child with a specific learning problem? We often cannot answer these last two questions without psychological testing.

Does every child who is like Billy need testing? We would say no, but whether a child does or does not need testing will depend on the opinion of the teacher and on our assessment. We are often asked to answer the question, "Is this neurological?" Our answer is always, "Yes. Learning problems are always neurological." Learning resides in the brain, not in the foot or heart. If a child isn't learning, it's because he can't or doesn't use his brain as expected. This does *not* mean that Billy has a neurological *problem* or that he needs to see a neurologist. It means that all of us (including the teacher) need to assess the situation carefully and find the best educational strategy to manage the situation.

Those are the suggestions we would give to *any* parents who received that note from their child's teacher. The only thing different about Billy is that he has had seizures and is on phenobarbital. Yes, they should tell the teacher about Billy's seizures. They might also ask her if she has seen any "daydreaming" or other evidence that he may have been having subtle seizures in school. We would also be concerned about the possible role of the phenobarbital. We would recommend checking the blood level of phenobarbital to see if it is too high and interfering with Billy's learning. We would probably recommend changing to another anti-convulsant (if Billy needed to continue medication) to see if his performance improved. *There is no way to be absolutely certain that the medication is not interfering with learning and behavior except to take the child off that medicine and, if necessary, change to another medicine.*

"This was the third time this fall that the teacher has called us in for a meeting. She says that Joshua is disruptive to the class. He bites, fights, and won't sit still. His reading is terrible, and I'm afraid that he is going to be expelled. What should we do? Can they expel someone from the second grade? I think that the real problem is that the teacher is afraid that he'll have a seizure in class and really just wants him out."

We would begin to analyze this problem by asking the parents to tell us more about Joshua. What sort of a child is he? Is he having these types of behavior problems at home? Are they new? When did they first start? Did he have similar problems last year in the first grade? Was there anything particular that might have caused them? What was the relationship of the onset of these problems to the onset of his seizures and to the initiation of his anticonvulsant medication?

Behavioral problems such as biting and fighting can come from many different sources. Any of the anticonvulsant medications can cause behavioral changes such as this. If the change began shortly after the start of a new anticonvulsant, then perhaps a different medication should be tried. However, behavioral changes rarely occur weeks or months after the child has been on the same medicine, unless there has been a change in the dose. New behavior problems can be caused by psychological disturbances initiated by problems at home or in school; they can be caused by the teacher's behavior towards the child and the child's reaction to his teacher's behavior. Does Joshua know about his seizures? Is he afraid or embarrassed by them? When people are anxious, they can be testy or lash out at others. Perhaps a careful explanation of his seizures would alleviate some of his fears, and this might allow him to be less aggressive in school.

Discussing the problems and the parents' concerns with the teacher (or the principal) and with their physician can help them to sort through these different causes. Whatever the cause, the recent change in Joshua's behavior certainly is reason for concern and investigation. It is a common symptom of problems that require solutions. It could be Joshua's unconscious way of asking for help.

"Martha's grades are terrible. She was a solid B student until her seizure, but since then she doesn't even finish her homework. Her last report card was C's and D's, and she now says that she wants to drop out of school and get a job. Could this be due to her medicine?"

In Martha's case, as in Joshua's, there are many potential sources for her problems. Puberty, boys, home problems, changes in school, depression, and concern and embarrassment over her seizures could all affect school work and should be explored in talking with Martha. We would check the blood level of her medication and lower it if it was high. If it wasn't, we would strongly consider changing to another medicine. While phenobarbital and phenytoin are the medications that most frequently affect learning, such effects can follow use of *any* of the anticonvulsant medications. Even as we were lowering or changing the medicine, we would explore with Martha what she knows about her seizures and her reaction to them. We would want to know how seizures have changed her lifestyle and her sense of self-esteem. We would ask about symptoms of depression and try to help her cope better with her epilepsy, whether or not this was the cause of her school problems. Perhaps she needs to talk with another teen who had similar problems with seizures.

"Circe's teacher called us this week because she is daydreaming in class. We had told the teacher to watch for seizures, and now she thinks that Circe is having absence seizures again. Should we increase her medicine?"

Circe could be having more absence seizures. Perhaps this alert teacher has identified the problem early. Have the parents seen any at home? Is Circe aware of missing things during class? Is it possible that the teacher is just watching too closely and misinterpreting things? Perhaps we should first check the blood level to be certain that she is taking the medication and taking enough. Perhaps we should see Circe and hyperventilate her to see if we can produce one of her spells. If we can't be sure in the office, we might want to have another EEG, to see if she is still having electrical spells. In this way we can sort out if Circe has a problem and the best approach to correcting it.

Learning problems, shyness, aggressive behavior, inattention, and reading problems are among the many school problems that can be related or unrelated to epilepsy. Your child will have some or many of the everyday ordinary problems that commonly occur during preschool, childhood, and adolescence. Keep track of your child's problems, but be careful that you do not attribute all of them to the medication or to epilepsy.

Learning problems are more common in children who have epilepsy. Early identification of a problem, if it exists, can assist in the development of strategies for compensation and lead to a far more successful school experience. However, learning problems can also be secondary to medication, to psychological stress, and to the school's and the teacher's reaction to the child and to epilepsy. Changes in school performance are best identified by the teacher, who, together with your physician, can also be your and your child's best ally in finding the cause and the best approach to a solution.

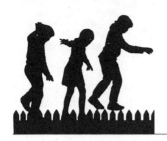

21. Routine Medical Care and Epilepsy

We are frequently called by parents, physicians, and dentists for advice about whether a medical procedure can be done safely on a child with seizures. They may be frightened by the potential effects of anticonvulsants or intimidated by the thought of a seizure's occurring during the procedure or while the child is under anesthesia.

Since anesthesia is the ultimate treatment for uncontrollable seizures, general anesthesia, used for an operation, will not cause seizures. If a child with epilepsy requires anesthesia, the only substantial concern is the inability of the child to receive his standard anticonvulsant medications by mouth. *If* the child is to receive nothing by mouth ("NPO") for 12 to 24 hours, it is advisable to give an extra dose of his regular medication prior to surgery. Routinely, pediatric anesthesiologists recommend that children take their regular medications, with just a sip of water, on the morning prior to surgery. If the child cannot receive anything by mouth for a long period of time after surgery, intravenous anticonvulsant medication may be necessary.

"Can my child be put to sleep for dental care?"

Yes. The standard anesthetics used for dental care will neither increase the likelihood of seizures nor affect the anticonvulsant's effectiveness. Some children continue to have seizures despite medication. Anyone performing a procedure on such a child should be capable of managing the seizure just as the parent would do at home.

"Is there anything different that should be done for the child who has epilepsy and requires anesthesia?"

No. If a child should have a generalized seizure, he will require an open airway. Therefore, posterior nasal packing (packing the back of the nose with gauze, to stop bleeding), sometimes done after a tonsillectomy or adenoidectomy, should be done with considerable caution and careful observation.

"What about cold medicines and cough syrups?"

Antihistamines and decongestants have been reported to decrease seizure threshold. It appears to us that some children may be quite sensitive to these medications. We have no ability to identify which children will react with a seizure when given these over-the-counter medications. There is no evidence that these medications actually alter the cold or flu; they merely ease the symptoms. It is said that a cold well treated lasts seven days; poorly treated, a week. So maybe just skipping these symptomatic medicines would be best.

If you feel that it is necessary to give your child one of the medications because the symptoms are very severe, and then your child has a seizure, the seizure may have been precipitated by the cold medication. On the other hand, it may have been precipitated by the illness. Or again, it could be coincidental. If your child repeatedly has seizures after receiving one of these medications, it would be prudent not to use them.

"Are there any other medications that my child should not receive?"

Stimulants such as Dexedrine and methylphenidate (Ritalin) are often useful in the management of the hyperactivity of attention deficit disorder. Although in the large doses occasionally used for psychiatric conditions (and in some animal models) these drugs have been reported to precipitate seizures, we have seen little evidence that they have an adverse effect in our children with epilepsy. When needed, their benefits clearly seem to outweigh any potential risks.

"Are vitamins beneficial?"

Except in the rare individual who has a clear vitamin deficiency there is no evidence that vitamins are beneficial (or detrimental) in treating epilepsy.

"Can my child receive routine immunizations?"

Yes, children with seizures and epilepsy can and should receive their immunizations, even the pertussis immunization. There may be a slight reaction to some of the immunizations, which may cause a fever, and that fever may be enough to precipitate a seizure, but *there is no evidence that current immunizations either cause epilepsy or make epilepsy worse. There is no evidence that immunizations are a cause of a* permanent encephalopathy.

But, when a young child has just begun to have seizures and the physician has not yet determined the cause of the epilepsy, *if* an infant is given an immunization *and* if there is a worsening of the seizures or a change in the child's rate of development, then parents are often convinced that the immunization caused the child's problems to get worse. It is often easier to defer the immunization for a few months until the course of the epilepsy and of the child's development becomes clearer. Then that child can be immunized. It is very clear that the immunizations currently recommended by the Academy of Pediatrics are far safer for the child than the diseases they are designed to prevent.

"Winnie developed a sore throat yesterday and her pediatrician started her on an antibiotic. Winnie is allergic to penicillin, so he put her on something called erythromycin. Today I can barely wake her up and she seems drunk. Do you think that this erythromycin is too strong for her?"

Winnie is on Tegretol for her seizures. Erythromycin interferes with the metabolism of Tegretol and makes the Tegretol level go very high. When a child on Tegretol is given erythromycin, one must reduce the amount of Tegretol by one-third. When the antibiotic is stopped, go back to the original dose.

Whenever a child is on an anticonvulsant medication and a new medication of *any* kind is given, ask your physician or pharmacist if the new drug has any interactions with the old one.

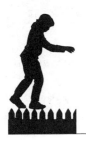

22. Sports and Epilepsy

Participation in sports is an important part of the process of growing up. There are, of course, marked variations in individuals' athletic ability, in children's stage of development, in their coordination, and in their interest in sports. Whether group play during recess, team sports like Little League, soccer, and football, or individual sports like swimming, tennis, and riding, sports are important to a child's personal and social development. They offer an opportunity to participate with others, to share, and to learn teamwork and self-discipline, skills important to the development of personality, self-esteem, confidence, and character. *No one should be deprived of those opportunities.*

Participation in organizations, such as Scouts, clubs, church groups, and so on, can also be important to the development of self-esteem and character. Children with epilepsy are less likely to be excluded from these organizations than they are from sports.

In society's paternalistic approach to children, and particularly its paternalistic approach to children with problems or potential problems, children are often restricted from opportunities for participation. Sports are one notable area of such restrictions. There is little reason for these restrictions. We should not paternalistically superimpose handicap on disability. Risk-benefit analysis is the principle that should govern decisions about a child's participation in sports.

No blanket statement about sports participation for persons with epilepsy is possible. Decisions about participation must be based on an individual's circumstances, the type of seizure, and his or her degree of seizure control. The decision must, further, be based on the risks of the particular sport and the accommodations that can feasibly be made for that individual.

The rules governing participation of children with epilepsy in sports should, in other words, be based on common sense! Each decision should be individualized.

"My son loves to play contact sports. He was a football player, on the freshman wrestling team, and played lacrosse. Now that he has had a seizure, the coach won't let him participate. He is crestfallen. What should we do?"

If your son has had a single generalized tonic-clonic seizure and your physician has found no reason for the seizure, there is probably no reason why he should not resume his sports. If he had a complex partial seizure, then this may have been the first recognized seizure in a young man who had been having unrecognized spells. Since he might have further complex partial seizures, which cloud consciousness and which might make him more prone to injury, his physician has probably started medication. Until he has adequate medication, it might be wise for him to practice with the team but refrain from game situations where a momentary lapse of attention might cause injury.

"Suppose my child continues to have seizures? Can she ever be part of the team again?"

It depends on the kind and the frequency of the seizures. Generalized tonic-clonic seizures could be embarrassing if they occurred during the game. Is this important to you or to your child? Is it important to the coach or to the team? More frequent partial complex seizures in which the child is confused may lead to embarrassing behavior on the field. Can your child cope with that? On some teams, the coaches and players have said that the player's participation was so important that they didn't care if she had seizures. These decisions involve negotiations among the coaches, the players, you, and your child.

"Does my son need to wear a special helmet to protect his head when he's playing?"

The brain of someone with epilepsy usually is no more sensitive or susceptible to injury than that of anyone else. In contact sports where headgear is required, that headgear should be sufficient for the child with epilepsy. Trauma to the head, which can occur in all of these sports, is unlikely to precipitate a seizure.

"The doctor had him hyperventilate in the office. It didn't cause a seizure, but could running hard and being out of breath cause a seizure while he is playing?"

No. Hyperventilation during exercise is balanced by changes in body chemistry and does not produce a seizure. We took care of one young woman who was so sensitive to hyperventilation that with only a few deep breaths she would experience seizures. The result was so reproducible that she participated in demonstrations for medical students every time she came to clinic for her check-up. Yet she was a long-distance bicycle rider and never had a seizure while riding.

"Jennifer wants to go on an Outward Bound trip this summer. We still haven't been able to get complete control of her absence seizures. They aren't frequent, but suppose one occurred while she was on one of those rope swings?"

If a spell occurred while she was on a rope, she could fall and hurt herself. On the other hand, anyone in the group who fell from the rope could injure himself, so the group leader should be quite careful. Perhaps you and Jennifer should talk with the leader. Maybe she could join the trip but avoid doing some of the most dangerous things. The independence taught by the trip and the benefits of being part of the group might be good for her and might also help her to realize that everyone has some limitations, at times. If her seizures were under control, her risks of injury would be little greater than those of others on the trip, and she could participate fully.

"Edith is eight and wants to go to one of those sports camps where they do gymnastics, work on the bars and the trampolines. Should I let her go?"

Everyone who uses a trampoline should be carefully supervised. If Edith is having frequent seizures, whether they are big seizures or staring spells, it's preferable that she not fall great distances. So she probably should not work on a high bar—or climb trees, either. However, if her seizures are controlled, if she continues to take her medicine, then her chances of injury are not much greater than the other children's. All child gymnasts need a soft place to land. It does not have to be softer for children with epilepsy. There should, of course, be mats and appropriate protection, for all the children, because anyone can make a mistake, as well as for the child who might have a seizure.

"Sherry wants to go out for cheerleading. They do all sorts of acrobatic stunts. What do you think?"

Surprisingly, cheerleading probably presents the greatest risk of injury of any high school sport. In the past there were no coaches, no training, no rules—and hard gym floors. The least coordinated individual used to be placed on the top of the pyramid! That's dumb, for the individual with epilepsy and for the one without. With adequate coaching and training, cheerleading should be no riskier for someone with controlled epilepsy than for someone who hasn't had seizures.

"Can David play soccer? Will hitting the ball with his head hurt him or cause a seizure?"

There is no evidence that hitting the soccer ball with one's head will injure the brain or precipitate seizures.

"What about water sports—swimming, rowing, and sailing?"

Water sports are all potentially dangerous. When anyone swims or dives there should always be adequate supervision. These sports present a minimally greater risk for the child with epilepsy, proportional to the frequency and the type of seizures. When these sports are competitive, the risk is probably decreased, since the competitors are being closely observed. In boating, anyone can capsize and tumble into the water. Any sailor can be knocked unconscious and into the water by the boom. All boaters should wear life jackets. Then they will be protected, even if they have seizures.

The same premise applies to all children. If a child could be injured in a sport, then there should be adequate protection to prevent or minimize an injury and adequate supervision to treat the injury if an accident occurs. For the child with seizures, the same is true. If a child has just started having seizures or has just started on new medication, then more supervision should be provided, and perhaps even a bit of overprotection, until the seizures are controlled or the degree of seizure control is ascertained. When the child has fewer seizures or no seizures at all, he doesn't need extra protection.

"My daughter is a competitive swimmer. She feels that her anticonvulsant medication slows her down, and she tends to skip it on the days before her meets. I'm afraid that she will have a seizure. What should I tell her?"

You should tell her that the medication is not likely to interfere with her performance but that a seizure *will* interfere. You should make a contract with her that if she is mature enough to take training and swimming seriously, then she is also mature enough to manage her seizures and to take her medication reliably. If she feels that the medications are slowing her down, she should discuss this with her doctor. Perhaps he can lower the dose. But your daughter should not do this on her own. Perhaps the medication could even be discontinued if she has been seizure-free for a sufficient period of time.

"We've just moved to a new town, and Todd hasn't had a seizure in almost a year. Should he tell his coach that he has epilepsy?"

Yes. That is the only way the coach can provide adequate supervision and be prepared if another seizure occurs. If the coach resists letting Todd participate, then you may have a battle to fight. It is important that you and your child be honest with the coach, just as you expect him to be honest with you.

"Would you let an adolescent with epilepsy participate in a marathon or in one of those triathlons? Does the stress of these increase the chance of seizures?"

In general, stress of this sort does not increase the chance of a seizure. The training for the event might provide a very good test. We would allow him to try. If the training seemed to increase the frequency of seizures, he should probably not compete. He may be distressed if he has a seizure during training, but it will probably be less distressing than not being allowed to try.

"It sounds as if you allow children with epilepsy to do almost anything that they're capable of. Is that correct?"

Yes. We think a little common sense goes a long way. The most common problems for children with epilepsy are the paternalistic worry of physicians and of society and the overprotection by families. Sports are an excellent way for your child to develop skills and self-confidence. These skills will be useful in adult life, whether or not the seizures are cured or controlled. Children with epilepsy have enough problems without being made to feel different because of the overprotectiveness of others who fear they will have a seizure.

We are far more permissive than many physicians. You or your doctor may put more restrictions on what your child, with or without epilepsy, can do. The risks of participation in a particular sport will vary with your child and his seizures. The benefits of a particular sport also vary with the child. Participation in a sport like football may or may not be very important to your child. You and your child will have to weigh both the risks and the benefits of participation. Your physician may be a good advisor.

Sports, particularly competitive sports, are about participation, about being a member of a team. They're about trying to be the best at something. They're about self-esteem. Sports seem to be good for most children; they are perhaps even more important for the child with epilepsy.

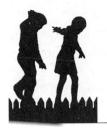

23. Driving and Epilepsy

Driving is risky business for everyone. The magnitude of the risk of driving is influenced by the driver's age, sex, and use of drugs or alcohol. Health problems such as diabetes, stroke, heart disease, and prior health-related incidents like head trauma and infections of the nervous system can also be risk factors. Epilepsy is only one health-related condition that constitutes a risk factor for driving.

Driving is considered by society to be a privilege, and, therefore, people are licensed to drive. In granting that privilege, society theoretically weighs the risks to the public of granting the license against the benefits to the individual of being able to drive. In the United States, a state grants or withdraws the privilege. What are the risks to society of someone driving who has epilepsy? What benefits does an individual lose when a license is not granted?

Because seizures are transient alterations of consciousness or of motor or sensory function, caused by electrical discharges from the brain, it is obvious that some of these alterations, particularly of consciousness, can lead to a motor vehicle accident if they occur while the person is driving. Not all seizures do involve loss of consciousness. Some are purely sensory. Some may be purely focal motor. Neither of these may interfere with control of the car. Some persons experience an aura (warning) before a seizure, which would allow them, if driving, to pull

Much information in this section was drawn from the excellent article by A. Krumholtz, R. S. Fisher, R. P. Lesser, and A. Hauser, "Driving and Epilepsy: A Review and Reappraisal," *JAMA* 265 (1991): 622–26.

off the road. Some seizures occur only during sleep. To be reasonable and sensible, we would recommend that licensing procedures should be guided by the type of seizure the individual has.

It is estimated that, while one in ten persons has a single seizure at *some time* during a lifetime, only a small proportion of these will have a second seizure; and even if an individual did have a second seizure, it would be unlikely to occur during the tiny fraction of his life that is spent driving. For most individuals who do experience a second seizure (epilepsy), seizures are controlled by medication; as long as the individual takes his medication, the risk of further recurrence remains low. Thus, there is even more reason to individualize rules about driving.

The chances of having a recurrence while driving will obviously be determined in part by the amount of time the person spends at the wheel. That risk is also affected by fatigue, lack of sleep, alcohol, use of other medications, and many unknown factors.

Thus, it is impossible to make any blanket statements about ALL *people with epilepsy and equally impossible to make blanket statements about the chance of a recurrence while a person with epilepsy is driving. The risks of recurrence and the risks of driving must be assessed individually.*

With these caveats, one study found that only one accident in 10,000 was due to a seizure while driving; six were due to natural death at the wheel. Alcohol was responsible for 2,500 of the 10,000 accidents studied. Some studies do suggest that the traffic accident rate may be higher for those with epilepsy, but studies also indicate that women *with* epilepsy have a lower accident rate than men *without* epilepsy. The rate of accidents for persons with epilepsy is no different from the rate for those with cardiovascular disease or diabetes. It has been estimated that, of accidents involving a person with epilepsy, in only one in five accidents was the accident the result of a seizure, and that those accidents, in fact, tended to be less severe, to involve only a driver's own vehicle, and to occur in less populated areas. Therefore, even when epilepsy might contribute to an accident, that accident appears to present, in general, less risk to others.

The risks and consequences of not being allowed to drive are also quite individual, depending on where the individual lives, the availability of alternative transportation, the need to drive to get to college or a job, and the social consequences of the resulting isolation. In this country, driving is often an economic and social necessity.

Although at one time few people with epilepsy were permitted to drive at all, in recent years there has been an increasing tendency to liberalize the restrictions and to individualize the limitations on driving. Laws regarding restrictions vary state by state in the United States and country by country. Some states have no restrictions, provided the physician gives permission to drive; in others a person with epilepsy must have been free of seizures for three months, in others one year, before driving. Most states have medical panels and appeals processes to review applications, but these panels often do not include neurologists or others with knowledge and experience with epilepsy.

Reporting requirements for seizures are confusing and differ from state to state. Very few states require the physician to report the name of an individual who has had seizures; however, when a physician feels that an individual presents a "substantial risk to others" because the individual is driving against medical advice, reporting may be necessary. Physicians with patients who continue to have seizures should warn them of the risks involved with continuing to drive and should document this warning in writing.

Persons with epilepsy should be aware of and obey the local regulations affecting their driving. Failure to follow regulations may result in accidents. Accidents occurring when the driver's epilepsy is unreported, even if the accident is unrelated to a seizure, can result in problems with insurance coverage. Check with your physician and your motor vehicle administration for applicable regulations. The most common regulation is that the individual be seizure-free for a designated period of time before driving. All of these time periods are arbitrary. Studies show that a person who is seizure-free for three months has an 85 percent chance of remaining seizure-free for the next year. Based on these studies, we recommend that the seizure-free interval be three months.

Seizures that are a result of changes in medication at a physician's direction should not necessarily limit driving privileges. If you had a seizure while your physician was decreasing your medicine, resumption of your previous dosage should reestablish seizure control and you should be able to continue to drive.

Individuals who have epilepsy controlled with medication and whose physicians are now recommending discontinuing medication pose special dilemmas for both the physician and the driver. Optimally, we would like to help patients be free of medication if possible. While in an ideal patient the risk of recurrent seizures is small, if they recur it is most likely to happen in the first three to six months after stopping medication. Most physicians recommend that the patient *not* drive during that period of increased risk. If driving is absolutely essential, then risks should be minimized by limiting the amount of time behind the wheel. Driving while tired or for long distances should be avoided during this period.

Persons who have a hemianopsia (loss of vision to one side) may not be allowed to drive. As Figure 2.6 shows, things to the right side of your body are perceived by the left part of each eyeball and are seen in the left occipital lobe. If there is a lesion in that occipital lobe, or if that occipital lobe is removed in epilepsy surgery, or if the pathway to it has been damaged, the person will not see things to the opposite side of their body. This usually does not cause a problem and the individual learns to avoid bumping into things. *But* if you can't see things to one side of your body, and are driving a car, you may bump into things with that side of your car. That is not good. Some states test for a hemianopsia and do not permit individuals whose vision is thus affected to drive. Others use big, convex mirrors to expand their fields of vision or prism glasses for the same purpose. Just be aware that a hemispherectomy may have consequences for your driving.

Clearly there is a need for better information on the risks of driving with epilepsy. Such information should assess the risks of recurrence of seizures and the factors which are predictive of such a recurrence, as well as the risks and hazards of accidents and of injuries to others. These risks should be placed in the perspective of other health-related disabilities. The driving risks represented by persons who use drugs and alcohol far outweigh the risks associated with epilepsy. These factors should be considered by the regulating agency when deciding whose driving should be restricted and for how long. The availability of restricted licenses that might permit an individual to drive to work or to school or only under certain circumstances might balance the public's risk of allowing some people with epilepsy to drive against the high cost of restricting the privilege.

While current laws in some states are, we believe, overly restrictive, it is the physician's responsibility to be aware of the laws in his state and to caution the patient also to be aware of the law.

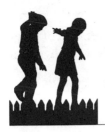

24. Marriage, Pregnancy, and Children

Parents rightly wonder and worry about their child's future. They hope that marriage and children will be part of their child's future. Not so long ago, marriage of persons with epilepsy was prohibited by law in many states. The eugenics movement, relying on a U.S. Supreme Court decision and on the principle that "one generation of imbeciles is enough," was able to implement these laws. Fortunately, the rationale behind these laws was proved to be erroneous, and the laws were abolished. Ironically, we are only now beginning to gain significant information about the genetics of the epilepsies. Many misconceptions and misbeliefs still abound, for example, about the effects of pregnancy on epilepsy and about the effects of epilepsy and its treatment on a fetus. Physicians themselves often give outdated answers to these questions.

Marriage and Parenthood

"Can I get married?"

Of course! If a person with epilepsy is competent to be a spouse, however that competence is defined, there is no reason why he or she should not get married.

"Can I have children?" "Would pregnancy make my seizures worse?"

Most women with epilepsy can bear children. Although pregnancy might affect your seizures, your risks during pregnancy are little different from the risks other women face. If you have questions about conditions that might have caused your epilepsy or about the effect of pregnancy on other health problems, you should check with your physician *before* you decide to become pregnant.

Your seizures may change during pregnancy. Therefore, your obstetrician needs to know about your epilepsy and your neurologist about your pregnancy. In about one-third of pregnant women, seizures get worse, in one-third they improve, and in one-third they are unchanged. Since we cannot predict which group you will fall into, your pregnancy should be monitored carefully.

"Can a person with epilepsy be a competent parent?"

The answer is clearly, "Yes!" Most people who have epilepsy are extremely competent parents, just as are most people without. Some are incompetent parents, just as are some without epilepsy. Individuals with epilepsy have personal strengths and weaknesses just as others do. You will have to ask yourself and your partner whether you as individuals have the ability, maturity, and judgment to be good parents. That is for you to decide, but a "no" decision should not be based simply on the fact that you have epilepsy.

"Can someone who still has seizures be a good parent?"

Absolutely, although the problems of being a parent with ongoing seizures may be more difficult, depending on the frequency of your seizures, their type, and even the time of day they occur. If your seizures are frequent and result in sudden loss of consciousness, you might drop or injure your child during a seizure. You may have to make arrangements for special help in the home or special arrangements for child care outside the home. But even so, you can be a good parent.

Risks of Pregnancy while Taking Anticonvulsant Drugs

"Should my epilepsy medication be reduced while I'm pregnant?"

Pregnancy, especially early pregnancy, is *not* a good time to be changing anticonvulsant medications or to be adjusting them. You and your physician should plan your treatment strategies together *before* you plan your pregnancy. Some medications are more likely to affect the fetus than others. Some women may no longer need to be on several medications, some may not need any medication. Whenever possible the woman should be on the least number of medications, on the lowest dose, before becoming pregnant.

Since blood levels change as your body chemistry itself changes during the pregnancy, blood levels of your medications should be monitored. We generally recommend that these levels be measured early in the pregnancy, then followed every month in the middle third of your pregnancy and every several weeks in the last trimester.

There are three principal reasons why seizures increase during pregnancy in almost one of three women with epilepsy. The first is that pregnant women are naturally fearful that taking drugs may affect the fetus and, therefore, they may fail to take their anticonvulsant medication according to schedule. A second reason is lack of sleep during pregnancy. A third cause of seizures during pregnancy is changes in the body's metabolism of drugs. Although such changes can cause blood levels to rise and thus cause toxicity, blood levels can also decline, leading to seizures. Your physician should closely follow your blood levels and provide appropriate adjustments.

Although there is little evidence that brief seizures injure the fetus, a prolonged seizure might affect your fetus and any seizures might cause injury to you. Therefore, we strongly urge that pregnant women with epilepsy who need medication for seizure control continue to take the drug that has been controlling their seizures.

"Are there risks to my baby when I am taking anticonvulsant drugs?"

Yes, if a pregnant woman is on anticonvulsant drugs, there are risks to the baby. Those risks vary with the drug and are usually small.

No pregnant woman should be on anticonvulsant medication if it is not needed.

Every pregnancy, with epilepsy or without, carries some risk of having an abnormal baby. Approximately 2 to 3 percent of all children will be born with some developmental abnormality. When a woman either has, or has previously had, epilepsy but is not taking medication during the pregnancy, the risk of a child with an abnormality is 4 to 8 percent (about twice as high as the baseline 3 percent). Thus, this woman has about a 95 percent chance of having a normal infant. Some studies suggest that this risk is not increased by taking anticonvulsants. Other studies say that the risk of abnormality if the mother is taking anticonvulsants could be as high as 7 to 17 percent. Even if we accept the highest estimate as correct, the chance of having a normal child is still 80 to 90 percent or more.

The chance of having an abnormal child is also increased if it is the father who has or has had epilepsy, although the risk is less high than when it is the mother.

Each medicine poses different potential risks to the fetus; some are more serious than others, and some are more likely to cause problems.

Abnormalities vary with the anticonvulsant and may be severe—such as spina bifida, congenital heart disease, or cleft palate—or minor abnormalities, as in the length of the fingers.

Trimethadione (Tridione) and paramethadione (Paradione). These drugs should never be used during pregnancy because of the very high incidence of serious malformations in babies of mothers taking them.

Phenytoin (Dilantin). This drug is believed by most people to carry an increased risk of cleft lip and palate, as well as of congenital heart disease. The risk of these problems is about 5 percent. Since these malformations occur during the first weeks of pregnancy, they cannot be prevented by stopping the drug after you realize you are pregnant. It is alleged that there is an increase in risk of "fetal hydantoin syndrome" when the mother has been taking phenytoin. In this syndrome, the infant has blunted fingers and toes and small fingernails, is of slightly short stature, and has a small head. Whether such children are intellectually disabled or not remains a matter of debate. Some people feel that the risk of this syndrome is perhaps 20 to 30 percent. Others feel that the significance of these minor abnormalities is greatly overstated. Similar features may be found in children of a mother with epilepsy who has taken phenobarbital (the fetal barbiturate syndrome) or one who has not been on medication at all.

Fetal hydantoin syndrome may be caused by the way certain women metabolize the drug. If you have had a baby who has the syndrome, your chances of having another affected child may be very high if you continue taking phenytoin (Dilantin) during your second pregnancy.

Other anticonvulsants. Phenobarbital and carbamazepine (Tegretol) may cause problems with the fetus that resemble the hydantoin syndrome. The risks for both drugs appear to be slightly less than for phenytoin. Valproic acid (Depakene, Depakote) increases the risk of neural tube defects (spina bifida). The risks to the fetus of newer anticonvulsant medications remain to be determined. *All women, but especially women on valproic acid or carbamazepine, should be taking folic acid, 0.4 mg per day, if they are intending to get pregnant or may become pregnant, and while they are pregnant.*

While all drugs are tested in pregnant animals before they are allowed to be sold, these tests are far from perfect in predicting the effects of the drug on the human fetus. Therefore, if you are considering becoming pregnant and are on any of the newer medications, discuss your plans with your physician *before* becoming pregnant. In general, we believe that the risk of abnormalities in the fetus of a woman on an anticonvulsant medication is 4 to 5 percent and that about 95 percent of pregnancies will be unaffected.

A woman who no longer needs medication should have it discontinued before she becomes pregnant. This should be done under a physician's supervision. For the woman in whom the need for continued medication is unclear, decision making can be complex.

It is likely that all anticonvulsant medications in pregnancy will pose some minimal risk to the fetus. Virtually all anticonvulsants may affect the metabolism of vitamin K in the newborn and may lead to bleeding. Therefore, the mother should receive vitamin K during the last week of pregnancy, or the infant should receive it immediately after birth.

❑ **Barbara was thirty-one and desperately wanted to have a child. She had recently been placed on phenytoin because of a single seizure. She had a dilemma. Should she get pregnant with the risks of medication to the fetus or should she stop the medication with the risks of a seizure to herself and the fetus? Although she realized that the risks of phenytoin (Dilantin) to her baby were small, she could not accept the guilt of potentially causing a problem. She was also fearful of having a seizure while she was pregnant and of possibly injuring the baby. She was much less concerned about the potential effects of a seizure on her own active life.**

We suggested a way out of her dilemma. Since she had had only a single seizure, the chances of her having another seizure were approximately 30 percent. If her medication was slowly discontinued, she could wait three to six months and see if another seizure occurred. After that time the risk of recurrence would be even smaller and she could become pregnant with greater security. If she had another seizure, then she would know that she needed an anticonvulsant medication and might try one with less potential risk to the fetus.

If you become pregnant while you are on anticonvulsants, you should be reassured that at least 80 to 90 percent of the babies will be normal. Pregnancy is not a good time to stop taking the medication or to switch to another drug, unless it is necessary for your seizure control.

Breastfeeding and Birth Control

"Can I breastfeed my baby?"

Yes. While all of the anticonvulsants will appear in the mother's breast milk, they are usually in such low concentrations that they do not affect the baby. However, if you are taking phenobarbital or phenytoin and the baby becomes too sleepy, then the baby's blood level should be checked. If the level is too high, breastfeeding might be stopped for a few days.

"What about birth control?"

Many anticonvulsants increase the metabolism of birth control steroids and make them less effective. Therefore, if you are using birth control pills, particularly the "mini-pill," and are taking anticonvulsants, you might have a higher chance of becoming pregnant. You should discuss the effects of your birth control pills on your anticonvulsant with your neurologist, and the effects of the anticonvulsant on the effectiveness of your birth control pills with your gynecologist.

"Will My Child Have Neurological Problems?"

"Since I have seizures, are there any risks of my child developing epilepsy?"

Yes, there is a small risk of your children developing epilepsy. The risk of epilepsy in the child whose mother or father has epilepsy is about twice as great as when neither of the parents has epilepsy but is still relatively small. The risk of anybody's child having epilepsy is 1 to 2 percent. If you or your husband has epilepsy, your child has a 3 to 4 percent chance of having epilepsy.

"If I have a child, will he or she be normal?"

No one can give you a warranty on your child. Some abnormalities are not detectable even by our most sophisticated prenatal and intrauterine screening. Some major problems are acquired at birth or are a consequence of later infection or trauma. Some genetic diseases cause epilepsy. Some risks are associated with anticonvulsants. There are some risks if you have previously had epilepsy.

If you are unwilling to take any risk, then you should probably not have a child. If you are willing to take a small risk, then you, as well as most people with epilepsy, can have healthy and normal children, unless you or your husband has epilepsy caused by one of the genetic diseases, such as tuberous sclerosis, or a metabolic condition. Some of the epilepsies, such as juvenile myoclonic epilepsy, are genetic. However, the vast majority of the epilepsies are of unknown cause and are not directly inherited.

At present, genetic testing of parents to predict the likelihood of epilepsy in their children remains for the future. If we were able to use DNA to make such a prediction, would you want to have the test?

Other Genetic Issues

Some people ask us about the risks for their child if other family members have epilepsy. Also, parents who do not have epilepsy themselves ask about risks for subsequent children when one of their children has had seizures. The answers to these questions require more detailed explanation.

Epilepsy may be a manifestation of some other disease. Some metabolic diseases, such as the aminoacidurias like phenylketonuria (PKU), and degenerative diseases, like Tay-Sachs and metachromatic leukodystrophy, may cause seizures. If one of your children has such a metabolic disease, the risk of a subsequent child's having it is one in four. That other child is also likely to have seizures. If your brother or sister had the condition and you did not, you might carry the gene. If you do, and if you were unlucky enough to marry someone else who also had the same abnormal gene, then the chance of your child's being affected could be as high as one in four. If you do not carry the abnormal gene, your chances of having an affected child are zero.

In a few diseases, such as tuberous sclerosis or neurofibromatosis, the recurrence rate may be as high as one in two. If you, as the parent, had tuberous sclerosis, for example, half of your children could also have the disease and may have seizures.

If one of your children has idiopathic seizures, seizures for which the cause cannot be identified, the chances of other children also having seizures is twice as high as in the general population. Thus, they would have a 3 to 4 percent chance of having epilepsy. If one of your children has a febrile seizure or a seizure after head trauma, the chances of brothers and sisters having similar seizures are also twice as high as the general population.

In summary, there is a genetic tendency to inherit epilepsy, but the risk is small both for the child of a person who has epilepsy and for her brothers and sisters.

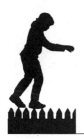

25. Support Services and Additional Information for People with Epilepsy and Their Families

All people with epilepsy and their families need information, help, and support when they receive a diagnosis of epilepsy. There are organizations they can turn to. The Internet (discussed below) can be another source of good information if used selectively.

National and Local Epilepsy Services

The Epilepsy Foundation national office (1-800-332-1000) is available to offer information and referral to individuals throughout the country. The national office provides information about seizure disorders and also tells people how to contact their local affiliates to obtain information about additional services and support. In addition, the national office of the Epilepsy Foundation provides legislative advocacy and supports epilepsy research at medical centers throughout the country.

Local affiliates of the Epilepsy Foundation in many regions are available to families, providing help and support. Among the services these organizations offer are:

• Epilepsy education
• Supported living
• Employment assistance

The available services vary from one affiliate to another according to the budgetary limitations of each. Many affiliates are able to offer only epilepsy education and support groups, while some of the larger ones are in a position also to provide:

- Employment support
- Advocacy for school inclusion
- Sibling workshops
- Cash assistance for services
- Support for independent living for adults
- Camps

The Epilepsy Foundation of the Chesapeake Region, our local agency, has become one of the larger affiliates in the country. Needless to say, we are very proud of what the group's leadership, and that of Leigh Kingham, its executive director, have achieved over the past many years. It is an example of what dedication, hard work, good staff, ingenuity, and good lobbying at the local, state, and regional levels can achieve. We are detailing some of its programs here as examples of what local services can be achieved by working diligently with your local affiliate.

This organization began in Baltimore City during the early 1970s with a small group of parents attempting to help support each other and obtain services for their children. Over the past thirty years, with each of the authors of this book (as well as many others) serving in leadership positions, the organization has grown, extending its services first to the surrounding county, then to most of the State of Maryland and now the region.

The Epilepsy Foundation of the Chesapeake Region now serves individuals with epilepsy—children and adults and their families—throughout Maryland, the District of Columbia, and Northern Virginia.

Education. We provide professional education to schools, police, emergency medical technicians, school nurses, and other service providers working with individuals with seizure disorders, and to medical professional such as EEG technicians and physicians. We also provide epilepsy education to school classes when the class includes a child with a seizure disorder, and to lay audiences.

Children's services. We have a program called Project ACT (All Children Together) which supports children with epilepsy with their social, emotional, and behavioral problems, so that they can fully participate in their local child care facilities. Although the program was originally designed for children with epilepsy, we found that similar problems are experienced by children with other disabilities, and we have expanded the program to include all children with disabilities. This innovative program provides individualized assistance to day care teachers and training for teachers and parents. Services are available for before- and after-school child care settings and for all-day child care.

Adult services. Our Community and Employment Partners group offers individualized employment placements and support for persons with disabilities in their communities. Counselors work closely with individuals to ensure that they get a job that will ensure the highest chance of employment success. Follow-up is provided for as long as the person needs assistance. Education is available for all employers, to allay any fears they may have about employing an individual with a disability.

Community Partners also provides assistance in many other areas. It will teach and assist in budgeting, socialization, even recreational involvement. Its goal is to assist people to live as independently as possible in the community of their choice.

Family support services. This program provides support groups for siblings and parents of people with epilepsy and other disabilities. Counselors offer advocacy and support to families whose children need additional services from the school system. When such services are provided, the children may be included in regular classrooms.

The staff is also able to offer financial assistance to families for services such as respite care and computers for children with disabilities, and to make it possible for parents to stay home with their children when necessary.

Most affiliates are not in a position to offer all of these services—now. The Epilepsy Foundation of the Chesapeake Region was not able to either, in the 1980s. But with the hard work of a dedicated board of community leaders and of those who have epilepsy in the family, as well as providers for those with epilepsy and a very dedicated staff, your organization can begin to provide some of these services, then more and more. It will take time.

You should join your local Epilepsy Foundation affiliate, not only for the services they can provide to you and yours, but for what you and your family can do for them and for others.

You might serve the organization as a member of the board to help with fund raising, to plan special events, to help assist in organizing support networks. Some parents tell us that they don't need a support network, that they can cope with their child's problems very well. If so, then the support network needs you for what you can provide to others.

If your child or his sibling is interested in volunteering, encourage them to become part of the peer network, to talk to other kids with seizures, to share experiences and feelings. Summer camps are wonderful experiences for children with epilepsy. There they can find that there are others just like them, see another child with a seizure; siblings can share and help each other.

These are just a few of the many ways you or your child can volunteer and build your local organization.

Getting Information

Epilepsy and the Internet

The Internet is a source of much good information about epilepsy and its treatments.

The Internet is a source of much misinformation about epilepsy and its treatments.

Both of these statements are true. This makes it difficult to decide whether the information you are finding is good or bad. You have to be your own filter. There is much good information in the various chat groups, but there are also many people who are biased, prejudiced, dissatisfied, and just plain unrealistic. We have not recommended any specific chat groups because they are so variable, depending upon who has signed on.

There are many potentially helpful web sites. Increasing numbers of physicians and medical centers have their own web sites. Some have very useful information, and some are primarily advertising. You will have to make your own decision about each. However, if your child has difficult-to-control epilepsy, you should seek out a comprehensive epilepsy center.

A *comprehensive epilepsy center* (or program) is defined as a group of individuals specializing in the treatment of epilepsy. Typically the group includes a neurologist specializing in epilepsy (preferably a pediatric neurologist if the patient is a child). The multidisciplinary team includes neurosurgeons, neuropsychologists, clinical nurse specialists, and social workers working together. To find a comprehensive epilepsy center, ask your family physician or your child's neurologist. If they don't know of one, they could inquire of their colleagues. There is not just one comprehensive epilepsy center, there are now many, and they are available in most areas of the country. However, not all centers are equal or equally appropriate for your child's problems. If you are looking for specialized services such as epilepsy surgery or the ketogenic diet, ask the center about how much experience it has with those treatments. Ask about their results, and don't be afraid to ask one center about another. Most centers and most specialists are willing to be of help and will be frank about the pluses and minuses of other centers.

There are many sources of information about epilepsy on the Internet. We have listed but a few that we have checked and can recommend. The list is far from exhaustive.

Reliable Sources of Information

The Epilepsy Foundation, the national (U.S.) voluntary organization, has a toll-free information line, 1-800-332-1000, and a web site, http://www.efa.org. To find one of the foundation's many affiliates across the United States, look in your local or regional phone book under Epilepsy Foundation. The EF maintains a national library that is the best single source of the latest information about epilepsy.

Many other countries have organizations similar to the Epilepsy Foundation. For example, Epilepsy Canada is the Canadian national voluntary organization that provides information, advocacy, and networking. It has province-oriented and local affiliates. Its telephone number is 1-514-845-7855, and its web site is http://www.epilepsy.ca.

Other web sites with useful and reliable information include http://www.stanford.edu/group/ketodiet, for information about the ketogenic diet (see also next section), and http://www.nih.gov, the National Institutes of Health site, which has some of the latest information about research as well as basic information about specific problems.

Selected Bibliography on the Ketogenic Diet

We did not place references about the ketogenic diet in the previous edition of this book because the information was changing rapidly and we did not want to provide information that was out of date. In the past few years, a consensus has been reached about many issues regarding the diet, and there is more general acceptance of the diet. Therefore we feel confident about providing the following references about the ketogenic diet (in order of publication):

T. D. Swink, E. P. G. Vining, J. M. Freeman, "The Ketogenic Diet," *Advances in Pediatrics* 44 (1997): 297–329.

J. M. Freeman, E. P. G. Vining, D. J. Pillas, P. L. Pyzik, J. C. Casey, M. T. Kelly, "The Efficacy of the Ketogenic Diet, 1998: A Prospective Evaluation of Intervention in 150 Children," *Pediatrics* 102 (1998): 1358–1363.

Blue Cross–Blue Shield Technology Assessment Program, "Ketogenic Diet for the Treatment of Children with Refractory Epilepsy," *TEC* 15 (1998): 1–27.

J. M. Freeman, E. P. G. Vining, "Seizures Rapidly Decrease after Fasting: Preliminary Studies of the Ketogenic Diet," *Archives of Pediatrics and Adolescent Medicine* 153 (1999): 946–949.

J. C. Casey, E. P. G. Vining, J. M. Freeman, et al., "The Implementation and Maintenance of the Ketogenic Diet in Children," *Journal of Neuroscience Nursing* 21 (1999): 294–302.

G. LeFever, N. Aronson, "Ketogenic Diet for the Treatment of Refractory Epilepsy in Children: A Systematic Review of Efficacy," *Pediatrics* 105 (2000): e46.

C. Hemingway, D. J. Pillas, P. L. Pyzik, J. M. Freeman, "The Ketogenic Diet: A 3- to 6-Year Follow-Up of 150 Children Enrolled Prospectively," *Pediatrics* 108 (2001): 898–905.

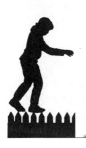

26. Insurance and Other Financial Issues

We could fill a book with discussion of insurance issues and some of the horror stories we have heard from patients. Therefore, we think it is important to pass on some of the tips we have collected over the years.

If you are about to change insurance companies or you are trying to have your child covered, you should do careful research before signing on with any insurance company or insurance plan. We recognize that many times you do not have any choice about the coverage, but you should try to optimize the benefit to your child. Find out about the following issues.

- Will the company allow you to go to the physician and hospital of your choice?
- Ask if your physician and hospital are in or out of the company's network, and find out what your proportion of financial responsibility or copay will be.
- Is there an out-of-pocket maximum for you, and will the insurance company then cover 100 percent of the medical costs? Often insurance companies will tell you that they pay 100 percent, but that is 100 percent of what *they* consider to be reasonable and customary. That can be misleading, and you can wind up with out-of-pocket expenses that you did not anticipate. For example, if a hospital charges $1,200.00 per day and your insurance company says the reasonable and customary charge is $800.00 per day, that leaves you with $400.00 *per day* out of

pocket, which can add up very quickly if your child is hospitalized for any length of time.

• *Before* signing on with an insurance company, get *in writing* any "promises" that the company makes to you, such as "You can see any doctor you choose" or "You may go out of state to any hospital you would like."

We recommend that you talk to the financial offices of your doctor or hospital to find out which insurances they accept and which ones they will bill directly, or whether you must pay out of pocket and then be reimbursed from your insurance. Paying out of pocket is prohibitive for most families, especially for ongoing treatment.

If your child qualifies for Medicaid in your state, consider carefully before you drop him from your insurance, because most hospitals do not accept Medicaid or Children's Medical Services from a state other than their own, and you may want to use the services of a doctor or epilepsy center out of state. In addition, many physicians do not accept Medicaid. The same premise holds true for children who go off to college and qualify for student insurance. They are only insured while actively enrolled, so if a child goes into the hospital for surgery and has to miss a chunk of time from school, he may not be covered. Most financial people will tell you that it is best to carry the child on your policy even if there is other coverage for him. Better overinsured than underinsured.

Very often you can enlist your primary care physician to help you get an appointment at an epilepsy center and to have it covered by insurance, by emphasizing that they are "specialists" in this area. Sometimes it is worth the financial investment, however it is paid, to go to an epilepsy center for a second opinion and then take those recommendations back to the physician who is caring for your child. Most physicians do not object to their patients' getting a second opinion.

If (or, unfortunately, more often when) coverage for epilepsy evaluation or treatment is denied, *appeal!* Insurance companies do not advertise their appeal process, but *all* companies have one. Decisions are often overturned on appeal. In insurance, as in life, it's the squeaky wheel that gets the grease.

You should not have to go into financial debt in order to get good care for your child. That generally is not necessary. There are many fine physicians around the country who are able to provide care for a child with a seizure disorder, and you should not feel that you have to move, mortgage your home, or take some other drastic measure to insure that your child's seizure disorder is adequately treated.

Another area of concern should be estate planning, particularly if you have a very disabled child. It is never too early to think about setting up the proper financial arrangements to be put in place once you and your spouse can no longer care for your child, or after your death. No one will be here forever, and you cannot, nor should you, assume that your other children will take on the role of caretaker after you are gone. You should find a lawyer who is familiar with estate planning, who can advise you on the options that you have and how to put them in place. If you make these arrangements early on, you will feel relieved that your child will be taken care of. Your other children will be able to breathe easier as well. It is wonderful for siblings to take an active part in their brother's or sister's life, but they are not the parent. It is amazing how quickly time passes. Your child will be an adult before you know it. Your time together will be more enjoyable for you both if you know that you have done what you can to plan for his or her future.

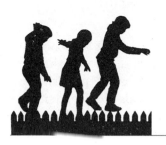

Conclusion

We're not sure why you have read this book. Perhaps it was because you were shocked, upset, or disheartened because your child has had a seizure or because she has been diagnosed as having epilepsy. Maybe you simply wanted to know more about seizures, their treatment, and their consequences. Whatever the reason, we hope that now you realize that epilepsy is not just a medical problem but affects many other aspects of your child's life and of your life. We hope that now, more familiar with what epilepsy is and what it is not, you will raise your child in a far more optimistic and accepting fashion.

We hope that your child grows up without handicap, or with as little handicap as possible, and that you accept him for whatever he may be, help him fulfill his genuine potential, and not impose handicaps. We hope that you have sensed our own personal involvement with each of our patients, that as you have read the stories of these children you have sensed how each of the children has affected us, too. We have learned from each of them, and we believe that you can as well. We know that you and your child will find your own ways of coping.

Acceptance of seizures and their uncertainties, or of associated handicapping conditions, does not come easily. And acceptance does not mean resignation. Optimism may at times be hard to find, but it is essential. We strongly believe that our optimistic approach is realistic. After all, most epilepsy will be controlled and outgrown. It would be a pity if anxiety and overprotection left your child truly handicapped. To achieve a full and normal life, you and your child must both become active, informed, optimistic participants. We hope that this book has helped and that your child will live a healthy, full, seizure-free life.

In the years since the earlier editions of this book were published we have received hundreds of letters and phone calls from parents expressing their thanks for our making this information and philosophy available. We wish to express our heartfelt thanks, in return, to all of you who have communicated with us. It is your words of appreciation that have inspired us to update our book and to continue our efforts on behalf of children with epilepsy and their families. Our philosophy is optimistic. We hope we have helped you to see the glass as mostly full, to keep your own hopes high, and to set the goals for your child realistically. We wish you and your child well.

Glossary

Absence seizure	A generalized seizure in which consciousness is altered, formerly called *petit mal,* a term now seldom used. They are usually brief; and occur many times in a day. The EEG pattern is three-per-second spikes and waves. Absence seizures are usually easily treated and usually outgrown.
Allopathic	A method of treating disease with remedies that produce effects different from those produced by the disease itself.
Ambulatory monitoring	The use of a cassette-like tape recorder to monitor the EEG while an individual is awake, at work, school, or play. The ambulatory monitoring device permits up to seventy-two hours of recording on tape. However, the amount of information produced about specific parts of the brain is limited. Since either the child or another observer must mark events thought to be seizures, and because the amount of EEG information is limited, ambulatory monitoring is useful only in special situations where it is important to clarify the nature of the spell (i.e., faint vs. seizure) and where quantification of spells is important. The procedure is far less expensive than video-EEG monitoring, but also less definitive.
Antiepileptic drug (AED)	Also called anticonvulsant drug. One of the drugs used to prevent recurrence of seizures. The particular drug chosen for a child depends on the type of seizures, the age of the child, and the type of side effect that might be expected.
Aplastic anemia	A decrease in the production of red and/or white blood cells, often due to the effects of a drug.
Association cortex	The part of the brain in the parietal lobe where vision, hearing, memories, and motor function come

together and where associations occur between sensations, movements, and thoughts.

Atonic seizure A form of generalized seizure in which body tone is suddenly lost and the child slumps to the ground or his head slumps forward. These difficult-to-control seizures often occur in Lennox-Gastaut syndrome. They may resemble the sudden seizure in which the child is thrown to the ground, often injuring his face or teeth. Atonic seizures and myoclonic seizures often occur in the same child, and the terms are often used interchangeably.

Atypical absence seizure A staring spell similar to an absence seizure but often with an atypical EEG. It may last longer than the typical absence seizure and may have other additional features (movement, falling, etc.). Atypical absence seizures may be more difficult to control with medications than typical absence seizures.

Aura The start of a seizure. It is usually described as a warning—a peculiar feeling, a sense of fear, a funny sensation in one part of the body. The neural activity indicated by these sensations can spread to other areas of the brain. If the seizure does not spread, the aura would be referred to as a simple partial seizure.

Automatism The complex and purposeless automatic movements that accompany a complex partial seizure. These movements often consist of smacking of the lips, chewing, picking at clothes, or wandering around in a confused fashion.

Autonomic nervous system The part of the brain that controls functions like heart rate, blood pressure, and skin temperature and color. Seizures from the temporal lobe can produce disturbances of autonomic function.

Axon The part of a neuron that resembles a telephone line and is responsible for the capacity of brain cells to communicate with one another.

Benign rolandic epilepsy A special form of seizures in children. It starts after three years of age. The seizure often begins with a sensation in the corner of the mouth, followed by local jerking of the muscles; it spreads to one side of the face, or one side of the body, and may become a generalized seizure. It has a typical EEG. These seizures occur more commonly during certain stages of sleep. They are usually outgrown.

Breathholding spell An episode in which the child does not breathe, turns blue, and may lose consciousness. These spells

	may, on occasion, result in a seizure. Breathholding spells are not serious and are not epilepsy. There are two forms: cyanotic (blue) and pallid (white).
Clonic seizure	The rhythmic jerking of an extremity or the whole body. Seizures that are only clonic are rare. Clonic seizures are usually the second component of tonic clonic seizures.
Complex partial seizure	A seizure that involves only part of the brain (usually the temporal or the frontal lobe) *and* that alters consciousness or awareness. It may be accompanied by automatisms. *Complex partial seizure* and *partial complex seizure* mean the same thing.
Consciousness	Alertness or awareness, the ability to interact normally with the environment. Consciousness is altered in generalized seizures or complex partial seizures but is usually not affected in simple partial seizures.
Convulsion	An older term for a seizure. It usually refers to seizures that have a motor component—jerking or stiffening. Other old terms for convulsion include *spell* and *fit*.
Convulsive syncope	A seizure that occurs in association with a fainting spell. The child experiences sweatiness, pallor, and dizziness, and faints and loses consciousness. A small percentage of people who faint will then have a brief tonic-clonic seizure. The fainting spell is termed syncope; when a tonic-clonic seizure is associated with it, it is called convulsive syncope. The convulsion of convulsive syncope is a benign seizure and does not require treatment.
CT or CAT scan	Computerized tomography, or computerized axial tomography, uses small doses of x-rays and computer analysis to produce a picture of the brain and allow the physician to see certain abnormalities.
Cyanotic breathholding spells	Breathholding spells in which the child starts to cry, then holds his breath and turns blue before losing consciousness. A seizure occasionally follows a breathholding spell.
Cysticercosis	An infection of the brain in which cysts within the brain become calcified and cause seizures. It is more common in underdeveloped than in developed countries.
Déjà vu	A sensation that you have seen something or someone before, whether or not you have. This sensation is normal and common, but when it occurs re-

	peatedly, it can be a manifestation of complex partial seizures emanating from the temporal lobe.
Dysgenesis	An abnormality of the development of the cortex (*dys* = abnormal, *genesis* = creation). There are many different possible abnormalities of cortical development, some of which may cause epilepsy. If the area of dysgenesis is in a place where it may be removed without causing deficit, surgery may cure the seizures.
EEG	The electroencephalogram records the electrical activity of the brain, or "brain waves." The EEG does not provide a diagnosis of epilepsy, but it assists physicians in clarifying the type or origin of seizures.
Eloquent	"Eloquent" areas of the cortex are areas that have critical function such as speech and motor function.
Encephalitis	Inflammation of the brain substance itself, due to bacterial or viral infection.
Epilepsies	Seizure patterns whose clinical manifestations and EEGs are sufficiently characteristic for a physician to be able to predict a patient's future course and to recommend specific medications. The term "the epilepsies" is also used to indicate that there are diverse forms of repeated seizures (epilepsy), not just one single type.
Epilepsy	Recurrent (two or more) seizures not provoked by specific events such as trauma, infection, fever, or chemical changes. Seizures may take many forms. Patterns of epilepsy that are similar and have a predictable outcome are termed epileptic syndromes.
Epileptic cephalalgia	The headache that follows some seizures. Seizures increase blood flow to the brain; resulting dilation of blood vessels may cause a postseizure headache. Migraine headaches can be mistaken for epileptic cephalalgia.
Epileptic syndrome	A pattern defined by seizure type, age at onset, characteristic EEG, and an expected outcome. Certain epileptic syndromes respond better to particular types of medications. Epileptic syndromes include infantile spasms, the Lennox-Gastaut syndrome, benign rolandic epilepsy, and others. The various epileptic syndromes make up the epilepsies.
Epileptogenic	Susceptible to a seizure. Areas of the brain more susceptible to seizures than other areas are considered

epileptogenic. The temporal and frontal lobes are usually more epileptogenic than other regions.

Febrile seizure
A seizure caused by fever. Febrile seizures are common in young children of six months to three or four years old, because of the lower seizure threshold of the young brain. Only rarely are they associated with later epilepsy. While frightening, they appear to cause little harm. They tend to occur in families. Physicians generally do not prescribe anticonvulsants to try to prevent these seizures.

Fit
A term still often used in England to refer to a seizure. Most American physicians prefer to avoid using that term to describe seizure episodes.

Focal resection
Surgical removal of one area or region of the brain.

Focal seizures
See simple partial seizure.

Focus
A local area of abnormality in the brain. These local abnormalities may be seen as spikes, or sharp waves, or as slowing on an EEG.

Generalized seizure
A seizure involving the whole brain. It may involve alterations of alertness or awareness, as during absence or complex partial seizures, or tonic-clonic movements of both sides of the body.

Grand mal seizure
The old term for a generalized tonic-clonic seizure.

Hemispherectomy
Surgical removal of one-half of the brain. There are several different types of hemispherectomy being performed.

History
The detailed medical story of previous events. The history establishes exactly what happened to the patient and explores the general state of a person's health.

Homeopathy
A system of treating disease with minute doses of a drug that in large doses produces symptoms similar to the disease itself.

Hyperventilate
To overbreathe. A physician may instruct your child to take a number of deep breaths for two to four minutes. This overventilation may cause an absence or complex partial seizure, which can then be observed by your doctor. Rapid breathing during exercise is rarely associated with a seizure. Anxiety may cause an individual to hyperventilate.

Hypsarrhythmia
A term used to describe the EEG frequently seen in children who have had infantile spasms. This characteristic EEG pattern is wildly chaotic, of very high voltage, with many spikes and slow waves. The terms *hypsarrhythmia* and *infantile spasms* are often, although incorrectly, used interchangeably.

Ictus	A Latin term for "stroke" or "event." A seizure, of whatever type, is referred to as an ictus.
Idiopathic	Of unknown cause. Seizures are called idiopathic seizures if no cause can be found. In more than half of the children experiencing seizures, causes cannot be found. Idiopathic seizures often have a better outcome than those that are symptomatic, that is, for which a cause can be found.
Infantile spasms	A special form of epilepsy that can occur in the first two years of life from multiple causes. The seizures consist of repeated episodes of flexion of the head onto the chest, the knees coming up, and the arms extending. Each episode lasts one to two seconds; episodes occur in a series of five to fifty, with a brief pause between each. The child may have many such series during each day. This form of epilepsy is commonly associated with significant mental retardation and requires prompt diagnosis and treatment with specific medication.
Intensive monitoring	Monitoring, using modern technology, of the characteristics of an individual's seizures and their correlation with an EEG. Monitoring may include ambulatory monitoring, prolonged EEGs, prolonged video-EEG monitoring, and use of depth electrodes or an electrode grid.
Interictal	Describes the period between episodes or seizures. (*See* ictus.)
Janz, juvenile myoclonic epilepsy of (JME)	A newly recognized syndrome that begins in late childhood with mild myoclonic jerks on going to sleep or awakening. This jerking may precede or be associated with absence seizures or generalized tonic-clonic seizures. It is often produced by sleep deprivation and commonly runs in families. The characteristic EEG and history make diagnosis of this condition easy, and treatment is usually very effective.
Lennox-Gastaut syndrome	A condition that includes two or more types of seizures, one of which is of the akinetic, atonic, falling-down type. Absence seizures and generalized tonic-clonic seizures, occurring particularly at night, are common. The EEG shows generalized slow spike or poly-spike and slow wave abnormalities. Mental retardation is common and often progressive. This is a severe seizure-type and one that is difficult to control.

Lobes	Parts of the brain. The principal lobes are the frontal lobes, important for personality and memory; the temporal lobes, which are responsible for speech, memory, and emotion; the parietal lobes, which integrate sensory function; and the occipital lobes, which are the site of vision.
Megalencephaly	Enlargement of the brain. Abnormalities of brain development may result in brain enlargement. When only one side of the brain is maldeveloped and enlarged (unilateral megalencephaly) and when the child has difficult-to-control seizures, a hemispherectomy may be useful.
Meningitis	Inflammation of the coverings of the brain, the meninges. Caused by bacterial or viral infections, meningitis may be accompanied by inflammation of the brain itself (encephalitis), resulting, on occasion, in seizures or brain damage.
Migraine	Migraine headaches, caused by changes within the blood vessels of the brain, are characteristically accompanied by paleness, nausea, vomiting, and sleep. They often last more than an hour. On rare occasions they can be confused with or associated with seizures. They tend to run in families.
Minor motor seizure	An old term, not part of the new classification, previously used to describe multiple types of spells, including both atonic and myoclonic varieties. Children with the Lennox-Gastaut syndrome generally experience multiple types of seizures, many of which are minor motor.
MRI scan	Magnetic resonance imaging scans, like CT scans, are used to identify structure and abnormalities within the brain. This new technique uses no x-rays and gives a clearer picture of brain structure than does the CT scan. It is more expensive and takes longer to do than the CT scan.
Myoclonic jerk	Sudden movement of arms or legs, most commonly occurring when a person is falling asleep. Myoclonic jerks during the day may be normal but if frequent could be part of one of the epilepsies.
Myoclonic seizure	Sudden jerks of muscle groups that resemble sudden jolts "like an electric shock." These jerks may be of a hand, a leg, a shoulder, or sudden flexion of the body forward or backward. While occasional myoclonic jerks may be normal, repeated myoclonic jerks can be a difficult-to-control form of epilepsy.

Neurofibromatosis	An inherited condition characterized by brown (café-au-lait, or coffee-colored) spots, mild mental retardation, and seizures. Small tumors on many nerves may compress surrounding tissue, causing pain, weakness, etc.
Neurons	The nerve cells of the brain.
Neurotransmitter	The chemicals released by the end (terminal) of an axon, they float across the space between cells and affect the "firing" of the next cell. Neurotransmitters may be excitatory or inhibitory to the next cell.
Pallid breathholding spell	Not true breathholding, but a sudden loss of consciousness due to slowing of the heart, usually occurring after mild trauma. It may, on occasion, result in a seizure. It is not epilepsy and rarely requires treatment.
Partial complex seizure	Another name for a complex partial seizure.
Partial seizure	A focal or local seizure in the brain.
Petit mal seizure	The old term, meaning "little spell," for an absence seizure. These spells usually include staring. Many kinds of seizures include staring, and they respond to different medications.
Photic sensitive seizure	A seizure caused by flashing lights, such as strobe lights or light shining through trees or a fence. In some "photic sensitive" individuals such stimuli may produce seizures.
Postictal	A Latin term meaning "after the seizure." (*See* ictus). Confusion, sleepiness, or weakness after the seizure is termed postictal since it occurs after the event.
Prognosis	Outcome or outlook of a medical condition.
Pseudoseizures	Events that resemble seizures but are not caused, as a seizure is, by electrical abnormalities in the brain. Pseudoseizures may be a child's conscious imitation of seizures, a way of coping with stress, or may be subconscious. Pseudoseizures often occur in persons who also have true seizures and may be difficult to differentiate from true seizures.
Rasmussen's syndrome	A rare, progressive condition that is characterized by unilateral seizures and progressive one-sided paralysis. Of unknown cause, this condition is best treated with hemispherectomy.
Recruitment	In physiologic terms, or in regard to epilepsy, recruitment refers to an enlisting of surrounding brain cells to fire simultaneously. Only when a certain number of cells are recruited to fire together will

	sufficient electrical activity be generated to appear as a spike on the EEG or as a clinical seizure.
Seizure	An episodic paroxysmal electrical discharge of nerve cells in the brain (neurons) resulting in alteration of function or behavior. There are many different forms of seizures, depending on where in the brain the electrical activity starts and the direction and rapidity of its spread in the brain.
Simple partial seizure	A focal or local seizure involving a single area of the brain. Since each area has particular functions, the typing of the seizure depends on which region is affected. Some are motor, involving the face, hand, or leg; some sensory, involving individual sensations in a part of the body; those involving a temporal lobe produce smells, tastes, fears, or memories. Unlike a complex partial seizure, consciousness is not altered during a simple partial seizure.
Sleep myoclonus	Sudden massive jerks of the body, often as someone is going to sleep. These are normal and are not epilepsy.
Spell	A term used to describe a seizure. The term is vague and is often used to refer to a seizure or a pseudoseizure if the nature of that episode is unknown.
Spike	A sharp abnormality on an EEG, it indicates an electrical discharge of a small number of neighboring brain cells. Recurrent spikes are electrical seizures and may spread to involve sufficient brain cells to cause a true change in function or behavior, that is, a clinical seizure.
Storage disease	One of the metabolic diseases in which some material, usually a breakdown product of normal tissue, cannot be further metabolized and is stored within nerve cells of the brain. This storage produces malfunction of the cells; it is commonly associated with progressive intellectual and neurologic deterioration and with seizures. Each of the various diseases has a name.
Sturge-Weber syndrome	Characterized by a birthmark (hemangioma or port wine stain) involving the forehead and variable parts of the face, often associated with vascular abnormality of the brain, seizures, progressive one-sided weakness, and progressive mental retardation.
Subpial transection	The pia is the covering of the brain that supplies blood to the surface of the cortex. Transection of it

	involves operating on the brain tissue below while preserving the pia; it is one way of surgically stopping seizures while not disrupting "eloquent" function.
Symptomatic	Indicating a defined cause. Seizures due to fever, meningitis, chemical abnormalities, or head trauma are called symptomatic seizures, or provoked seizures.
Synapse	The tiny space between the end of the axon and the body of the next neuron.
Syncope	Fainting. The characteristics include a feeling of dizziness associated with pallor and sweatiness, followed by loss of consciousness. When this benign condition is followed by a brief tonic-clonic seizure it is termed convulsive syncope.
Syndrome	A collection of signs or symptoms that together form a condition with a known outcome, or which requires special treatment.
Threshold	The susceptibility of a single neuron to fire or of the brain to have a seizure. Many factors may lower the brain threshold and precipitate a seizure. Anticonvulsant drugs raise the threshold and make seizures less likely.
Tics	A sudden, episodic, repetitive movement, most commonly involving eye-blinking or movements of the face and head, but sometimes of other parts of the body. These complex movements are not associated with alterations in consciousness, and they can usually be stopped consciously for periods of time. They are not associated with EEG abnormalities and are not seizures.
Todd's paralysis	Weakness occurring in one limb or one side of the body after a focal or unilateral seizure. This paralysis, while often thought of as exhaustion of the brain, actually results from inhibition of the seizures and of the normal function of the brain on that side. Todd's paralysis after a seizure is usually resolved in one to two hours but may, on occasion, continue for several days. It always disappears completely.
Tonic-clonic seizure	The generalized seizures people often think of when they think of epilepsy, formerly called grand mal seizures. They are characterized by stiffening and then rhythmic jerking movements of the body.
Tonic seizure	A seizure that involves stiffening of the arms, legs, and back and loss of consciousness. The stiffening

	may last several seconds to a minute. Most tonic seizures go on to a clonic component. Tonic seizures are uncommon except as the first part of the tonic-clonic seizure.
Toxoplasmosis	A chronic infection, often acquired by a fetus *in utero,* that affects multiple organ systems. It can cause mental retardation, scarring of the brain, and seizures.
Tuberous sclerosis	A disease characterized by skin lesions (white spots, thickened patches, etc.), seizures, and mental retardation. Because it is caused by abnormal development of cells, many other organs of the body (e.g., eyes, heart, kidneys) experience changes or tumors.
Unilateral seizure	A seizure involving one side of the body, usually the face, arm, or leg. A unilateral seizure involves or spreads through a single half of the brain.
Video EEG	The use of video cameras to capture visually the onset and characteristics of seizures or episodes while simultaneously monitoring the EEG to see electrical changes. Video-EEG monitoring permits a physician to identify whether a seizure is associated with an EEG change, that is, whether it is a real seizure or a pseudoseizure. It will often allow physicians to identify the areas in the brain where the individual's seizures are beginning.

Index

Abnormalities, contributive physical, 74
Absorption, and therapeutic range, 149.
   See also Medications
Acceptance, 259–61, 263–64, 275, 322;
   challenge to, 290; learning, 373; realis-
   tic, 319–20
Acidosis, 191
ACT (All Children Together), Project, 364–
   65
Activation procedures, 105. *See also* Electroencephalogram
Adjustments, spinal, 203–4
Adrenocorticotropic hormone (ACTH), for
   infantile spasms, 120
AIDS, 129
Allergic reactions, 137; baseline studies for,
   137–38; to phenobarbital, 150–51; to
   valproic acid, 156–57
Allopathic therapy, 196, 375
Alternative therapies, 194–98; biofeedback, 207; cerebellar stimulation, 206–
   7; Chinese, 196, 200–202; chiropractic,
   203; craniosacral therapy, 204; homeopathy, 202–3; massage, 205; osteopathy, 204–5; oxygen, 205–6; phytotherapy, 202; theoretical basis for, 199–200;
   transcranial magnetic stimulation, 207;
   vagus nerve stimulation, 207
Ambulatory EEG monitoring, 109–10. *See
   also* Monitoring
American Academy of Pediatrics, 343
Aminoacidurias, 361
Anemia, aplastic, 154, 375
Anesthesia, 220, 341
Anger, parental, 259, 321
Angiomas, 74, 126–27, 126 (fig.), 127 (fig.)
Anticonvulsant medications, 19, 82–83,
   136, 176, 360; allergic rashes from,
   137; and alternative therapies, 194–95,
   197; and behavioral problems, 338;
   blood levels of, 143–47; depression

due to, 305; vs. diet, 182–83; FDA evaluation of, 158–59; on ketogenic diet,
   191; and mental retardation, 284; in
   mother's breast milk, 360; pharmacoki-
   netics of, 136–42; "proper" dose for,
   135; in Rasmussen's syndrome, 130;
   and risks of pregnancy, 356–60; side
   effects of, 335; sports and, 349; therapeutic range for, 143, 144 (table), 145–
   47
Anticonvulsant medications, specific: carbamazepine, 153–55; ethosuximide,
   156; felbamate, 159–60; gabapentin,
   160; lamotrigine, 160–61; levetiracetam, 161; mephobarbital, 151; phenobarbital, 150; phenytoin, 152–53; primidone, 152; tiagabine, 161; valproic
   acid, 156–58; vigabatrin, 161–62
Antiepileptic drug (AED). *See* Anticonvulsant medications
Antihistamines, 342
Anxiety, 315, 373; coping with, 277–79; of
   parents, 272, 315–16
Aplastic anemia, 154, 375
Aroma therapy, 195
Arteriovenus malformations, 124
Association for Retarded Citizens (ARC),
   294
Attention deficit disorder (ADD), 333–34
Attention problems, 333–35
Aura: defined, 22, 23, 376; and driving,
   351–52
Autism, 123, 174
Automatism, 38, 376
Autonomic nervous system, 41, 376
Axon, 13, 14 (fig.), 376

Barbiturates, and mental retardation, 284
Batten's disease, 131
Behavioral disturbances, paroxysmal, 59–
   60

Library of Congress Cataloging-in-Publication Data

Freeman, John Mark.
Seizures and epilepsy in childhood / John M. Freeman, Eileen P. G. Vining,
Diana J. Pillas.—3rd ed.
     p.   cm.
Includes bibliographical references and index.
ISBN 0-8018-7050-X (hc. : alk. paper) — ISBN 0-8018-7051-8 (pbk. : alk.
paper)
     1. Epilepsy in children—Popular works.   2. Convulsions in children—
Popular works.   3. Health education—Popular works.   I. Vining, Eileen
P. G., 1946–   II. Pillas, Diana J., 1940–   III. Title.

RJ496.E6 F7 2002
618.92'853—dc21   2002070074